CREATIVE INTERVENTIONS
WITH TRAUMATIZED CHILDREN

CREATIVE ARTS AND PLAY THERAPY

Cathy A. Malchiodi and David A. Crenshaw,
Series Editors

Creative Arts and Play Therapy for Attachment Problems
Cathy A. Malchiodi and David A. Crenshaw, Editors

Play Therapy:
A Comprehensive Guide to Theory and Practice
David A. Crenshaw and Anne Stewart, Editors

Creative Interventions with Traumatized Children,
Second Edition
Cathy A. Malchiodi, Editor

Music Therapy Handbook
Barbara L. Wheeler, Editor

Creative Interventions with Traumatized Children

SECOND EDITION

Edited by

Cathy A. Malchiodi

Foreword by Bruce D. Perry

THE GUILFORD PRESS
New York   London

© 2015 The Guilford Press
A Division of Guilford Publications, Inc.
72 Spring Street, New York, NY 10012
www.guilford.com

Printed in the United States of America

This book is printed on acid-free paper.

Last digit is print number: 9   8   7   6   5   4   3   2   1

The authors have checked with sources believed to be reliable in their efforts to
provide information that is complete and generally in accord with the standards
of practice that are accepted at the time of publication. However, in view of the
possibility of human error or changes in behavioral, mental health, or medical
sciences, neither the authors, nor the editors and publisher, nor any other party
who has been involved in the preparation or publication of this work warrants that
the information contained herein is in every respect accurate or complete, and
they are not responsible for any errors or omissions or the results obtained from
the use of such information. Readers are encouraged to confirm the information
contained in this book with other sources.

Library of Congress Cataloging-in-Publication Data

Creative interventions with traumatized children / edited by Cathy A.
Malchiodi.—Second edition.
     p. ; cm.—(Creative arts and play therapy)
   Includes bibliographical references and index.
   ISBN 978-1-4625-1816-6 (hardcover : alk. paper)
   I. Malchiodi, Cathy A., editor.   II. Series: Creative arts and play therapy.
   [DNLM: 1. Stress Disorders, Post-Traumatic—
therapy. 2. Adolescent. 3. Child. 4. Creativity. 5. Sensory Art
Therapies—methods.   WM 172.5]
   RJ506.P66
   618.92'8521—dc23

                                                                2014014447

About the Editor

Cathy A. Malchiodi, PhD, ATR-BC, LPAT, LPCC, REAT, is an art therapist, creative arts therapist, and clinical mental health counselor, as well as a recognized authority on art therapy with children, adults, and families. She has given more than 350 presentations on art therapy and has published numerous articles, chapters, and books, including *Understanding Children's Drawings*; *Handbook of Art Therapy, Second Edition*; and *Creative Arts and Play Therapy for Attachment Problems* (with David A. Crenshaw). A faculty member at Lesley University, Dr. Malchiodi is founder of the Trauma-Informed Practices and Expressive Arts Therapy Institute and President of Art Therapy Without Borders. She is the first person to have received all three of the American Art Therapy Association's highest honors: Distinguished Service Award, Clinician Award, and Honorary Life Member Award. She has also received honors from the Kennedy Center and Very Special Arts in Washington, DC.

Contributors

Susanne Carroll Duffy, PsyD, RPT-S, Pleasant Point Health Center, Eastport Health Care, Inc., and By The Sea Seminars, Perry, Maine

Lennis G. Echterling, PhD, Department of Graduate Psychology, James Madison University, Harrisonburg, Virginia

Cornelia Elbrecht, MA, AThR, School for Initiatic Art Therapy, Apollo Bay, Victoria, Australia

Claire M. Ghetti, PhD, LCAT, MT-BC, CCLS, Elizabeth Seton Pediatric Center, New York, New York; The Grieg Academy, University of Bergen, Bergen, Norway

Amber Elizabeth Gray, MPH, MA, LPCC, BC-DMT, NCC, Restorative Resources Training and Consulting, Santa Fe, New Mexico

Craig Haen, PhD, RDT, CGP, LCAT, FAGPA, private practice, White Plains, New York

Mary Pellicci Hamilton, MSAT, ATR-BC, LPC, Art for Therapy, LLC, Westport, Connecticut

Russell E. Hilliard, PhD, LCSW, LCAT, MT-BC, CHRC, Seasons Hospice and Palliative Care, Rosemont, Illinois

Laura V. Loumeau-May, MPS, ATR-BC, LPC, Journeys Program/Valley Home Care, Inc., Paramus, New Jersey; Art Therapy Graduate Program, Caldwell University, Caldwell, New Jersey; Contemporary Arts Division, Ramapo College, Mahwah, New Jersey

Cathy A. Malchiodi, PhD, ATR-BC, LPAT, LPCC, REAT,
Trauma-Informed Practice and Expressive Arts Therapy Institute, Louisville,
Kentucky; Department of Expressive Therapies, Lesley University,
Cambridge, Massachusetts

Margaret M. McGuinness, MA, MEd, ATR-BC, private practice,
Southfield, Michigan

Laury Rappaport, PhD, MFT, REAT, ATR-BC, Focusing and Expressive
Arts Institute, Santa Rosa, California; Department of Psychology, Sonoma
State University, Rhonert Park, California; and Integrative Psychotherapist,
Sutter Health, Institute for Health and Healing Santa Rosa, California

Bart Santen, PsyD, Focusing Institute, New York, New York; Mental Health
Care Group, Neurofeedback Institute, Utrecht, The Netherlands

Kathy J. Schnur, MEd, RN, CTS, ATR-BC, private practice,
Detroit, Michigan

Ellie Seibel-Nicol, MA, ATR-BC, Family Study Center,
Danbury, Connecticut

Anne L. Stewart, PhD, Department of Graduate Psychology, James Madison
University, Harrisonburg, Virginia

Madoka Takada Urhausen, MA, LMFT, ATR-BC, private practice and
The Guidance Center, Long Beach, California

Annette M. Whitehead-Pleaux, MA, MT-BC, Shriners Hospitals
for Children, Boston, Massachusetts; St. Mary-of-the-Woods College,
St. Mary of the Woods, Indiana

Foreword

There are among us healers. This has been true for thousands of generations. These individuals are needed to help those in pain; kind-hearted and good people, they listen, watch, and then act. And in all cultures and across thousands of years, despite hundreds of explanations about the "cause" or source of the pain, healing always involves rhythm, relationship, and reason. Activities or interactions that restore regulatory rhythms in movement, sleep, eating, and interacting with others help heal. The relationship is the agent of change in every human activity, including healing; a cognitive "explanation" or narrative regarding the pain/disease (whether physiologically accurate or not) helps us cope and heal.

Seven years ago, the first edition of this classic book was published. Each chapter was by a healer discussing some aspect of his or her work. It was a unique collection of creative and compassionate healers sharing their experience and wisdom. The present edition expands upon this. Over the last decade, there has been a slow and steady accumulation of evidence examining the neurobiological mechanisms that may underlie the effectiveness of many of the creative and performance arts in the healing process; further, outcome studies are demonstrating the effectiveness of many of the therapeutic modalities that were once considered outside the mainstream of "evidence-based" practice. The scientific method is, in many instances, "proving" what the elders and healers, in some ways, have always known.

Helping maltreated and traumatized children is the focus of this book. In the Foreword to the first edition, I tried to outline the value of this book and its special role in our field. Rather than diluting this perspective, I choose to include it in this Foreword; sadly, the fundamental challenge and context for this second edition has not changed over the last decade. The way we choose to help these children is still a disgrace; and this book—with all of its healing wisdom—is still a beacon of hope.

*   *   *

Childhood is, and always has been, a vulnerable time. Every generation from the Stone Age through thousands of cultures to the modern era has been challenged with war, famine, plague, murder, and rape— and always the most vulnerable, particularly children, have suffered the most. In early generations, trauma was pervasive; in many cases, it was more pervasive than in the relatively safe and stable world we try to create for our children today. Yet while we like to think we protect, nurture, educate, and enrich our children better than our ancestors did, in actuality, many children's lives are still filled with threat, violence, loss, and trauma, as seen in domestic violence, the death of a loved one, physical abuse, sexual abuse, or natural disasters. Today, fully one-third of adults have experienced multiple forms of significant adverse childhood events—often traumatic in nature. And we are now more aware that these adverse and traumatic experiences change us in many ways; after trauma, our bodies and minds, our hearts and souls are seared and then twisted and modified to help us survive.

The cost of childhood trauma is enormous, not only economically in the hundreds of billions of dollars spent in treating it each year, but also in the lost potential of creativity and productivity when a child's humanity is shattered. All too often, children are diminished by the trauma they have experienced. Yet this need not be. A traumatized child *can* heal and grow stronger and wiser by facing, coping with, and overcoming trauma and its aftermath. This is the promise of effective healing from trauma, of true therapeutic experience.

Unfortunately, in our compartmentalized, "evidence-based practice," buzzword world of therapies, dominated by a reductionist medical model, we are not providing the majority of our traumatized children with true therapeutic experiences. The small percentage of traumatized children being served by our mental health system is a national disgrace. Those who enter the system receive fragmented, ineffective, often impersonal services. We are decidedly not helping traumatized children effectively cope and heal.

While much of the field looks ahead for solutions to these challenges, hoping that we will find the right neurobiological system to target with the right prophylactic drug to prevent posttraumatic stress disorder; or that we will find the subset of the most genetically vulnerable individuals to target with our interventions; or that we will be able to put all traumatized children into a one-size-fits-all, easy-to-export, 20-session group treatment protocol, I would suggest that, instead, we look back. There is something to be learned from our ancestors.

Our ancestors had to learn to cope with trauma in order to survive; somehow traumatized people had to find ways to continue to sustain family, community, and culture and move forward. What did they do to cope with trauma? Are there clues in what they did that may help us today? Examination of the known beliefs, rituals, and healing practices for loss and trauma that remain from aboriginal cultures reveal some remarkable principles. Healing rituals from a wide range of geographically separate, culturally disconnected groups converge into a set of core elements related to adaptation and healing following trauma. These core elements include an overarching belief system—a rationale, a belief, a reason for the pain, injury, loss; a retelling or reenactment of the trauma in words, dance, or song; a set of somatosensory experiences—touch, the patterned repetitive movements of dance, and song—all provided in an intensely relational experience with family and clan participating in the ritual.

The most remarkable quality of these elements is that together they create a total neurobiological experience influencing cortical, limbic, diencephalic, and brainstem systems (not unlike the pervasive neurobiological impact of trauma):

- Retell the story.
- Hold each other.
- Massage, dance, sing.
- Create images of the battle, hunt, and death.
- Fill literature, sculpture, and drama with retellings.
- Reconnect to loved ones and to community.
- Celebrate, eat, and share.

These aboriginal healing practices are repetitive, rhythmic, relevant, relational, respectful, and rewarding; they are experiences known to be effective in altering neural systems involved in the stress response in both animal models and humans. The remarkable resonance of these practices with the neurobiology of trauma is not unexpected. These practices emerged because they worked. People felt better and functioned better, and the core elements of the healing process were reinforced and passed on. Cultures separated by time and space all converged on the same general approach.

The beauty of this book, *Creative Interventions with Traumatized Children*, is that it draws on these ancient practices. It describes modern versions of the most effective, time-honored, and biologically respectful therapeutic practices created by our ancestors. It is important, however, that these innovative therapeutic practices now carry forward and refine these time-honored principles. While these therapeutic practices may not at first seem "biological," be assured that they are not only likely to change the brain, but they will assuredly provide the patterned, repetitive stimuli required to specifically influence and modify the impact of trauma, neglect, and maltreatment on key neural systems. The neural systems altered by trauma originate in the lower parts of the brain (e.g., dopaminergic, serotonergic, and noradrenergic neural networks). These brainstem and midbrain systems will only be modified effectively by patterned repetitive neural activity that gets to the brainstem and midbrain from primary somatosensory experiences—rhythmic auditory, tactile, visual, and motor–vestibular stimulation—such as massage, music, dance, and repetitive visual and tactile stimuli (e.g., eye movement desensitization and reprocessing).

Amid the current pressure for "evidence-based practice" parameters, we should remind ourselves that the most powerful evidence is that which comes from hundreds of separate cultures across thousands of generations independently converging on rhythm, touch, storytelling, and reconnection to community—all of which are included in this book—as the core ingredients to coping with and healing from trauma.

BRUCE D. PERRY, MD, PhD
The ChildTrauma Academy, Houston, Texas
Northwestern University, Chicago, Illinois

Preface

Since the publication of the first edition of *Creative Interventions with Traumatized Children*, there have been many significant developments in trauma intervention with children, adolescents, and families. Simultaneously, an understanding of how creative arts therapies (art, music, dance/movement, and drama) and play therapy enhance reparation and recovery in traumatized children has dramatically increased. Expanded knowledge of neurobiology, developmental trauma, sensory-based approaches, and posttraumatic stress has informed both how we define trauma as well as what constitutes effective and neurodevelopmentally appropriate intervention. Additionally, not only creative arts therapists and play therapists apply creative strategies in work with children, but also a growing number of counselors, psychologists, marriage and family therapists, and other mental health and health care professionals are embracing the value of sensory-based, action-oriented approaches with young clients.

There are many situations that may constitute a traumatic experience for children. A traumatizing event can be the death of a parent or sibling, divorce, placement into foster care, relocation, an accident, or a medical illness. For others, it can be exposure to bullying, domestic violence, physical or sexual abuse, a catastrophic natural disaster, or terrorism and war. Unfortunately, some children encounter repetitive stressful circumstances throughout their lives, increasing their suscep-tibility to adverse psychosocial and developmental problems through-out the lifespan. Depending on the child, the degree of exposure to distressing events, and other factors, trauma can be an experience that is mentally, emotionally, and physically exhausting, terrifying, and con-fusing.

Throughout my work as an art therapist, expressive arts therapist, and mental health counselor, I have always been intrigued that children relive their traumas not only in their minds but also through their bod-ies. Today, experts on neurobiology and mind–body responses to trauma underscore that in treating psychological trauma, helping professionals must first address the body's responses to distress. While we can provide children with cognitive strategies to cope with traumatic stress, we must also use developmentally appropriate, sensory-based interventions that reach children in brainwise ways. Creative arts and play therapies are one way to do this, by establishing a relationship between therapist and child that involves activities that emphasize "right-brain to right-brain" communication and relational, action-oriented strategies (Malchiodi, 2013, 2014).

Arts and play also offer unique possibilities for nonverbal expres-sion and meaning making. The seminal work of Judith Herman (1992) underscores that when individuals experience psychologically trauma-tizing events, they often are unable to verbally express or describe what has occurred, yet they have a need to articulate the unspeakable. Chil-dren intuitively use expressive arts and play to act out what they are reliving and what they may find unspeakable; this premise is at the heart of this book. This second edition of *Creative Interventions with Trau-matized Children* explores this premise, taking the reader more deeply into the sensory processes inherent in arts and play therapy that effect change in children and allow them to make meaning of trauma and loss. Throughout the book, experienced practitioners from the fields of creative arts therapies and play therapy explain and demonstrate action-oriented, creative interventions grounded in sensory-based, neurobiol-ogy-informed principles and practices. Helping professionals are intro-duced to a variety of cutting-edge approaches in work with children and adolescents, including art therapy, music therapy, drama therapy, dance/ movement therapy, and play therapy methods that integrate expressive arts, storytelling, and sandtray. But in particular, this volume provides new information on the creative arts therapies and play therapy in three areas of interest to trauma specialists: neurobiology and neurodevelop-ment, self-regulation, and resilience and posttraumatic growth.

NEUROBIOLOGY AND NEURODEVELOPMENT

Since the publication of the first edition, neurobiological and neurodevelopmental principles have become an essential part of the effective practice of creative arts and play therapy. Chapter 1 provides updated coverage of key neurobiology principles central to creative intervention with traumatized children and explains why trauma-informed practice is a neurodevelopmentally relevant strategy. Specific approaches that are based in current neurobiology and somatically based practice are also demonstrated; for example, Chapter 3 describes and illustrates how art therapy complements and enhances the widely applied method of eye movement desensitization and reprocessing with children, explaining the importance of integrating art and imaginal techniques within this approach. Similarly, Chapter 6 presents an art-based approach that describes a somatic perspective and the technique of "body mapping" to address childhood dissociation. Chapter 9 presents a neurodevelopmental, somatically based overview of the sensory properties of clay and how clay can be used with children who have experienced developmental trauma.

SELF-REGULATION

Authors in this volume also underscore the self-regulating capacities of the creative arts therapies and play-based approaches. Self-regulation refers simply to the ability to moderate emotions and somatic responses to stress. Hyperarousal is a common response to traumatic events, and young clients who have been exposed to distressing situations often have difficulties with self-regulation. Experiences with art, music, movement, and other activities can provide a comforting and calming effect that decreases anxiety and fear.

Throughout this book, specific applications of creative arts therapies and play therapy are illustrated and demonstrated as key methods to help deactivate arousal and stimulate the body's relaxation response. Chapter 14 highlights a focusing-oriented approach to expressive arts therapy as well as mindfulness as an essential component of intervention in work with traumatized children and adolescents. Similarly, music therapy is an effective and widely used strategy for stress reduction and self-regulation with hospitalized children who are experiencing both physical and emotional distress (Chapter 15). Finally, applications of arts and play therapies are central to self-regulation in children who have experienced interpersonal violence, helping them develop adaptive coping skills, self-empowerment, and stress reduction (Chapter 12).

RESILIENCE AND POSTTRAUMATIC GROWTH

The importance of enhancing children's capacity for resilience and posttraumatic growth is highlighted throughout this book. Resilience is often defined as the ability to bounce back from adverse events; posttraumatic growth refers to positive psychological change as the result of experiencing distressful or challenging circumstances. Trauma-informed practice embraces the concept that children can experience a sense of being capable and that they can be encouraged to take part in their own recovery. The creative arts and play therapies are ideal approaches because they naturally introduce opportunities for self-empowerment and active participation that engage participants on a sensory level. For many children, the use of creative interventions provides a way to experience mastery over the events that have disrupted their lives, leading to enhanced resilience.

Finally, while children have always been exposed to crises, there is increasing global attention to understanding the effects of trauma on children who have experienced large-scale man-made and natural disasters and violent events in neighborhoods, schools, and communities. In recent decades, high-profile incidents such as Hurricane Katrina and the Southeast Asia tsunami, the war in Iraq, terrorist threats and attacks, and gun violence in schools have received intense media coverage, as well as public and professional interest. Even children not directly exposed to these incidents have been affected by these crises, especially those who have previously experienced trauma or loss. Many of those who experienced these types of traumatic events continue to struggle with reactions such as anxiety, depression, or posttraumatic stress disorder.

Because so many practitioners are often confronted with helping young survivors cope with tragedy on a large scale, Chapter 5 provides an overview of art therapy and creative interventions for those who have experienced a mass disaster, in particular the Sandy Hook Elementary School shooting and the aftermath of the terrorist attacks on September 11, 2001. Mass man-made and natural disasters call upon helping professionals' capacity to both practice empathy with child survivors and their families and use creative strategies to normalize distress and help establish a sense of safety and self-empowerment.

Because psychological trauma produces a "felt sense" of fear, worry, and confusion in many children, the self-soothing nature of the expressive arts and play become particularly important in effectively addressing somatic reactions after a large-scale traumatic event and in crisis intervention with families (Chapter 10).

The contributing authors in this volume, each of whom uses action-oriented, creative interventions in his or her work with traumatized children, all agree on one thing: Sensory-based, hands-on methods are an essential part of effective treatment in cases of trauma. For those children who are withdrawn or fear disclosure of abuse or violence, the sensory nature of creative activities allows expression of the unspeakable and circumvents "talk" that may be difficult or temporarily impossible. For others, the use of creative interventions provides the opportunity to immediately engage in experiences of mastery over the events that have disrupted their lives. For helping professionals, the approaches and methods described throughout this book capitalize on metaphor and symbol as ways to help even the most distressed child clients depict, regulate, and control what cannot be told with words alone. Being able to communicate "what happened" through pictures, play, movement, sound, and other media allows for emotions, events, and memories to be witnessed by others, and is a powerful first step in addressing the needs of any trauma survivor.

We all endure trauma and loss at one point or another as adults; unfortunately, many of the children we see in treatment have had to endure the suffering that trauma brings throughout their young lives. In the first edition of this book, I cited a belief that has guided my work with traumatized individuals of all ages. It is the third noble truth of Buddhism, which states that all human suffering can be ultimately transformed and healed. In more pragmatic terms, this means that recovery from trauma is possible in all individuals, including our child clients. All children have the potential to reenact and retell their experiences through creative expression, particularly when their therapists recognize and utilize the power of the creative arts and play to transform suffering and to help them recapture health and hope for the future.

ACKNOWLEDGMENTS

It is with great respect that I take this opportunity to acknowledge individuals in the field of trauma who have helped to make this book possible.

First, I want to thank Bruce D. Perry, whose seminal contributions to the field of child trauma and neurodevelopment are wide-reaching, influential, and inspirational to literally thousands of helping professionals. There is no one more worthy of writing the Foreword to this book than Dr. Perry because of his lasting commitment to the importance of somatosensory interventions in work with children and his writings on the interface between neurobiology and trauma.

I next thank each of the contributors for agreeing to write chapters for this text. Their expertise not only addresses and illuminates the scope and potential of creative methods in work with children and families, but also has expanded the collective knowledge of just how to apply creative arts and play to trauma intervention. I feel very fortunate to have encountered each of these contributors at this juncture, and I am grateful that they have shared their wisdom and experience throughout this book.

Finally, bringing together an edited book is a collaborative effort between editor, contributors, and publisher. I extend a special thanks to Senior Acquisitions Editor Rochelle Serwator, copy editor Margaret Ryan, Art Director Paul Gordon, and Senior Production Editor Laura Specht Patchkofsky for facilitating yet another pleasurable editorial experience and production process. I thank The Guilford Press for having the foresight to launch the Creative Arts and Play Therapy series, highlighting the importance of action-oriented, "brainwise" methods of therapy. I am delighted that this second edition is part of this series and grateful that creative interventions are being increasingly recognized as valuable and effective approaches to treatment by mental health professionals.

REFERENCES

Herman, J. (1992). *Trauma and recovery*. New York: Basic Books.

Malchiodi, C. A. (2013, September 9). Creative art therapy and attachment work. *Psychology Today*. Retrieved from *www.psychologytoday.com/blog/arts-and-health/201309/creative-art-therapy-and-attachment-work*.

Malchiodi, C. A. (2014). Creative arts therapy approaches to attachment issues. In C. A. Malchiodi & D. A. Crenshaw (Eds.), *Creative arts and play therapy for attachment problems* (pp. 3–18). New York: Guilford Press.

Contents

PART I

Creative Interventions and Children

Basics of Practice

CHAPTER 1

Neurobiology, Creative Interventions, and Childhood Trauma

Cathy A. Malchiodi

Children may be in therapy for a variety of reasons related to trauma. Some children experience the death of a parent, survive a serious accident, or lose their home or possessions due to a natural disaster. Others may experience several traumatic events during their young lives or be subjected to chronically stressful situations such as abuse, neglect, or multiple foster care environments. Although some children are not permanently affected by these experiences, others may suffer serious symptoms that interfere with normal emotional, cognitive, or social development.

Terr (1990) notes that "trauma does not ordinarily get better by itself. It burrows down further and further under the child's defenses and coping strategies" (p. 293). Children who are traumatized often feel helpless, confused, and ashamed and are afraid to trust others or their environment. Therapists who encounter these children must form a productive relationship with them to enable them not only to revisit painful experiences, but also to overcome intrusive memories, make meaning, and find hope. In order to reach these children effectively, therapists must use both developmentally appropriate methods and interventions that address traumatic memories and provide emotional relief.

In recent years recognition has grown that trauma is an autonomic, physiological, and neurological response to overwhelming events or experiences that creates a secondary psychological response (Perry, 2009; Rothschild, 2000). This recognition has reframed how therapists intervene with individuals who have symptoms of stress, and it acknowledges that these symptoms are the body's adaptive reactions to distressing events. There is an increasing consensus that intervention must also employ techniques that focus on the sensory impact of trauma.

This chapter provides an overview of trauma from a neurobiological view and a foundation for understanding why sensory-based, creative interventions such as arts therapies and expressive methods are effective and often necessary in work with traumatized children. For therapists who are not familiar with these modalities, a brief description of creative arts therapies and expressive therapies is offered along with general information on the nature of traumatic events and their impact on children.

DEFINING TRAUMA

For the purpose of this book, "trauma" is defined as an experience that creates a lasting, substantial, psychosocial, and somatic impact on a child. Traumatizing events can be single occurrences such as an accident or witnessing an injury to another or several experiences that become traumatic in their totality. Extensive exposure to neglect or abuse; experience of terrorism or war; or survival of a disaster and subsequent loss of home, possessions, and/or family members are examples of repeated or chronic trauma experiences. Terr's (1981, 1990) seminal work with child survivors of the Chowchilla kidnapping incident offers some of the first reports on the complexity of traumatic experiences and posttraumatic symptoms. As a result of the Chowchilla study and subsequent investigations, Terr identified many of the characteristics commonly seen in traumatized children, including behaviors seen in art and play activities and influences on cognitive and emotional development. She also described two forms of traumatic events: acute or Type I trauma (single event) and chronic or Type II trauma (multiple or cumulative events). In either type of traumatic event, children may encounter physical and/or emotional disruption and suffer bodily trauma and/or psychological effects.

Therapists who work with traumatized individuals now understand that a number of factors actually mediate how single or multiple traumas affect children and how these factors may predispose young clients to more serious problems. Posttraumatic stress disorder (PTSD) is well known to most mental health professionals; the current definition and criteria are found in the fifth edition of the *Diagnostic and Statistical Manual of Mental Disorders* (DSM-5; American Psychiatric Association, 2013). Characteristics similar to PTSD in children were described as early as the 1930s, reflecting the currently accepted symptom cluster in assessment of PTSD. It was not until 1987, in DSM-III-R (American Psychiatric Association, 1987), that specific features of children's PTSD emerged that account for developmental differences between young clients and adults. The current DSM-5 criteria for PTSD can be summarized in the following general reactions and responses:

- *Alterations in arousal.* Hyperarousal is common, including intense psychological distress and/or physiological reactivity when exposed to something that resembles an aspect of the traumatic event. This excessive arousal may cause difficulties with concentration, sleep problems such as difficulty falling or staying asleep, hypervigilance, and irritability or outbursts of anger. Children may also exhibit hypoarousal, including dissociation, when exposed to situations or experiences that stimulate sensory memories of a traumatizing event.

- *Reexperiencing.* Children may suddenly feel as though a traumatic event is recurring in the present, have intrusive thoughts about the event, and experience nightmares that include sensory or declarative aspects of the event. Reminders of the traumatic event come in the form of auditory, visual, olfactory, vestibular, and other sensory cues as well as anniversaries of events.

- *Avoidance.* Children may attempt to avoid thoughts or feelings associated with the traumatic event or to be unable to recall aspects of the event. They may attempt to avoid activities or situations that evoke memory of a trauma, detach from family and friends, have difficulty sleeping due to nightmares associated with the event, have decreased interest in previously pleasurable activities, and experience a foreshortened sense of the future.

- *Negative cognitions and mood.* Children may have a persistent and distorted sense of self-blame or may have a decreased interest in activities they previously enjoyed.

- *Developmental problems.* Children may experience developmental delays such as emotional and cognitive problems or attachment disorders if traumatic events disrupt relationships with parents or caregivers. This particular aspect of posttraumatic stress in children is believed to be the result of multiple traumatic events, particularly interpersonal violence during childhood (a summary of developmental trauma is provided later in this chapter), and underscores the close association between repeated trauma exposure and disruptions in normal development in children.

DSM-5 includes a new subtype of PTSD, called *preschool subtype posttraumatic stress disorder*. In brief, more behaviorally and developmentally sensitive criteria are used to identify posttraumatic stress in younger children; for example, play can be used as a way to identify PTSD because very young children do not have the capacity to verbalize what they are feeling in response to traumatic experiences. Additionally, the criteria underscore that very young children may not display extreme or overt distress at the time of traumatic events, and their trauma reactions may become apparent in the form of impaired relationships with parents, caregivers, siblings, peers, or teachers.

In preschool children, school-age children, and adolescents, the duration of trauma reactions must exceed 1 month and cannot be attributed to another medical condition or other influence. A number of factors also affect how children respond to traumatic events and if they go on to exhibit emotional disorders, including PTSD. Biological aspects, temperament, resiliency, developmental stage, attachment to parents or caregivers, abilities and adaptive coping skills, and available social support are related to individual susceptibility to PTSD (U.S. Department of Health and Human Services, Administration for Children and Families, Administration on Children, Youth and Families, Children's Bureau, 2012), acute stress reactions, and mood or behavioral disorders. Children directly exposed to a traumatic event, such as a violent crime, death, or disaster, who do not have adequate social support in the form of family, caregivers, or community or who experience multiple crises are more susceptible to trauma and may require additional, long-term treatment. These children have a higher risk of PTSD and other stress-related disorders, although the prevalence rates vary depending on the research study (National Child Traumatic Stress Network, 2014; Silva, 2004). In brief, a number of characteristics and experiences contribute to how trauma affects children and whether or not children suffer long-lasting and disruptive symptoms.

Fortunately, only a portion of children exposed to stressful events go on to develop PTSD or other serious disorders, but it is widely accepted that vulnerability and resiliency factors (see Malchiodi, Chapter 2, and

Part IV, this volume) impact the development of symptoms that require ongoing treatment. Most children need a minimum of intervention and usually return to normal personal and social functioning in a short time. In these cases, interventions that incorporate psychoeducation, debriefing, prevention strategies, and brief therapies may lessen the initial distress, identify social supports, and enhance adaptive coping skills.

Developmental Trauma

Bessel van der Kolk (2005) proposes the term *developmental trauma disorder* (DTD) to describe children who have experienced multiple traumatic events, such as chronic neglect or abuse. DTD is a concept intended to underscore the impact of chronic trauma on children's affect regulation, neurological functioning, and self-concept. Developmental trauma may disrupt children's capacities to play (Tuber, Boesch, Gorking, & Terry, 2014) and engage in creative expression, thus making it difficult to reach these young clients even through sensory-based interventions. Children who have experienced developmental trauma are often wary of relationships, even with a trusted therapist, because of early, repeated experiences of interpersonal violence and neglect. Chronic traumatic stress may overwhelm children's abilities to self-soothe, preventing retrieval of positive attachment experiences and sensations (Malchiodi & Crenshaw, 2014). Many have highly developed adaptive coping strategies that protect them from emotional closeness, readiness to learn, and imagination (Lieberman & Knorr, 2007). Although not formally a category in DSM-5, helping professionals often utilize the lens of developmental trauma when evaluating child clients who have experienced repeated incidences of abuse, neglect, violence or war, abandonment, and/or foster care.

THE NEUROBIOLOGY OF TRAUMA

In response to a greater understanding of the neurobiology of trauma, there is now wide agreement that trauma reactions are both psychological (mind) and physiological (body) experiences. In order to help children who have been traumatized, it is first important to have a working knowledge of the neurobiology of trauma, know how the brain is organized, and understand how the body and mind react to traumatic events. This section does not intend to provide in-depth explanations of human physiology and how trauma affects the brain; this material is widely available and is covered in numerous contemporary texts. Instead, the purpose here is to provide a basic overview that summarizes major concepts pertaining to trauma intervention as an introduction to creative interventions with traumatized children.

The Triune Brain

The human brain is often described as consisting of three basic parts: the brainstem, the limbic system, and the cortex. The brainstem is the first area to mature and is, from an evolutionary standpoint, the oldest area of the brain. It is responsible for regulating basic functions such as reflexes, the cardiovascular system, and arousal. The cerebellum is connected to the brainstem and coordinates motor, emotional, and cognitive functioning. The brainstem and cerebellum are often referred to as the "reptilian brain" because they are like the brain of reptiles (Levine & Klein, 2007).

The limbic system includes a group of structures—the hypothalamus, amygdala, and hippocampus—that forms a ring around the brainstem. The limbic system is often referred to as the "emotional brain" because it is the source of urges, needs, and feelings. Its primary functions involve self-preservation, the fight, freeze, or flight response, and implicit memory—learned associations that link sensations with context. The limbic system, in a sense, evaluates experiences for emotional significance and reacts to these experiences in ways that are learned by the individual over time.

The cortex and neocortex are referred to as the "thinking brain" because they are the parts of the brain where reasoning, communication, and planning occur. They contain the capacity for language and consciousness and the ability not only to think thoughts, but also to think *about* thoughts, behaviors, and emotions. Despite the more complex levels of functioning mediated by this region of the brain, the lower parts of the brain also have a significant impact on actions and responses.

Trauma reactions are believed to occur when responses of the limbic system, activated to mobilize oneself in the face of personal threat, are not utilized in a productive way. Essentially, children who experience an event such as physical abuse, disaster, terrorism, or any other distressing occurrence may go into what can be considered a "survival mode." In other words, if the energy normally used for fighting, freezing or fleeing is not expended, the emotional activation is held in the nervous system and not dissipated or released (Levine, 2012). In the case of traumatic stress, even though the nervous system is still highly activated, children may experience a disruption or impairment in normal functioning and develop habitual responses such as explosive emotions, noncompliant behavior, psychological numbness, cognitive problems, or other reactions depending on personality factors and the type and extent of distress.

Consider 8-year-old Mark, a child who is currently in treatment at a local psychiatric facility. He has a long history of severe physical abuse, sexual abuse, and neglect and has lived in multiple foster homes. Mark has very little ability to control his impulses; in the classroom and play therapy room, he often initiates arguments with other children, steals, sets fires, and is prone to tearful outbursts when under even minimal stress. He finds it difficult to focus his attention on any one game or toy for more than a minute and reacts to fear-inducing situations with psychological numbing and withdrawal, frozen and unable to move. Mark is also developmentally delayed, behaving like a much younger child and drawing human figures at a 4-year-old level (Figure 1.1).

How the brain reacts to repetitive traumatic experiences may explain many of Mark's current responses to others and his environment. As an individual who is profoundly or chronically distressed,

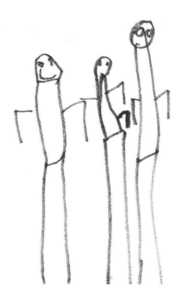

FIGURE 1.1. Human figures by Mark, age 8 years.

Mark reacts with little self-control because he is unable to regulate his emotional responses. His behavior may be a survival response involving fighting (arguing) and sometimes freezing (psychological numbing and withdrawal), depending on the perceived threats in his environment that cause fear, terror, or feelings of helplessness. He may have learning disabilities due to years of distress that have affected his cognitive and social functioning. In contrast to Mark, healthy, capable, and resilient children can use problem-solving skills, available sources of social support, and other resources to overcome stressful events; those who have traumatic stress reactions cannot engage in healthy forms of functioning and go on to develop symptoms of PTSD or other emotional disorders.

The Mind–Body Connection

It is well accepted that the body often mirrors emotions. Different parts of the brain may become active when we look at sad faces or happy faces, imagine a happy or sad event or relationship, or hear a particular song or sound. These emotions are connected to a variety of hormonal fluctuations as well as cardiovascular and neurological effects (Sternberg, 2001). In fact, the physiology of emotions is so complex that the brain knows more than the conscious mind can reveal—that is, one can display an emotion without being conscious of what induced it (Damasio, 2000, 2011).

In the case of traumatic events, sensory experiences related to the crises (e.g., images, touch, sound, and smell) may become learned associations that resurface when one encounters a different, yet similar, set of stimuli. For example, when Mark feels insecure around other children, he automatically reacts with uncontrollable rage, recapitulating his early relationships with an abusive sister; if he feels threatened by an adult, he becomes hypervigilant and immobilized as his body prepares for physical violence or punishment. There is general agreement that traumatic events similar to the ones Mark has experienced take a toll on the body as well as the mind. After a significant trauma, the "body remembers" (Levine, 2012; Rothschild, 2000), and, as van der Kolk (1994) notes in the title of his classic book, "the body keeps score" of emotional experiences.

Memory Storage

The way in which memory is stored is also important to understanding how the brain is impacted by traumatic events. In brief, there are two types of memory: explicit and implicit. Explicit or declarative memory is conscious memory and is composed of facts, concepts, and ideas; one has access to language to describe what one is thinking and feeling. Explicit memory allows conscious processing of information, reasoning, and meaning making, thereby helping individuals define and make sense of their experiences.

Implicit memory stores sensory and emotional components and is related to the body's learned memories. Riding a bicycle is a good example of implicit memory, whereas narrating the chronological details of the event (getting on the bike, pedaling to the park) is an example of explicit memory. In implicit memory, there is no language; the senses *are* the memory—what we see, what we hear, sensations of smell, touch, and taste become the implicit containers of that experience.

Many trauma specialists believe that posttraumatic stress reactions may result when implicit memory of trauma is excluded from explicit storage (Rothschild, 2000); that is, an individual may not have access to the context in which the emotions or sensations arose. Additionally, language (a function of explicit memory) is not generally accessible to trauma survivors after a distressing event. In particular, Broca's area, a section of the brain that controls language, is affected, making it difficult to relate the trauma narrative, leading to difficulties in identifying and verbalizing experiences (van Dalen, 2001). Van der Kolk observes that when an individual is about to speak about a traumatic event, "[there] is a problem with verbalization . . . the Broca's area shuts down" (Korn, 2001, p. 4).

Perhaps this inability to verbalize one's responses to trauma relates to the human survival response; when an experience is extremely painful to recall, the brain protects the individual by literally making it impossible to talk about it. Because trauma is stored as somatic sensations and images, it may not be readily available for communication through language, but may be available through sensory means such as creative arts, play, and other experiential activities and approaches (Malchiodi, 2012a).

CREATIVE ARTS THERAPY AND PLAY THERAPY WITH TRAUMATIZED CHILDREN

In addition to having a working knowledge of the physiology of trauma reactions in children, it is also important to understand the variety of therapeutic approaches that use creativity, imagination, and self-expression as their core. Creative interventions have been formalized through the disciplines of art therapy, music therapy, dance/movement therapy, drama therapy or psychodrama, poetry therapy, and play therapy, including sandtray therapy. Each discipline has been applied in psychotherapy and counseling with individuals of all ages, particularly children, for more than 60 years. Art, music, dance, drama, and poetry therapies are referred to as *creative arts therapies* because of their roots in the arts and theories of creativity (National Coalition of Creative Arts Therapies Associations, 2014). These therapies and others that utilize self-expression in treatment are also called *expressive therapies* (Malchiodi, 2005, 2013, 2014). Expressive therapies are defined as the use of art, music, drama, dance/movement, poetry/creative writing, bibliotherapy, play, and/or sandplay within the context of psychotherapy, counseling, rehabilitation, or medicine. Additionally, expressive therapies are sometimes referred to as *integrative* when purposively used in combination in treatment. These individual approaches are defined as follows:

• *Art therapy* is the purposeful use of visual arts materials and media in intervention, counseling, psychotherapy, and rehabilitation; it is used with individuals of all ages, families, and groups (Edwards, 2004; Malchiodi, 2012b).

• *Music therapy* is the prescribed use of music to effect positive changes in the psychological, physical, cognitive, or social functioning of individuals with health or educational problems (American Music Therapy Association, 2014; Wheeler, 2015).

• *Drama therapy* is the systematic and intentional use of drama/theater processes, products, and associations to achieve the therapeutic goals of symptom relief, emotional and physical integration, and personal growth. It is an active approach that helps the client tell his or her story to solve a problem, achieve catharsis, extend the depth and breadth of his or her inner experience, understand the meaning of images, and strengthen his or her ability to observe personal roles while increasing flexibility between roles (National Association for Drama Therapy, 2014).

• *Dance/movement therapy* is based on the assumption that body and mind are interrelated and is defined as the psychotherapeutic use of movement as a process that furthers the emotional, cognitive, and physical integration of the individual. Dance/movement therapy effects changes in feelings, cognition, physical functioning, and behavior (American Dance Therapy Association, 2014).

• *Poetry therapy and bibliotherapy* are terms used synonymously to describe the intentional use of poetry and other forms of literature for healing and personal growth.

• *Play therapy* is the systematic use of a theoretical model to establish an interpersonal process wherein trained play therapists use the therapeutic powers of play to help clients prevent or resolve psychosocial difficulties and achieve optimal growth and development (Crenshaw & Stewart, 2014; Webb, 2007).

• *Sandplay therapy* is a creative form of psychotherapy that uses a sandbox and a large collection of miniatures to enable a client to explore the deeper layers of his or her psyche in a totally new format; by constructing a series of "sand pictures," a client is helped to illustrate and integrate his or her psychological condition.

• *Integrative approaches* involve two or more expressive therapies to foster awareness, encourage emotional growth, and enhance relationships with others. This approach is distinguished by the practice of combining modalities within a therapy session. Integrative approaches are based on a variety of orientations, including the use of arts as therapy, as psychotherapy, and for traditional healing (Estrella, 2005; Knill, Levine, & Levine, 2005).

It is important to clarify that although some practitioners define art, dance/movement, music, or drama therapies as play therapies (Lambert et al., 2007), creative arts therapies and expressive therapies are not merely subsets of play therapy and have a long history as distinct approaches in mental health and health care. While the art activities may sometimes be a form of play, encouraging children to express themselves through a painting, music, or dance involves an understanding of the media beyond the scope of play. In brief, the arts therapies are different from play therapy because they integrate knowledge of art with principles of psychotherapy and counseling.

In addition to the disciplines and approaches mentioned above, many therapists integrate activities that enhance relaxation as part of trauma intervention. Relaxation techniques often include creative components such as music (see Hilliard, Chapter 4, this volume), movement, or art making. Guided imagery or visualization, meditation, yoga, and other methods of stress reduction are also used with children who have experienced traumatic events (Murdock, 2013; Willard, 2010).

Art, music, and dance/movement therapies and other creative interventions such as play have sometimes been incorrectly labeled as *nonverbal* therapies. However, verbal communication of thoughts and feelings is a central part of therapy in most situations. In fact, most therapists who use these methods integrate them within a psychotherapy approach, including, but not limited to, psychodynamic, humanistic, cognitive, developmental, systems, narrative, solution-focused, and other approaches. For example, practitioners who describe their work with children in this book utilize specific frameworks to facilitate therapy with children based on current knowledge of best practices in trauma intervention. There are also creative interventions that specifically focus on verbal communication and self-expression as part of treatment, such as drama therapy, creative writing and poetry therapy, and bibliotherapy.

UNIQUE CHARACTERISTICS OF CREATIVE INTERVENTIONS WITH TRAUMATIZED INDIVIDUALS

In a now classic article on trauma and creative interventions, Johnson (1987) observed that creative arts therapies have a unique role in the treatment of trauma-related disorders, noting that individuals who experience traumatic events have difficulty with verbal expression. He underscored the point that creative arts therapies are effective interventions with psychological trauma in children, individuals with mental illness or developmental delays, and older adults with neurodegenerative disorders or speech problems. Johnson's observations were made almost a decade before the fields of neurobiology, psychiatry, and psychology confirmed that trauma has profound effects on the part of the brain that controls language, and before the roles of explicit and implicit memory in trauma-related disorders were more fully identified.

For young trauma survivors with limited language or who may be unable to put ideas into speech, expression through art, music, movement, or play can be a way to convey these ideas without words and may be the primary form of communication in therapy. Creative interventions involving art, play, music, movement, or other modalities add a unique dimension to treatment because they have several specific characteristics not always found in strictly verbal therapies used in trauma intervention. They are also "brainwise" (Badenoch, 2008) interventions because they are compatible with what we know about how traumatic experiences affect the brain. The brainwise characteristics of these approaches include, but are not limited to, their ability to facilitate (1) externalization, (2) sensory processing, (3) right-hemisphere dominance, (4) arousal reduction and affect regulation, and (5) relational aspects.

Externalization

In trauma intervention, externalization of trauma memories and experiences is considered central to the process of relief and recovery. All therapies, by their very nature and purpose, encourage individuals to engage in a process of externalizing troubling thoughts, feelings, and experiences. Creative interventions encourage externalization through one or more modalities as a central part of therapy and trauma intervention. Gladding (2012) notes that using the arts in counseling may speed up the process of externalization and that expressive modalities allow people to experience themselves differently. Early studies by Terr (1990) identify specific ways that children externalize their trauma experiences through play in repetitive, abreactive, and corrective actions.

Externalization through visual means, play activity, movement, or other modalities may help shift traumatic experiences from the present to the past (Collie, Backos, Malchiodi, & Spiegel, 2006). In art therapy, for example, trauma memories can be externalized through the creative process of making or constructing an image or object. Self-expression through a painting, movement, or poem can relate past experiences, but this is only one benefit of how creative expression externalizes trauma. In fact, most therapists using creative arts or expressive therapies in trauma intervention capitalize on the ability of art, music, play, and other comparable methods of expression to *contain* traumatic experiences rather than encourage cathartic communication of raw emotions or mere repetition of troubling memories. Essentially, child clients are encouraged to use creative self-expression as a repository for feelings and perceptions that can be transformed during the course of treatment, resulting in emotional reparation, resolution of conflict, and a sense of well-being. When verbal communication is limited after traumatic experiences, it may be that some other form of externalization must be used in addition to verbal therapies such as cognitive-behavioral or other accepted approaches to trauma relief.

Sensory Processing

In many approaches to trauma intervention, therapists encourage individuals to explore the trauma narrative—the story of what happened when the trauma occurred and the feelings associated with the event—at some point during treatment. The goal is to help traumatized individuals process what is distressing; transform disturbing behaviors, thoughts, and feelings; and ultimately find relief. With children, however, expressing the trauma story with words is not always possible for developmental reasons, and, as previously mentioned, for severely traumatized clients, words may not be accessible when it comes to describing trauma memories. In many cases, it may be counterproductive to ask young trauma survivors, particularly those who have experienced interpersonal violence, to describe or directly revisit traumatic events.

Expressive and creative arts therapies are defined by psychology as "action" or "experiential" therapies (Weiner, 1999) because they are action-oriented methods through which individuals explore issues and communicate thoughts and feelings. Art and music making, dance and drama, creative writing, and all forms of play are participatory and sensory and require individuals to invest energy in them. For example, art making, even in its simplest sense, can involve arranging, touching, gluing, stapling, painting, forming, and many other tangible experiences. All creative methods focus on encouraging clients to become active, empowered participants in the therapeutic process.

Creative interventions not only serve as a catalyst for individuals to explore thoughts, feelings, memories, and perceptions, they also involve visual, tactile, olfactory, auditory, vestibular, and proprioceptive experiences. Creative activity can also be used with verbal therapies in trauma intervention with children to enhance communication. Drawing, for example, facilitates children's verbal reports of emotionally laden events in several ways: by reducing anxiety, helping the child feel comfortable with the therapist, increasing memory retrieval, organizing narratives, and prompting the child to tell more details than in a solely verbal interview (Gross & Haynes, 1998; Lev-Weisel & Liraz, 2007).

Because highly charged emotional experiences such as trauma are encoded by the limbic system as a form of sensory reality, expression and processing of sensory memories of the traumatic event are necessary to achieve successful intervention and resolution (Rothschild, 2000). Action-oriented activities tap the limbic system's sensory memory of the event and may help bridge implicit and explicit memories of it

(Malchiodi, 2012a; Steele & Malchiodi, 2012) because the brain creates images to contain all the elements of traumatic experience—what happened, emotional reactions to it, and the horror and terror of the experience. When memory cannot be expressed linguistically, it may remain at a symbolic level where there are no words to describe it. In brief, to retrieve that memory so that it can become conscious, it must be externalized in its symbolic form.

Many trauma specialists believe that sensory expression may make progressive exposure of the trauma story and expression of traumatic material tolerable, helping patients overcome avoidance and allowing the therapeutic process to advance relatively quickly (Collie et al., 2006). Active participation and progressive sensory exposure through creative methods may also help reduce the emotional numbing that occurs with PTSD by allowing children to actively imagine, to experiment with or reframe an event, or to rehearse a desired change through self-expression. That is, creative methods involve tangible objects, play activities, movements, or other experiences that can be physically altered. The role of imagination in expressive therapies is illustrated throughout this book, but in essence these therapies assist children in moving beyond preconceived beliefs through experimentation with new ways of communication and sensory activities that involve "pretend."

Right-Hemisphere Dominance

In the field of attachment, it is widely accepted that what happens early in life in terms of relationships affects brain development and is essential to secure attachment (Perry, 2009). *Neuroplasticity* is the brain's ability to renew and, in some cases, even rewire itself to compensate for deficits. Brain plasticity is greater earlier in life, a fact that underscores the importance of intervening with young children to enhance not only their attachment, but also their affect regulation, interpersonal skills, and cognition.

The right hemisphere of the brain is particularly active during early interactions between very young children and caregivers, and when early interactions have been positive, it stores the internal working model (Bowlby, 1988/2005) for secure attachment relationships and healthy affect regulation (Schore, 2003). Siegel (2012) and Schore (2003) note that interactions between baby and caretaker are right-brain mediated because during infancy the right cortex is developing more quickly than the left. Siegel proposes that the output of the right brain is expressed in "non-word-based ways" such as drawing a picture or using a visual image to describe feelings or events. Although creative arts therapies are whole-brain activities, there is substantial evidence that they have right-hemisphere dominance in terms of engaging spatial, sensory, and other nonverbal aspects of experience and communication (Malchiodi, 2014). In brief, current thinking about trauma in general supports the effect of childhood trauma on right–left brain integration (Teicher, 2000) and that sensory-based interventions, such as art and play, may be more effective than language-based interventions because they are right-brain dominant (Klorer, 2008).

Arousal Reduction and Affect Regulation

The reduction of arousal or hyperarousal in young clients is a central goal in trauma intervention. Children who have been victims of interpersonal violence are particularly at risk for problems with hyperarousal, hypoarousal (dissociative states), and affect regulation. On an implicit level, these children's worldviews often include feelings of abandonment and lack of safety; in order to stay safe, they often react with rage at anyone who is perceived as a threat, or they disengage (dissociate) from adults because they have learned that caregivers abandon or hurt children.

For this reason, most forms of trauma intervention begin with a focus on regulation of emotions, stress reduction, and restoration of feelings of safety. Art therapy and music therapy, for example, can be used to activate the body's relaxation response to soothe and reduce stress reactions. In my earliest work with children from violent homes, I learned that art and other expressive activities had a soothing, hypnotic influence and that traumatized children were naturally attracted to these experiences when anxious or suffering posttraumatic reactions (Malchiodi, 1990). Creative arts therapies in general seek to help individuals find activities that are effective in tapping their positive sensory experiences, which can then be practiced over time and eventually become resources for self-regulation of overwhelming emotions. In trauma intervention, recalling memories of positive events that can reframe and eventually override negative ones is helpful in reducing posttraumatic stress, particularly if a sensory experience of "remembered wellness" or safety is included. Simple activities such as drawing a picture of a pleasant time or hearing a soothing, familiar song, story, or rhyme appear to be effective because of the capacity of image making to elicit sensory memories and details of positive moments (Malchiodi, Riley, & Hass-Cohen, 2001). Both music therapy (Wheeler, 2015) and art therapy (Malchiodi, 2013) have demonstrated reductions in autonomic responses such as blood pressure, heart rate, and respiration.

Relational Aspects

Interpersonal neurobiology (Siegel, 2012; see also Badenoch, 2008) refers to an overarching theory that brings together many concepts that have emerged from attachment research, neurobiology, and developmental and social psychology. It is based on the idea that social relationships shape how our brains develop, how our minds perceive the world, and how we adapt to stress throughout the lifespan. In brief, all psychotherapy and counseling are relational approaches because the outcome of intervention is dependent on the core relationship between the therapist and client.

Creative arts therapies are inherently relational therapies because they involve an active, sensory-based dynamic between practitioner and individual; all creative arts therapies that involve mirroring, role play, enactment, sharing, showing, and witnessing are relational approaches to treatment (Malchiodi, 2005, 2012b, 2014). They may be helpful in tapping early those relational states that existed before words became dominant, allowing the brain to establish new, more productive patterns (Malchiodi, 2012a; Riley, 2002). Additionally, being an attuned and focused witness to a child's efforts to complete a hands-on task and assisting those efforts, when appropriate, mimics the neurobiological relationship between a caring adult and child. For some children, repetitive experiential and self-rewarding experiences that include a positive and attuned witness are central to repairing developmental trauma (Perry, 2009).

Although all the creative arts therapies can be used with a goal of enhancing relationships, dance/movement therapy is most often used to address relational issues because it focuses on the body. For example, *mirroring* is commonly used to establish and enhance the relationship between the individual and the therapist. The goal of mirroring is not imitation of movements, postures, facial expressions, and gestures, but to achieve a sense of connection and understanding between the client and practitioner. Mirroring is also a form of nonverbal, right-hemisphere communication that naturally occurs in secure attachment relationships through the gestures, postures, and facial expressions that transpire between a caregiver and child (for more information, see Gray, Chapter 8, this volume).

Relational aspects are evident in art, music, and drama therapies also. In art therapy, a therapist is a provider of materials (nurturer), assistant in the creative process, and active participant in facilitating visual self-expression. Music therapy provides similar experiences through interaction with music making; it also has the potential to tap social engagement and communication when collaboration or simultaneous instrument playing is involved. Finally, drama therapy offers multisensory ways to establish relationship through role play, mirroring, and enactment and often includes other creative arts and play to reduce stress and assist trauma integration.

CONCLUSION

Applying creative interventions in trauma intervention has enormous potential, as demonstrated in this chapter and throughout the applications and cases described in this book. For children in general, creative activities in therapy offer many benefits: pleasure in making, doing, and inventing; play and imagination; and enhancement of self-worth through self-expression. There are additional reasons to consider integrating creative arts therapies, play therapy, and other action-oriented approaches for children who are traumatized. For these young trauma survivors, creative expression (1) offers a way to contain traumatic material within an object, image, story, music, or other art form; (2) provides a sense of control over terrifying and intrusive memories; (3) encourages active participation in therapy; (4) reduces emotional numbness; and (5) enhances reduction of hyperarousal and other distressing reactions. When verbal techniques fail to ameliorate trauma memory in children, art, play, music, or movement can provide the necessary means to reenact the feelings and sensations associated with traumatic experiences. In subsequent chapters, these and other advantages of creative activities, as used in intervention with traumatized children, are described to demonstrate in detail how these approaches facilitate emotional reparation, relief, and recovery.

REFERENCES

American Dance Therapy Association. (2014). What is dance therapy? Retrieved January 23, 2014, from *www.adta.org/about/who.cfm*.

American Music Therapy Association. (2014). Music therapy makes a difference: What is music therapy? Retrieved January 22, 2014, from *www. musictherapy.org*.

American Psychiatric Association. (1987). *Diagnostic and statistical manual of mental disorders* (3rd ed., rev.). Washington, DC: Author.

American Psychiatric Association. (2013). *Diagnostic and statistical manual of mental disorders* (5th ed.). Arlington, VA: Author.

Badenoch, B. (2008). *Being a brain-wise therapist: A practical guide to interpersonal neurobiology*. New York: Norton.

Bowlby, J. (2005). *A secure base*. New York: Routledge. (Original work published 1988)

Collie, K., Backos, A., Malchiodi, C., & Spiegel, D. (2006). Art therapy for combat-related PTSD: Recommendations for research and practice. *Art Therapy: Journal of the American Art Therapy Association, 23*(4), 157–164.

Crenshaw, D. A., & Stewart, A. L. (Eds.). (2014). *Play therapy: A comprehensive guide to theory and practice*. New York: Guilford Press.

Damasio, A. (2000). *The feeling of what happens*. New York: Harcourt.

Damasio, A. (2011). *Self comes to mind: Constructing the conscious brain*. New York: Vintage.

Edwards, D. (2004). *Art therapy*. London: Sage.

Estrella, K. (2005). Expressive therapy: An integrated arts approach. In C. A. Malchiodi (Ed.), *Expressive therapies* (pp. 183–209). New York: Guilford Press.

Gladding, S. T. (2012). Art in counseling. In C. A. Malchiodi (Ed.), *Handbook of art therapy* (2nd ed., pp. 263–274). New York: Guilford Press.

Gross, J., & Haynes, H. (1998). Drawing facilitates children's verbal reports of emotionally laden events. *Journal of Experimental Psychology, 4*, 163–179.

Johnson, D. (1987). The role of the creative arts therapies in the diagnosis and treatment of psychological trauma. *Arts in Psychotherapy, 14*, 7–13.

Klorer, P. G. (2008). Expressive therapy for severe maltreatment and attachment disorders: A neuroscience framework. In C. A. Malchiodi (Ed.), *Creative interventions with traumatized children* (pp. 43–61). New York: Guilford Press.

Knill, P., Levine, E., & Levine, S. (2005). *Principles and practice of expressive arts therapy: Towards a therapeutic aesthetics*. London: Jessica Kingsley.

Korn, M. L. (2001). Trauma and PTSD: Aftermath of the WTC disaster—an interview with Bessel A. van der Kolk, MD. *Medscape General Medicine*

3(4) [formerly published in *Medscape Psychiatry and Mental Health eJournal* 6(5), 2001]. Available at *www.medscape.com/viewarticle/408691.*

Lambert, S. F., LeBlanc, M., Mullen, J. A., Ray, D., Baggerly, J., White, J., et al. (2007). Learning more about those who play in session: The national play therapy in counseling practices project (Phase I). *Journal of Counseling and Development, 85*(1), 42–46.

Levine, P. (2012). *In an unspoken voice: How the body releases trauma and restores goodness.* Berkeley, CA: North Atlantic Books.

Levine, P., & Klein, M. (2007). *Trauma through a child's eyes: Awakening the ordinary miracle of healing.* Berkeley, CA: North Atlantic Books.

Lev-Weisel, R., & Liraz, R. (2007). Drawings versus narratives: Drawing as a tool to encourage verbalization in children whose fathers are drug abusers. *Clinical Child Psychology and Psychiatry, 12*(1), 65–75.

Lieberman, A., & Knorr, K. (2007). The impact of trauma: A developmental framework for infancy and early childhood. *Psychiatric Annals, 37*(6), 416–422.

Malchiodi, C. A. (1990). *Breaking the silence: Art therapy with children from violent homes.* New York: Brunner/Mazel.

Malchiodi, C. A. (Ed.). (2005). *Expressive therapies.* New York: Guilford Press.

Malchiodi, C. A. (2012a). Art therapy and the brain. In C. A. Malchiodi (Ed.), *Handbook of art therapy* (2nd ed., pp. 17–26). New York: Guilford Press.

Malchiodi, C. A. (Ed.). (2012b). *Handbook of art therapy* (2nd ed). New York: Guilford Press.

Malchiodi, C. A. (Ed.). (2013). *Art therapy and health care.* New York: Guilford Press.

Malchiodi, C. A. (2014). Creative arts therapy approaches to attachment issues. In C. A. Malchiodi & D. A. Crenshaw (Eds.), *Creative arts and play therapy for attachment problems* (pp. 3–18). New York: Guilford Press.

Malchiodi, C. A., & Crenshaw, D. A. (Eds.). (2014). *Creative arts and play therapy for attachment problems.* New York: Guilford Press.

Malchiodi, C. A., Riley, S., & Hass-Cohen, N. (2001). *Toward an integrated art therapy mind–body landscape* (Cassette Recording No. 108-1525). Denver: National Audio Video.

Murdock, M. (2013). *Spinning inward: Using guided imagery with children for learning, creativity, and relaxation.* Boston: Shambhala.

National Association for Drama Therapy. (2014). Frequently asked questions about drama therapy: What is drama therapy? Retrieved January 23, 2014, from *www.nadt.org/faqs.html.*

National Child Traumatic Stress Network. (2014). Facts and figures. Retrieved January 4, 2014, from *www.nctsn.org/resources/topics/facts-and-figures.*

National Coalition of Creative Arts Therapies Associations. (2014). Definition of professions. Retrieved January 22, 2014, from *www.nccata.org.*

Perry, B. D. (2009). Examining child maltreatment through a

neurodevelopmental lens: Clinical applications of the neurosequential model of therapeutics. *Journal of Loss and Trauma, 14,* 240–255.

Riley, S. (2002). *Group process made visible: Group art therapy.* Philadelphia: Brunner-Routledge.

Rothschild, B. (2000). *The body remembers: The psychophysiology of trauma and trauma treatment.* New York: Norton.

Schore, A. (2003). *Affect regulation and the repair of the self.* New York: Norton.

Siegel, D. J. (2012). *The developing mind: How relationships and the brain interact to shape who we are* (2nd ed.). New York: Guilford Press.

Silva, R. (2004). *Posttraumatic stress disorders in children and adolescents.* New York: Norton.

Steele, W., & Malchiodi, C. A. (2012). *Trauma-informed practice with children and adolescents.* New York: Taylor & Francis.

Sternberg, E. (2001). *The balance within: The science connecting health and emotions.* New York: Freeman.

Teicher, M. D. (2000). Wounds that time won't heal: The neurobiology of child abuse. *Cerebrum: Dana Forum on Brain Science, 2*(4), 50v67.

Terr, L. (1981). Psychic trauma in children: Observations following the Chowchilla school-bus kidnapping. *American Journal of Psychiatry, 138,* 14–19.

Terr, L. (1990). *Too scared to cry.* New York: HarperCollins.

Tuber, S., Boesch, K., Gorking, J., & Terry, M. (2014). Chronic early trauma as a childhood syndrome and its relationship to play. In C. A. Malchiodi & D. A. Crenshaw (Eds.), *Creative arts and play therapy for attachment problems* (pp. 215–226). New York: Guilford Press.

U.S. Department of Health and Human Services, Administration for Children and Families, Administration on Children, Youth and Families, Children's Bureau. (2012). *Child maltreatment 2011.* Available from *www.acf.hhs.gov.*

van Dalen, A. (2001). Juvenile violence and addiction: Tangled roots in childhood trauma. *Journal of Social Work Practice in the Addictions, 1,* 25–40.

van der Kolk, B. (1994). *The body keeps the score.* Cambridge, MA: Harvard Medical School.

van der Kolk, B., (2005). Developmental trauma. *Psychiatric Annals, 35*(5), 401–408.

Webb, N. B. (Ed). (2007). *Play therapy with children in crisis: Individual, group, and family treatment* (3rd ed.). New York: Guilford Press.

Weiner, D. J. (1999). *Beyond talk therapy: Using movement and expressive techniques in clinical practice.* Washington, DC: American Psychological Association.

Wheeler, B. L. (2015). *Music therapy handbook.* New York: Guilford Press.

Willard, C. (2010). *Child's mind: Mindfulness practices to help our children be more focused, calm and relaxed.* Berkeley, CA: Parallax Press.

CHAPTER 2

Ethics, Evidence, Trauma-Informed Practice, and Cultural Sensitivity

Cathy A. Malchiodi

Creative interventions, like any therapeutic approach, require that therapists use them appropriately and effectively in practice. Creative arts therapies and expressive therapies provide the foundation for a variety of useful techniques with traumatized children, but these approaches cannot be applied without a rationale and understanding of basic principles, trauma-informed practice, and experience. Because so many therapists intuitively use creative approaches in their work with children, they may take for granted that a large and formalized body of knowledge on the use of these approaches already exists.

Although therapists cannot possibly know every aspect of creative arts therapies and expressive therapies, there are several areas with which they should become familiar before applying these therapies in trauma work. First and foremost, using any of these interventions with traumatized children involves unique ethical issues related to each expressive modality and should include knowledge of evidence-based practice. Trauma-informed principles and cultural sensitivity about play, toys, music, props, and art materials in therapy is also requisite to work with young clients, particularly those from diverse backgrounds. This chapter provides a brief overview of these ethical, cultural, evidence-based practice, and special issues, with an emphasis on aspects relevant to the use of creative arts therapies and expressive therapies with traumatized children.

ETHICAL PRACTICE OF CREATIVE INTERVENTION

Knill, Levine, and Levine (2005) observe that creative approaches used in therapy have distinct characteristics that set them apart from strictly verbal techniques and from each other. For example, visual expression is conducive to more private, isolated work and introspective exploration; music often taps feelings and may lend itself to socialization when people collaborate in song or in simultaneously playing instruments; and dance/movement offers opportunities to interact and form relationships. Play incorporates many forms of creative expression and may involve a wide range of individual or interpersonal interventions. All creative arts therapies and expressive therapies utilize tactile, kinesthetic, and auditory experiences in various ways, depending on the activity. Each form of creative expression has its unique properties and roles in therapeutic work depending on its application—the practitioner, the client, and the setting—and objectives.

The differences inherent in each modality inform the ethical practice and application of creative interventions in work with traumatized children. Although all mental health professionals abide by the ethical codes of their specific disciplines, creative arts therapists and play therapists have ethical standards for practice that address issues specific to the use of these methods with clients (see the Appendix at the back of this book for websites of organizations where these standards can be found). Familiarity with the content of these codes enhances therapists' applications of these approaches and helps them develop a clearer understanding of the purpose and characteristics of the methods they are using. Although it is impossible to become an expert on all aspects of all therapies, therapists should have hands-on experience with, and a working knowledge of, the modalities they employ and a rationale for their use in trauma intervention.

The ethical codes of creative arts therapies and play therapy underscore important aspects of practice not found in the ethics codes of counselors, psychologists, social workers, and other mental health professionals. The field of play therapy emphasizes the ethics of "touch" in therapy because of the nature of the relationship between therapists and children in the playroom (Sprunk, Mitchell, Myrow, & O'Connor, 2007). Play therapists also underscore the importance of informed consent before touch is introduced or occurs in play sessions and recommend that therapists give parents or caregivers and children examples of types of touch that might happen in play therapy and initiate discussion about physical safety and sexual boundaries. For example, touch is not automatically ethically eliminated from play therapy just because a client has experienced "bad touch"; children who have been physically or sexually abused often need to experience safe and positive touch in order to reestablish trust and attachment.

Art therapists stress sensitivity to specific ethical issues when it comes to introducing art expression in treatment (Malchiodi, 1998, 2012). Art therapy involves the creation of a product that constitutes part of clients' confidential treatment record, just as written documentation, audiotapes, or videotapes of sessions would be confidential. In other words, therapists who ask child clients to make drawings, paintings, or other art must consider how they will record, store, and, in certain situations, retain original artworks produced in therapy. Digital cameras have made it possible to store photographic copies more easily, allowing children to keep their products, but, in some cases, such as those involving abuse or neglect, it is often necessary to retain the actual artwork for legal deposition. In all cases, children's art expressions are defined as part of therapeutic records and are shared or displayed only with permission of parents or guardians and child assent for specific purposes; records of art expressions (digital or otherwise) are kept on file according to state laws, institution and agency regulations, and current standards of professional practice.

Finally, therapists, even those who are skilled in one or more creative arts therapy, are careful not to interpret creative expressions based on their own intuition or projections. In general, creative arts therapists, expressive arts therapists, and play therapists do not seek to interpret individuals' drawings, movement, poems, or play, but facilitate those individuals' discovery of personal meaning and understanding of such expressions. They use verbal techniques to help young clients explore their feelings and perceptions rather than relying solely on interpretation. As with any form of therapy, therapists listen to and respect what young clients are communicating through self-expression and flexibly apply techniques that are best suited to clients' needs and treatment objectives.

EVIDENCE AND CREATIVE INTERVENTIONS

Using creative methods in counseling or psychotherapy comes with the responsibility of learning established and emerging information on the use of these approaches with children and trauma. The term *evidence-based practice* refers to a body of scientifically established knowledge about specific clinical interventions or treatments (Hoagland, Burns, Kiser, Ringeisen, & Schoenwald, 2001). In brief, for an intervention or treatment to be classified as *well established*, two or more studies must demonstrate that it is better than placebo, medication, or alternative treatment or that it is equal to another established intervention. Interventions or treatments are classified as *probably efficacious* if at least one study demonstrates their superiority to placebo or shows efficacy via other accepted methods. Evidence-based practice not only advances therapists' knowledge of which protocols and techniques are most effective, but also helps ensure that clients receive the best treatment based on current knowledge.

The Substance Abuse and Mental Health Services Administration (SAMSHA), a U.S. agency, lists evidence-based trauma intervention protocols submitted by researchers on a national registry (National Registry of Evidence-Based Programs and Practices [NREPP], 2014). Therapists relying on this list as a resource should realize that although this database provides some guidance in choosing effective methods, these protocols are not endorsed by SAMSHA; for example, some of the protocols on the database are the result of research studies that do not include control groups or multiple trials. Trauma-focused cognitive-behavioral therapy (TF-CBT; Cohen, Mannarino, & Deblinger, 2006) is one approach in the NREPP list that continues to demonstrate strong evidence for trauma intervention with children, according to SAMSHA's guidelines. TF-CBT mentions the use of "artistic narrative" within its protocol, indicating that art and play approaches can be applied during this particular evidence-based intervention with children.

Common practices in art therapy, music therapy, and play have not yet been studied extensively to determine if they qualify as evidence-based practices in the field of trauma intervention with children. For example, a study of short-term art therapy did not demonstrate significant relief of posttraumatic stress in pediatric patients (Schreier, Ladakakos, Morabito, Chapman, & Knudson, 2005). However, even evidence-based trauma intervention protocols based on CBT include some form of art expression and/or play because children require developmentally appropriate strategies such as drawing, games, props and toys, and role play.

"Best practices" in creative arts therapies have been identified in an effort to establish which methods show promise and demonstrate reliable outcomes when compared to other treatments. *Best practices* are different from *evidence-based practices* in that they are derived from clinical data on practitioners' particular applications or commonly used protocols within a discipline. Limited research studies that demonstrate their effectiveness with other disorders and populations exist, but there is a rapidly growing interest in producing more outcome studies of expressive therapies in general. The International Society for Traumatic Stress Studies (ISTSS; 2014) recognizes that creative arts therapies and play therapy fulfill a significant role in trauma intervention with children and adolescents, underscoring their sensory aspects in the amelioration of stress reactions, including posttraumatic stress, and as methods of nonverbal processing.

Gil (2006) makes an important point in reference to current evidence-based practices in trauma intervention and the use of art and play within those protocols. Like evidence-based approaches, creative arts therapies and expressive therapies employ gradual exposure and work with affective material related to traumatic experiences. Gil notes that, unlike in models such as TF-CBT, which have a specific agenda and set of instructions, expressive activities "are initiated by children or facilitated by clinicians and employed at their pace, within the context of a therapy relationship, and with respect for children's need to utilize their defensive mechanisms in a fluid fashion" (p. 102). In other words, children are allowed to set their own pace for self-expression through play and art, depending on needs for adaptive coping, the nature of the trauma, children's individual temperament and cultural values, and other factors. Creative approaches may be less likely to be evaluated because they include both nondirective (spontaneous or authentic self-expression) and directive (specific activities) approaches. Nevertheless, therapists who use these methods should regularly review the available literature on evidence-based practice.

TRAUMA-INFORMED PRACTICE

Although there are many approaches to trauma intervention that are effective in work with children, some are more compatible with creative arts and play than others. *Trauma-informed* practice is one such approach. It (1) emphasizes knowledge of how the mind and body respond to traumatic events; (2) recognizes that symptoms are adaptive coping strategies rather than pathology; (3) acknowledges clients' cultural sensitivity to values, perceptions, and worldviews of illness and treatment; and (4) maintains the belief that individuals are not only survivors, but also "thrivers" (Malchiodi, 2012). Trauma-informed practice is not only applied to trauma intervention; it is used as a model for systems, institutions, and organizations that assist individuals, groups, and families with a variety health challenges (Steele & Malchiodi, 2012). In brief, it is a strengths-based, resilience-enhancing framework for helping people of all ages and with many different emotional, interpersonal, cognitive, and physical problems.

Trauma-informed expressive arts therapy (Malchiodi, 2012) is an example of an arts-based approach that utilizes trauma-informed practice as a framework for intervention. It is based on the idea that the creative arts therapies are helpful in reconnecting implicit (sensory) and explicit (declarative) memories of trauma and in the treatment of posttraumatic stress disorder (PTSD) (Malchiodi, 2012). In particular, it is an approach used to assist the individual's capacity to self-regulate affect and moderate the body's reactions to traumatic experiences, thereby setting the stage for eventual trauma integration and recovery. It includes a neurosequential approach that capitalizes on the expressive therapies continuum (Lusebrink, 2010) and neurodevelopment (Perry, 2009) in applying appropriate creative arts therapies and integrative interventions. Throughout this book, authors describe additional trauma-informed strategies to help young clients recover the "creative life" (Cattanach, 2008), reinforce a sense of safety, and build strengths through experiences of mastery and enhance resilience.

Three aspects of a trauma-informed expressive arts therapy approach are central to effective practice with traumatized children: (1) sensory-based methods, (2) posttraumatic play, and (3) culturally sensitive intervention. Whether applying trauma-informed principles or other strategies, these aspects are central to all creative interventions.

Sensory-Based Methods

As discussed in Chapter 1, creative approaches are sensory-based methods because they tap tactile, auditory, visual, and kinesthetic experiences to facilitate nonverbal levels of processing. These methods can assist individuals in expressing sensory aspects of traumatic experiences, help reduce hyperarousal through stress reduction, and may be useful in bridging declarative and nondeclarative memories. In using these approaches, practitioners have the opportunity to apply art, play, music, movement, stories, and dramatic enactment in treatment both to ease trauma-related symptoms and to facilitate the expression and resolution of trauma narratives.

In order to be effective, therapists should have a clear understanding of why and how creative approaches support sensory work with children. For example, creative arts therapies can be useful in helping children recognize body reactions to stress and trauma-related memories. Asking a child to indicate through colors, shapes, and lines on a body outline "where you feel the fear/worry/anger/sadness in your body" begins the process of identifying how the child reacts to an intrusive memory or distressing event. Similarly, a child could be asked to use sound or a musical instrument to communicate a feeling or express it through movement. Therapists serve as facilitators of self-expression and, more important, as empathetic, attuned individuals who encourage children to use creative methods to transform fear, worry, anger, and sadness and help them identify their own healing responses through sensory experiences. Because this sensory work with children is both directive and nondirective, therapists should be prepared to face the challenge of trauma intervention with both flexibility and sensitivity to the application of various media.

Because trauma-related symptoms may include intrusive memories, anxiety, and hyperarousal, which can be psychologically paralyzing for some individuals, helping young clients take small steps toward expression of feelings and experiences is a necessary skill. Rothschild (2000), Levine (2012), and others refer to this as *titration*, a trauma-informed process of helping individuals slowly release distressing emotions, memories, and thoughts in small amounts. Rothschild compares titration to shaking up a bottle of soda and then carefully unscrewing the top to slowly release the contents. If done correctly, only a small *fizz* is heard and no liquid escapes the bottle; however, if the top is removed too quickly, the contents of the bottle will explode. Rothschild's analogy effectively demonstrates the point that therapists must consistently provide interventions that help their clients safely release troubling feelings and memories at an appropriate pace.

Applying the titration principle when using creative approaches involves an understanding of materials, props, toys, stories, music, and movement and how to modulate their use in relation to children's needs and degree of symptoms. In particular, it is important to know that a material, prop, or method can be productive (leading to self-soothing, affect regulation, or corrective experiences) or nonproductive (leading to distress). For example, large paper and watery paint can provide an experience of free play and expression but may not be appropriate for some traumatized children who need structure, safety, and consistency. In using music or sound, it is important to understand how rhythm, affect, and content may influence the pace of a session, promote relaxation, or stimulate positive emotions. Similarly, toys and props should be selected for a specific purpose, based on knowledge of how children who have been traumatized may react. If therapists have not had experience with and preparation in the creative methods they plan to use, they may not be able to appropriately and gradually assist children in finding relief and recovery.

Expressive methods can and do stimulate the flow of traumatic memories, either in the form of trauma narratives (stories about the event) or implicit experiences (sensory memories of the event) because of the tactile, kinesthetic, auditory, olfactory, or visual aspects inherent in creative activities. For example, in an art therapy group of four children from the same family, the youngest child, 6 years old, attempted to clean his brush in a plastic water jar and accidentally knocked it over, spilling water everywhere. At that moment, he reacted with a freeze response to an anxiety-producing situation, intensely watching the therapist for a reaction. In the same moment, two of the children jumped from their seats and ran to the door (a flight response). The fourth child hid (flight) beneath the table, becoming silent and watchful (freeze). These children reacted to the sights and sounds of the water spilling just as they would if someone accidentally spilled milk at their dining table at home and risked physical punishment for their actions. The spilled water jar triggered implicit memories of fear, anxiety, and responses that included hypervigilance, escape routines, and other physical strategies for survival (e.g., hiding under the table or running for the door). In this family, each child had developed automatic survival-based reactions when threatened by the possibility of retaliation from an adult who was verbally and physically abusive.

Creative expression can also become a way to rehearse adaptive coping skills and positive experiences of safety, stability, attachment, and self-esteem. Many children, if given a safe environment and opportunity, will intuitively use creative expression for pleasure and to self-soothe. Some children may find relief through cuddly toys (tactile); some through brightly colored tissue paper, glitter, and paints (visual); and others may respond positively to dance or movement (kinesthetic) or making or listening to music (auditory). In other situations, therapists can use directive approaches to help children experience positive forms of self-expression; for example, an activity such as creating a safe place for an animal (Malchiodi, 2006), in which children select or are given small plastic or soft toy animals and are encouraged to use a box or other materials to make a place where the animal feels safe and gets all its needs met. Through imaginative caretaking of the toy animal and constructing a safe place for it, issues of protection and nurturance can be explored and practiced in a tangible, sensory way, with help and prompting from the therapist if needed.

Finally, the sensory nature of creative approaches can evoke self-soothing experiences common to childhood—rhythmic movements and sounds, tactile and visual pleasure, and imagination and fantasy. Imagination and fantasy are the first adaptive coping strategies children have available to them, especially during the preschool years. By using imagination, children can formulate a more appealing narrative for what has happened or divert themselves from it momentarily. Art making, play, drama, music, stories, and movement allow children to escape their fears, worries, and sadness, if only during the time they are engrossed in an activity. The experience of losing oneself in a pleasurable activity can induce feelings of relaxation and self-satisfaction and reinforce positive sensations—but, as described in the previous section on posttraumatic play, becoming engrossed in an activity in a nonproductive, rigid way that leads to feeling worse afterward is not helpful to children over time. In providing activities to traumatized children, therapists are consistently challenged to observe their young clients' responses to these expressive interventions and to reevaluate whether interventions are providing the sensory experiences necessary for emotional restoration, resolution, and eventual recovery.

Posttraumatic Play and Art Expression

Rosa was 7 years old when she, her mother, and a younger brother arrived at a shelter for battered women and their children. Rosa's mother, Tasha, had been only 15 years old when she gave birth to Rosa, and Rosa's biological father abandoned them at that time. For the next 7 years, Rosa lived in public housing in a large Midwestern city in an environment regrettably dominated by drug abuse, neighborhood violence, and poverty. In addition, Tasha and Rosa were often physically abused by various boyfriends Tasha brought into the home; reports made to child protective services indicated that Rosa was sexually abused on several occasions, but the details and types of abuse remained unclear. Social services and law enforcement documented numerous incidents of domestic violence to Rosa and her mother, and in each case Rosa became both a child witness and a victim of physical brutality.

When Rosa was 5 years old, her mother could no longer afford to pay rent, and they became homeless. Rosa's life was chaotic and nomadic during her first years in elementary school, limiting her attendance at school to only a few months each year. Tasha gave birth to a son whose biological father also abandoned the family, adding to the stress of continued poverty, homelessness, domestic violence, and abandonment. During this time, Rosa became increasingly anxious, withdrawn, and preoccupied. Fortunately, Tasha realized that she could no longer manage her family's situation by herself, called a domestic violence helpline, and was taken to a local shelter.

Although Rosa received some limited intervention from school counselors, it was not the type of regular treatment needed to ameliorate the effects of the multiple traumatic events she had experienced. She now exhibited many of the classic signs of PTSD, including avoidance, hyperarousal, and recurrent memories of multiple abuses to herself and her mother. She could no longer sleep through the night, had frequent nightmares, and developed phobias of school because she feared separation from her mother. The birth of her brother exacerbated the stress she experienced, and she became increasingly aggressive when her mother directed her attention to her sibling and away from Rosa.

Like many children who have encountered multiple traumas, Rosa presented a repetitive narrative in her art and play during early therapy sessions. Over the course of several meetings, Rosa related the following story in drawings and spontaneous narrative:

> "A little girl is being hurt by a man who hits her with a baseball bat and sometimes his hands. He hurts the mother, too. The mother and the little girl try to run. He keeps hurting them with the bat. He hits the little girl really hard and hurts her face. There is blood on the mother. They get into the bathroom and close the door [Figure 2.1]. The little girl is real afraid that the man will get in. The little girl's face is hurt and there is blood [Figure 2.2]. The mother

I am __9__ years old and in the __3__ grade.

I was __9__ years old when __I was hurt__.

This is a picture of me:

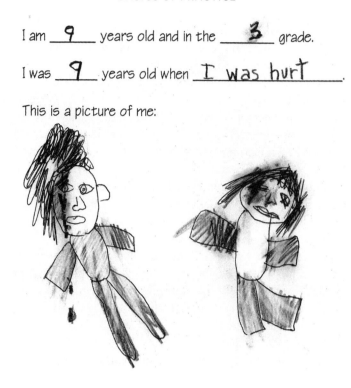

FIGURE 2.1. Rosa's drawing of "what happened" to a "little girl and her mother" during domestic violence.

takes the little girl to the hospital and she gets a bandage put on. She is still real afraid."

Rosa spontaneously related an important personal story about "what happened" through her artwork, but she is not getting relief from telling her story through art and play. Like many children who are affected by significant traumatic experiences, Rosa often reexperiences these events through repetitive and intrusive thoughts. She also reenacts the traumatic events through art expression or play; in Rosa's case, the story is specific to events she experienced, but for other children these themes can be nonspecific and symbolically related to traumatic events. For example, children who survived Hurricane Katrina in the Gulf Coast region of the United States created miniature towns inundated by rising floodwaters in sandplay with toy figures, whereas others constructed sandtrays with monster themes or battle scenes.

This is a picture of what happened **To my face:**

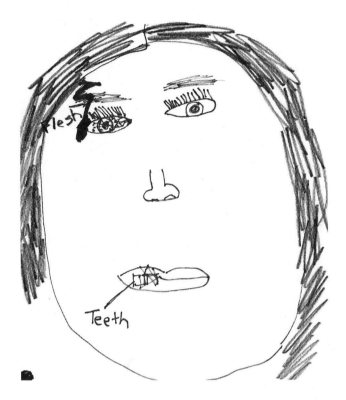

FIGURE 2.2. Rosa's self-portrait depicting the face of a "little girl" after being hurt.

Posttraumatic play and posttraumatic art expression are important adaptive coping strategies used by children who have experienced serious emotional trauma or loss. The term *posttraumatic play* is used to describe both the recurrent memories and the reenactment common to children who are distressed by single-incident or chronic traumas. Terr (1979, 1990) first used the term to describe the play activity of children who have experienced traumatic events but not the resolution of the emotions associated with those events. In contrast to normal play, which leads to pleasure, satisfying expression, problem solving, and learning, posttraumatic play is often anxiety-ridden and constricted, repetitive, rigid, and without resolution. For example, a child may consistently attempt to destroy a toy house, repeatedly saying, "House goes boom," to describe the devastation experienced during a tornado. For the child engaged in this type of play, mastery over the event is not possible, and emotional relief from play is unavailable. During the first several weeks of treatment, Rosa unproductively repeated the story of a particularly brutal incident of domestic violence involving physical abuse and terror without receiving needed relief from her fears and anxiety. It also conveyed her hopelessness and lack of belief in rescue and resolution of her situation; in Rosa's initial art expressions, no one is able to save her mother and her from "hurt" and "blood." At this stage of intervention, it is important for Rosa to communicate what happened and her feelings about it, but her art expression is stagnant, stuck, and unproductive in finding solutions to her trauma experiences, without hope of support from caregivers or other adults.

Gil (2006) provides an excellent summary (see Table 2.1) of the differences between "stagnant posttraumatic play" and what she defines as "dynamic posttraumatic play." According to Gil, the stagnant version of posttraumatic play may leave the child retraumatized, dissociative, in a state of hyperarousal, or feeling hopeless and helpless. In contrast, children who engage in dynamic posttraumatic play are less rigid, interact more freely with the therapist, take a more active role on their own behalf, and are generally more emotionally relieved by the experience. Their play leads to helpful, empowering adaptation and resolution of trauma reactions. The differences between the two types of play are subtle but discernible with careful observation over time. These differences are important to detect for all therapists who observe traumatized children's play, art, or other expressive work because, as Gil notes, the lack of positive resolution is a signal that a child may need more directive, purposeful intervention.

Because play encompasses a number of forms of self-expression, including movement, dramatic enactment, and storytelling, therapists should have a solid understanding of what differentiates posttraumatic play from healthy play activity. Art expressions, too, may be rigid and repetitive and contain unresolved narratives about trauma. In all cases, the challenge is how to help children find corrective, self-soothing, and productive experiences through creative approaches. Creative activity in and of itself does not necessarily lead to positive resolution, no matter how carefully selected. Therapists should be prepared to make both appropriate creative and verbal interventions to assist children in this process; the goal is to facilitate play and other forms of expression that help children explore feelings and experiences but do not reinforce

TABLE 2.1. Differences between Dynamic and Stagnant Posttraumatic Play

Dynamic posttraumatic play	Stagnant posttraumatic play
• Affect becomes available.	• Affect remains constricted.
• Physical fluidity becomes evident.	• Physical constriction remains.
• Interactions with play become varied.	• Interactions with play remain limited.
• Interactions with clinician become varied.	• Interactions with clinician remain limited.
• Play changes, or new elements are added.	• Play stays precisely the same.
• Play occurs in different locations.	• Play is conducted in same spot.
• Play includes new objects.	• Play is limited to specific objects.
• Themes differ or expand.	• Themes remain constant.
• Outcomes differ, and healthier, more adaptive responses emerge.	• Outcomes remain fixed and nonadaptive.
• Rigidity of play loosens over time.	• Play remains rigid.
• After-play behavior indicates release or fatigue.	• After-play behavior indicates constriction/tension.
• Out-of-session symptoms may remain unchanged or peak at first, but then decrease.	• Out-of-season symptoms are unchanged or increase.

Note. From Gil (2006, p. 160). Copyright 2006 by The Guilford Press. Reprinted by permission.

traumatic memories. This process includes actively helping children transform these memories by providing creative activities to enhance relaxation and self-soothing abilities and to assist in finding solutions and reframing traumatic stories.

Culturally Sensitive Trauma Intervention

Trauma-informed practice dictates that practitioners be culturally sensitive in choosing interventions, designing treatment, and particularly in communicating with clients. Sue and Sue (2012) define *cultural competence* as the recognition of individuals' cultures and the development of skills, knowledge, and procedures that enables practitioners to provide effective services to those individuals. In trauma intervention with children, cultural competence includes knowledge of how culture may affect traumatic reactions in young clients, based on a variety of factors, including, but not limited to, ethnicity; degree of acculturation; location (rural or urban); region (e.g., northern vs. southern United States); family, extended family, and peers; socioeconomic status (SES);

gender; development; and religious or spiritual affiliation. The National Child Traumatic Stress Network (NCTSN; 2014) cites "cultural identity"—the culture with which someone identifies and looks to for accepted standards of behavior—as a factor in the treatment of childhood trauma. Cultural factors also may impact frequency of exposure to traumatic events; for example, children and adolescents from minority backgrounds are at increased risk for trauma exposure (NCTSN, 2014). Disasters additionally pose substantial risks for children of ethnic minorities and in developing countries because of socioeconomic and political conditions, increasing the likelihood of more severe symptoms. In brief, many aspects come together to determine children's worldviews and cultural preferences for participation and disclosure in therapy.

Diversity issues and worldview influence how children perceive toys, props, and play, depending on cultural background or experiences. Gil and Drewes (2005) provide one of the few comprehensive overviews of how cultural influences specifically affect children's play within therapy. They note that there are some obvious ways that therapists who use play activities, toys, and props can enhance intervention with attention to diversity issues. They underscore that therapists serious about using play in treatment should maintain an organized collection of toys and props that are developmentally, gender, and culturally diverse. For example, toy animals differ among cultures, so it is important to provide figures that are typical to many different cultural groups and that have distinctive cultural meanings. Similarly, the selection of books, dolls, games, and props should take diversity issues into consideration. For example, Kao (2005) notes that the most traditional and preferred toys in Asian cultures fall into five distinct categories: social, intellectual, seasonal, physical, and gambling.

Therapists should have on hand art materials that support and nurture creativity for children of various cultures, such as crayons, felt-tip markers, and clay in a range of tones that approximate different skin colors. Photo collage materials should reflect a variety of cross-cultural images, including various ethnicities, family configurations, lifestyles, and beliefs. Craft materials such as fabric, yarn, beads, or other objects may be helpful in stimulating some children whose experiences with art evolved around fabric decoration, jewelry making, or traditional needle arts (Malchiodi, 2005).

Generally, children's self-expression is influenced by what they are exposed to in their communities, but also by the media (Malchiodi, 1998, 2005). Television, movies, videogames, Internet and social media, and print material are extremely important elements of culture that have a powerful and often direct impact on children's view of themselves. Exposure to media is one of the strongest sources of images and stories, and children adopt those images and stories that have had a significant impact on them. One of the most memorable examples in recent years involves the events of September 11, 2001; any child who saw the repeated footage of the planes hitting the World Trade Center buildings reenacted that image in drawings and play activities for weeks, months, and, in the case of those most severely affected through traumatic loss, years (Malchiodi, 2002; TEDxOverland Park, 2012). In addition to significant events, television, movies, and the Internet are powerful influences that shape children's adoption of clothing and fashion as well as language, behaviors, and worldviews. These influences are recognizable in children's drawings that reference cartoon characters, popular film or music stars, or movie, television, or videogame plots; older children and adolescents may include cultural conventions from peer groups, such as graffiti, gang symbols, or tattoo art (Riley, 1999).

In providing culturally sensitive creative intervention, therapists must be flexible in how they initiate creative expression as therapy with children. Art, music, movement, and play provide a means of communication that bypasses language to some extent, and in situations where verbal communication is difficult, the use of creative approaches may be preferable; however, this does not automatically mean that any method or activity is culturally appropriate in all cases. In fact, creative approaches have not been sufficiently examined within a cultural framework. Mental health professionals who use these approaches with children must continually appraise how cultural factors may impact clinical applications of creative arts therapies and expressive therapies with traumatized clients.

Many cultures expect individuals to contain and regulate their feelings, implying that sharing emotions or personal experiences is a sign of immaturity. For example, for some children, a nondirective approach ("Draw anything you want to" or "Improvise a movement from your imagination") may be threatening, perceived as intrusive, or counterproductive to developing trust and establishing a safe, comfortable environment for creative expression. Children may prefer the security of copying images or the familiarity of learning dance steps, practicing a song, or hearing a story to creating something original, particularly if their cultural identity dictates the former as the preferred way to experience art, music, or dance. This preference should be accepted and understood as part of who the child is because it may elicit positive memories of success or high self-esteem in children.

Therapists must also be especially sensitive to the preferences, values, and worldviews of parents, caregivers, and other family members of child clients when employing creative approaches. For example, parents of school-age children may question the use of play, toys, art, or props, possibly misunderstanding free expression as a technique to help ameliorate traumatic symptoms. Adult family members may not fully comprehend why play or art is being used as a primary method, may see the use of these modalities as frivolous or unproven, or may simply be uncomfortable with creative interventions because of personal or cultural reasons. Families often want to know that their children will get some immediate benefits or may even see the therapist as ineffective if there is not immediate change in their children's emotional distress. Because children's parents or caregivers are usually involved in the treatment of their children's trauma symptoms, culturally sensitive, trauma-informed therapists must help them understand the creative interventions that will be used. Therapists should ask parents or caregivers what indicators of change they expect to see in their children, respecting their opinions and views about the content and their desired outcome of intervention. When participating in any therapy, including interventions involving creative approaches, all children and their families want to be treated with respect, to know that their concerns and preferences are heard, and to feel that their opinions are important, valued, and accepted.

Therapists using culturally sensitive, creative methods in trauma-informed treatment consider biological, psychological, social, and cultural perspectives when discerning how children appraise their experiences and cope with events. In addition, therapists also consider developmental factors and children's capacity and preference for creative expression as a means of intervention. Finally, therapists evaluate child clients for risk and resilience in choosing activities and goals and base their choices on cultural aspects.

CONCLUSION

Therapists with an understanding of ethical, evidence-based, and trauma-creative approaches are in a unique position to do effective and rewarding work with traumatized children. Practitioners who use creative approaches also must continually learn how to recognize post-traumatic play, art, and other similar expressions; to capitalize on sensory aspects of creative arts and expressive therapies in treatment; and to maintain cultural sensitivity and respect for diverse worldviews about therapy, trauma reactions, and creative interventions. Learning these concepts is an ongoing process that forms the foundation of successful and effective treatment and advances the range of therapeutic skills that professionals can offer their child clients.

REFERENCES

Cattanach, A. (2008). Working creatively with children and families: The storied life. In C. Malchiodi (Ed.), *Creative interventions with traumatized children* (pp. 211–225). New York: Guilford Press.

Cohen, J. A., Mannarino, A. P., & Deblinger, E. (2006). *Treating trauma and traumatic grief in children and adolescents.* New York: Guilford Press.

Gil, E. (2006). *Helping abused and traumatized children: Integrating directive and nondirective approaches.* New York: Guilford Press.

Gil, E., & Drewes, A. A. (Eds.). (2005). *Cultural issues in play therapy.* New York: Guilford Press.

Hoagland, K., Burns, B., Kiser, L., Ringeisen, H., & Schoenwald, S. (2001). Evidence-based practice in child and adolescent mental health services. *Psychiatric Services, 52*(9), 1179–1189.

International Society for Traumatic Stress Studies. (2014). Guideline 17: Creative arts therapies for children. Retrieved January 22, 2014, from *www.istss.org/AM/Template.cfm?Section=PTSDTreatmentGuidelines&Template=/CM/ContentDisplay.cfm&ContentID=2337.*

Kao, S. C. (2005). Play therapy with Asian children. In E. Gil & A. Drewes (Eds.), *Cultural issues in play therapy* (pp. 180–194). New York: Guilford Press.

Knill, P., Levine, E., & Levine, S. (2005). *Principles and practice of expressive arts therapy: Towards a therapeutic aesthetics.* London: Jessica Kingsley.

Levine, P. (2012). *In an unspoken voice: How the body releases trauma and restores goodness.* Berkeley, CA: North Atlantic Books.

Lusebrink, V. (2010). Assessment and application of the expressive therapies continuum. *Art Therapy: Journal of the American Art Therapy Association, 27*(4), 166–170.

Malchiodi, C. A. (1998). *Understanding children's drawings.* New York: Guilford Press.

Malchiodi, C. A. (2002). Editorial. *Trauma and Loss: Research and Interventions, 2*(1), 4.

Malchiodi, C. A. (2005). The impact of culture on art therapy with children. In E. Gil & A. A. Drewes (Eds.), *Cultural issues in play therapy* (pp. 96–111). New York: Guilford Press.

Malchiodi, C. A. (2006). *The art therapy sourcebook* (2nd ed.). New York: McGraw-Hill.

Malchiodi, C. A. (2012). Art therapy in practice: Ethics, evidence and cultural sensitivity. In C. A. Malchiodi (Ed.), *Handbook of art therapy* (2nd ed., pp. 42–51). New York: Guilford Press.

National Child Traumatic Stress Network. (2014). Culture and trauma. Retrieved January 22, 2014, from *www.nctsn.org/resources/topics/culture-and-trauma*.

National Registry of Evidence-Based Programs and Practices. (2014). Home page. Retrieved January 22, 2014, from *http://nrepp.samhsa.gov*.

Perry, B. (2009). Examining child maltreatment through a neurodevelopmental lens: Clinical applications of the neurosequential model of therapeutics. *Journal of Loss and Trauma, 14,* 240–255.

Riley, S. (1999). *Contemporary art therapy with adolescents.* London: Jessica Kingsley.

Rothschild, B. (2000). *The body remembers.* New York: Norton.

Schreier, H., Ladakakos, C., Morabito, D., Chapman, L., & Knudson, M. M. (2005). Posttraumatic stress symptoms in children after mild to moderate pediatric trauma: A longitudinal examination of symptom prevalence, correlates, and parent–child symptom reporting. *Journal of Trauma and Acute Care Surgery, 58*(2), 353–363.

Sprunk, T. P., Mitchell, J., Myrow, D., & O'Connor, K. (2007). Paper on touch: Clinical, professional, and ethical issues. Retrieved February 16, 2007, from *www.a4pt.org/download.cfm?ID=9971*.

Steele, W., & Malchiodi, C. A. (2012). *Trauma-informed practice with children and adolescents.* New York: Taylor & Francis.

Sue, D. W., & Sue, D. (2012). *Counseling the culturally diverse: Theory and practice* (6th ed.). New York: Wiley.

TEDxOverland Park. (2012). Art therapy: Changing lives, one image at a time: Cathy Malchiodi at TEDxOverlandPark. Retrieved from *www.youtube.com/watch?v=yHu6909NTTc*.

Terr, L. (1979). Children of Chowchilla. *Psychoanalytic Study of the Child, 34,* 547–623.

Terr, L. (1990). Childhood trauma: An outline and overview. *American Journal of Psychiatry, 148,* 10–20.

PART II

Applications with Children and Adolescents

CHAPTER 3

Eye Movement Desensitization and Reprocessing and Art Therapy with Traumatized Children

Madoka Takada Urhausen

This chapter describes an innovative approach of treating children with trauma by combining art therapy and eye movement desensitization and reprocessing (EMDR). In recent years EMDR has been identified as a preferred practice in the treatment of traumatized adults, including veterans of war and those afflicted by human-made or natural disasters (American Psychiatric Association, 2004; Chemtob, Tolin, van der Kolk, & Pitman, 2000; U.S. Department of Veterans Affairs and U.S. Department of Defense, 2010; van der Kolk, 2008). The Substance Abuse and Mental Health Services Administration (SAMHSA) indicates that EMDR's efficacy is based on exposure and desensitization (*www.mentalhealth.samhsa.gov*).

Developing a definitive methodology to implement EMDR with traumatized children, however, has been challenging due to the number of variables involved in this population. Some of the diversity issues include varying developmental stages, cultural and social constructs of trauma, different environments and support systems, and prevailing numbers of comorbid presentations. Most recently, one of many evidence-based practices widely utilized in the United States, managing and adaptive practice (MAP; *www.practicewise.com*), has added EMDR to its own Web-based database as "good support or better practice" for children with posttraumatic stress disorder (PTSD) as it referenced its protocol summary on the research conducted by Ahmad, Larsson, and Sundelin-Wahlsten (2007) and Kemp, Drummond, and Mcdermott (2010).

This chapter is not intended to introduce techniques to be applied with this population unless the reader has had adequate training in both modalities (see the section "Ethical Practice of Creative Intervention" in Malchiodi, Chapter 2, this volume). Sources for training in art therapy and EMDR are listed at the end of this chapter and in the "Trauma-Related Resources" section of the Appendix. This chapter is dedicated to readers who are interested in the use of these approaches for psychotherapeutic application with children who have witnessed or experienced trauma, including life-threatening or deeply distressing events.

EMDR AND TRAUMA RESOLUTION

Although EMDR is often defined as a cognitive and exposure therapy, it is also a strength-based, psychodynamic, and humanistic approach to treatment. It addresses cognitive distortions and their lasting damaging effects on self-concept and the subsequent adapted perceptions, attitudes, and behavioral choices stemming from historical events. It is also unique in its application of bilateral stimulations (BLS) of the right and left hemispheres of the brain to access the affective and sensory states that are associated with memories of significant events. The core working assumption of EMDR is that all people have the ability to heal themselves if the factor that gets in the way of natural healing can be removed or its negative effects diminished. This framework of resilience as inherent in each person is based on Shapiro's proposed adaptive information processing model (AIP) that has been validated by current studies of neurobiology (Shapiro, 2001, 2011; Tinker-Wilson & Tinker, 2011). Shapiro (1995, 2001; Shapiro & Laliotis, 2011) hypothesizes that the integration of distinctly separate memories in the left and right hemispheres allows the individual to bridge and reorganize personal experiences of a traumatic event without additional damaging effects of the trauma.

Desensitization and reprocessing are enhanced by administration of BLS, which facilitate access to a series of targets, including deeply held negative beliefs about self as a result of unprocessed trauma. BLS are employed typically in the form of eye movement; tapping of body parts such as palms, shoulders, or knees; or having a client hold an alternately pulsating device or listen to alternating sounds. Furthermore, EMDR emphasizes a present-moment focus by cultivating mindfulness in order to hold internal resources during reactivation of disturbing memories. Resources are identified as personal strengths and protective factors, such as the individual's positive attributes, skill sets, supportive relationships, and dreams and inspirations, as well as preferred sensory modes or objects that yield a certain level of comfort and can be enlisted as assets for self-regulation. A carefully designed protocol with BLS assists the client to safely revisit distressing events while enabling access to a relaxed state. The purpose is to optimize the executive functioning of the neocortex and thereby allow for objective observation of thoughts, feelings, and sensations to facilitate the reorganization of fragmented and distorted experiences. This dual attention toward present and past experiences encourages the client to question previously held negative beliefs that are usually not easily negotiable due to psychological and physiological reactivity, leading to cognitive restructuring.

ADAPTING EMDR FOR TREATMENT WITH CHILDREN

Using EMDR with children is an emerging practice; modifications to the standard protocol are suggested by researcher-practitioners such as Adler-Tapia and Settle (2008), Gomez (2011, 2013), and Parnell (2013). Adler-Tapia and Settle follow the standard eight-phase protocol of EMDR more closely than others working with this population. Their treatment manual for children (Adler-Tapia & Settle, 2008) encourages the use of tools from other disciplines, including "play therapy, art therapy, sandtray, and any other techniques that the therapist determines helpful for clients to express themselves" (p. ix). Applications of art expressions are practical as well as effective in facilitating EMDR protocol and provide a perfect synergy to the working model of EMDR with its intent to provide rational voices to symptomatic behaviors in order to bring forth sensory, affective, and cognitive integration. In particular, sensory integration is an important part of recovery in working with traumatized individuals of any age, increasing the sense of relief that comes with mastery over their bodies' trauma reactions (Levine, 2002).

TRAUMA-INFORMED ORIENTATION IN SENSORY WORK

Children's responses to traumatic events depend on many mitigating factors, including the response of caregivers, the degree of secure attachment, availability of support systems, and their own resilience (Perry, 1999). Regardless, somatic symptoms are very common among children (Levine & Kline, 2007; Malchiodi, 1990; Rothschild, 2000). Ruling out organically based disorders, symptomatic somatic issues may be caused by hyperarousal and tension in a body that is flooded with fear and anxiety; children may also become hypoaroused or experience dissociation. Unresolved trauma may cause children to fluctuate between states of freeze, fight, flight, or fall with minimal provocation (Levine, 1997). EMDR attempts to reconcile these chronic, dissonant experiences. Graphic images can also aid children to restore a sense of temporal order and other nonverbal implicit memories (Gantt & Tinnin, 2008).

EMDR emphasizes the multidimensional aspects of traumatized children's experiences and appreciates their unique expressions as attempts to cope. Consequently, this approach honors the pace of each client's treatment as well as the style in how he or she associates freely with sensations, feelings, and thoughts. Sensory dysregulation is viewed as a survival strategy to experience only as much as is tolerable of painful traumatic memories. This understanding is aligned with polyvagal theory (Porges, 2011), which articulates that the neural regulation system creates hierarchy in neural platforms to organize various functions of the body and physiological experiences as adaptive strategies to stressful events. When offering various resources, opportunities arise to recontextualize and integrate traumatic events; mind–body integration is key to effective resolution of the trauma. Perry and Szalavitz (2006) encourages therapists to adopt a "bottom-up" approach as opposed to the "top-down" approach of traditional cognitive therapy. Art therapy enables children to access different senses in a concrete manner via choice of art material, movement, and the environment in which it is practiced. EMDR, combined with art therapy, is relevant to trauma-informed practices (TIPs), endorsed by Steele and Malchiodi (2012), which prioritize survivors' safety, choice, and control and engage them through sensory-based methods and collaboration. The value of combining these two modalities lies in therapists' ability to tailor intervention to the unique experiences and requirements of each child.

ATTACHMENT WORK, EMDR, AND ART THERAPY

Maladaptive beliefs about self and a nonsupportive environment obstruct the natural healing process of the child client. In the treatment of children, therapists' positive relationships with primary caregivers and their environments are essential. Therefore, establishing a strong therapeutic alliance with both child and caregivers is vital for emotional safety prior to proceeding to reprocess trauma. The therapist aims to provide corrective experiences while facilitating EMDR interventions. EMDR inherently involves a very intimate process that requires the therapist's use of self, with BLS directly administered to the client, often via touch, and by ongoing attunement to the client's nuances in facial expressions and to physical, emotional, and sensory responses.

Parnell (2013) claims that the efficaciousness of EMDR is greatly due to its relational component and the degree to which it fosters attunement to support and ensure progress. Based on advancements in neuroscience research and today's emphasis on the impact of attachment on the brain's structural development, Siegel (1999, 2011) illuminates the importance of working within the interpersonal relationships to effect changes in the brain that create healing. Siegel coined the term *attachment-focused EMDR* for Parnell's EMDR-based method because Parnell departs significantly from the standard EMDR protocol by emphasizing enhancement of attachment and resource building.

Gomez (2013) addresses EMDR treatment of complex PTSD and attachment and dissociative symptoms with children who exhibit pervasive emotional dysregulation. She examines attachment injuries of children as ways to initially assess and conceptualize cases for a better outcome. Korn (2011) sees attachment style as a factor that determines under- or overregulation. She discusses how disorganized attachment, for example, presents as difficulty with self-regulation, an inability to modulate the level of emotional and physiological response experienced while relating to personal issues, resulting in alternating between hyper- and hypoarousal. Korn resonates with Fosha's (2003) concept of metaprocessing—the ability to reflect on the process itself—by having the client observe and note the changes within the self and in the relationship with the therapist. The dyadic nature of attachment-focused interventions can support the improvement in affect regulation and lessen the sense of vulnerability to trauma (Fosha, 2003; Schore, 2003).

Whenever possible, forming an ongoing relationship with caregivers is advisable. The treatment should be paced according to the needs of the child and his or her support system, as consolidating the support system is another important task when working with children. Lovette (1999) notes that using EMDR with children is not effective or suitable when there is unresolved trauma in the family and the environment is unstable. Dausch (personal communication, October 2013), who specializes in adoption, substantiates the value of providing EMDR to adoptive parents for the first 6 months of the treatment prior to offering therapy to children. She suggests that this practice solidifies treatment for adoptive children because their parents increase their capacity to tolerate the challenges of dealing with the children's trauma and to able to attend to the children's treatment without being triggered themselves. Dausch also reports having parents tap on their children's shoulders to support BLS. This is a beautiful and tactful practice in reinforcing and enhancing secure attachment.

The level of therapeutic connection forged in EMDR, in the framework of attachment-focused practice, through witnessing, attending, understanding, and intervening in clients' personal stories of trauma and healing is akin to trauma work involving art therapy wherein metaphors and symbols provide venues to a client's expressions. "Metaphors are the language of the right brain" and facilitate access to healing (Gomez, 2013). Riley (1997) also identifies metaphor as a basic tool and a central component of art therapy. In her seminal comprehensive guide to art therapy, Landgarten (1981) dedicates the book to those art therapists who have listened with their eyes. I would further elaborate that the attachment-focused practitioners of EMDR and art therapy listen with their whole being.

MECHANICS OF EMDR:
A CHILD-FRIENDLY APPROACH

After taking a thorough history, the EMDR therapist prepares the child client for the mechanics of BLS by using helpful metaphors. Frequently, the metaphor of riding a train or watching a movie is used, with images, thoughts, or senses coming up for a child to notice, report, and reprocess. Some children may relate better to the metaphor of flipping through the information via smartphones, only on autopilot. Picture books are available that explain the EMDR process to children and can serve as bibliotherapy (Gertner, 2008; Gomez, 2007).

Increasing coping skills and installing resources are built into the preparation phase. Korn (2011) delineates different domains—behavioral/mastery, sensorimotor, relational/attachment, and imaginal—from which memories and experiences can be elicited as resources for clients. Of these, the imaginal realm, because it encompasses spiritual and interpersonal aspects of human experience, can be accessed to provide children with strengths outside of what is readily available in their environment. When a child cannot access a safe or calm place as a resource, the imaginal realm can be explored by the use of stories, music, or symbols from dreams and spiritual connections to evoke positive experience. Identifying figures from TV or other media as allies for the child may also be helpful. The value of utilizing resources across all stages of EMDR treatment is corroborated by most contemporary practitioners of EMDR but emphasized particularly by those who work with traumatized children (Gomez, 2013; Korn, 2011; Parnell, 2013). A natural progression for child-friendly EMDR practice is to incorporate art processes that could provide comfort and nurturing as well as grounding support.

Once the child becomes familiar with the use of resources to address autonomic nervous system responses to triggers and to maintain engagement with intervention without dissociating, he or she can also learn to self-administer BLS via a preferred sensory modality. Possible materials include therapeutic toys such as play dough, held in both hands and squeezed alternately; practicing butterfly hugs with crossed arms to tap alternate arms in a slow and even pace of a resting heart beat; or using slow and smooth finger painting alternately with left and right hands. Some art therapists including McNamee (2003, 2004) and Talwar (2007) have suggested drawing with alternating hands as a BLS method to work with trauma, but I have found the repeated process of stopping to draw cumbersome and distracting. Ultimately, it derails the processing of the important free associations that pass so quickly, and it is not conducive to desensitization or reprocessing.

Next, assessment helps to narrow down the "target" with specific procedural steps to make the process palatable to the child. EMDR lends itself naturally to expressive arts-based assessment with initial inquiry of "What picture do you get when you think of the event?" and "What do you notice in your body when you bring up that picture?" Distilling certain disturbing events into a picture and giving voice to the physiological and emotional responses triggered by the memory can help the child identify the problematic area to target.

It is then helpful to assist clients with the process of identifying negative cognitions (NCs) about self and positive cognitions (PCs—those that the child would rather believe about him- or herself). Mindfulness is cultivated by providing empathy in response to emotions, thoughts, and physical sensations, which are measured via scaling questions. Scaling questions used with adults are generally too abstract and confusing for most young children or adolescents with cognitive challenges or with those who lack an integrated memory of trauma. Nonverbal means such as art expressions are recommended instead, and negative and positive scales can be implemented and monitored by using a visual scaling chart. Showing children how to identify their distress level by using a fear ladder, emotion thermometer, or a scale of hurt or pain (with various facial expressions in different colors) can be productive at this stage; for example, as a child shifts energetically from being a make-believe sloth to a cheetah, from a dull to a bright color, from a less defined shape to a fully filled circle, and so forth. Gomez (2013) uses opposite animal attributes to portray and monitor the condition, for example, "tall and proud as a giraffe versus small [and insignificant] as a mouse."

The simplest example of a visual scale to measure subjective units of disturbance (SUDs) is a worksheet with five circular facial expressions ranging from scared to brave or sad to happy. To measure validity of cognition (VoC), a pie chart or an outline of a heart shape can be filled with varying colors delineating the percentage of how true the child feels the positive statement about self is. Scanning the body for any discomfort associated with traumatic memory is also a part of an assessment and can easily be facilitated by drawing or sculpture that can later be used to reevaluate any shifts of sensations to reflect changes and transformations. Finally, therapists can align themselves with clients by utilizing the same language as that of their young clients, whose communication is typically articulated through metaphor.

In modifying EMDR for children, Parnell (2013) eliminates many of the cognitive strategies such as scaling questions and identifying preferred PCs prior to processing. She explains that making these modifications ensures that clients stay connected with right-brain memory systems without interference from left-brain cognitive activity. She does keep the final phase of body scan, however, to review how the child has shifted energetically and "tap in" resources by the BLS of tapping (Parnell & Phillips, 2013).

In preparation for the desensitization phase, it is essential for the child to develop strategies to remain focused on the target to process.

Art expressions allow children to hold on to a concrete image while processing via BLS. Schmidt (1999) observes that the clients stay attuned to the feelings associated with their drawing and its possible benefit includes faster trauma resolution with EMDR. The drawing, for example, can literally be placed in front of them as it reflects the worst part of the picture and elicits associated memories. However, in order for successful processing to take place the therapist must keep the children's response to activating reminders of disturbing events within their threshold of tolerance to maintain their engagement. Prior to desensitization and reprocessing, children review their support systems, strengths, and coping skills. The resourcing BLS activities previously exercised are reinforced to increase a sense of control over their bodies. An act of art-making can serve as a grounding technique. At times, children may be asked to contain their difficult feelings using art in order to keep their threshold of tolerance within manageable range. Caulfield (personal communication, September 2013) reflects on an EMDR session in which she asked a client who was demonstrating feeling stuck to draw a container for her anger to which the client responded with a house-shape that she filled vigorously with heavy crayon marks.

When it is determined that the child's range of tolerance indicates a readiness for exposure, the therapist can then proceed to offer desensitization and reprocessing via BLS. Several sets of BLS in the modality of choice are administered to process the original picture with its emotions, cognitions, and sensations, and subsequent shifts or changes that are noticed. The goal is to help the child client assimilate and integrate distressful memories and sensations toward successful resolution of the targeted trauma.

ABREACTION AND INTERWEAVE

Abreaction refers to the experience of reliving an event or interaction in order to release emotions; it is sometimes defined as a form of catharsis. Therapists should use caution and have various "interweave" techniques available to provide support for the child in the event of abreactions or explicit expressions of difficulties that are often released during the desensitization phase. The term *interweave* in this context means to weave together alternative and often opposing ideas about one's experiences. There are different types of interweaves; for example, a cognitive interweave elicits factual information so that insight can be developed and assimilated into the child's memory of the event. Asking the child "How big was the perpetrator compared to you?" or "Was there anything you could have done to prevent the disaster?" facilitates new understanding that it was not the child's fault that the bad thing happened. During the interweave, it may also help to bring out the grounding image that the child drew during the earlier preparation phase, have the child breathe in and out while looking at the drawing, and do slower sets of BLS or the butterfly hug. Frequently, children ascertain and embrace this type of self-awareness without the therapist's intervention of an interweave. Therapists typically intervene only when clients are repeating negative thoughts and distress reactions or when their "stuckness" is evidenced through repetitive symptomatic play. The purpose of using interweaves is to shift the dynamic and offer relief from ongoing abreactions.

Children with complex trauma respond particularly well to additional interventions that offer a supportive stance in the form of a relational interweave. The therapist's use of self, attunement, and empathy provide faith in the process. Prior to the emergence of a full-blown abreaction, the therapist can heed the pace of the client's responses by titrating BLS (adjusting the speed or changing the modality) to alleviate distress. For example, facilitating self-soothing, sensory-oriented BLS, such as having clients stroke something soft, even a pet or therapy animal, or make a structured drawing of something or someone that provides comfort, in combination with the therapist's tapping, can be helpful in redirecting clients to resources before continuing the desensitization process.

INSTALLATION AND CLOSING

The installation phase of EMDR provides the enhancement of the positive gains made in earlier phases that yielded adaptive resolutions of memory networks. The resources are continually built up during the stabilization of the client (Korn & Leeds, 2002). Gomez (2013) discusses the opportunities available with installation to utilize developmentally appropriate modalities such as singing a song or other creative avenues to amplify the strengths of newly adapted positive cognitions. Installation is generally followed by body scan, closure, and reevaluation; the procedure prompts therapists to continue to assess and work on any unresolved targets to desensitize. Reevaluation can be as simple as having a child draw a safe place (Zaghrout-Hodali, Ferdoos, & Dodgson, 2008) and compare it with the original safe place that the child drew in the preparation phase.

CASE EXAMPLES

Trauma survivors engaged in EMDR often report expedient recovery from debilitating symptoms of anxiety and depression stemming from unresolved trauma. They gain corrective experiences via reexposure in the context of a therapeutic relationship. Likewise, child survivors engaged in art therapy often report comfort and relief from their art therapists' earnest attempt to understand their stories through art expressions (Tanaka & Urhausen, 2012). The combined use of EMDR and art therapy is a multimodal approach that is not possible in cognitive therapy alone. Clients' styles of attachment play a critical role in determining how therapists apply these approaches. The following case studies illuminate this point.

In the next several sections, case examples demonstrate the use of art therapy in combination with EMDR. The first case involves a single-incident trauma and the second case, complex chronic trauma. Finally, an example of group work with children dealing with an incident of historical trauma is presented. Pseudonyms and other alterations are made to protect the confidentiality of these clients, who honored me with the ultimate gift of trust in their own healing journeys and to educate others through this chapter.

Alex: Involving the Caregiver

Alex, an 11-year-old boy with biracial Hispanic and Caucasian heritage and mild autistic spectrum features, was brought to psychotherapy by his father for his volatile mood and the behavioral issues that impacted his relationships at home and at school. According to his father, Alex was isolative and "moped around and acted like everyone was against him." The father's primary concern was that Alex displayed an agitated mood and was verbally aggressive toward his younger stepsiblings because they "annoyed him." In response, his father and stepmother would become stern and redirect him instead. Alex was prone to feeling dismissed as a problem, and his needs went perpetually unmet. Additionally, Alex would question the judgment of his non-English-speaking stepmother and was openly defiant toward her. This behavior infuriated the father and caused the stepmother to further disengage from Alex.

Alex reportedly lived with his mother and her then boyfriend, whom he called "Stepdad," until 4 years ago. After his parents separated, his father remarried and two younger siblings were born prior to Alex coming to live with the family. Alex worried about his mother incessantly and looked forward to visitations with her, which occurred inconsistently.

Due to complex family and psychosocial history, I spent much time during the assessment phase meeting with various family members in different units to determine family dynamics, their strengths and resources, and exclusively utilizing art therapy to facilitate an open dialogue among family members. Promoting art-based interactions also served to remove communication barriers with family members who were at different developmental levels and communicated in two different primary languages. In this way, the father was also excused of the role of acting as interpreter and mediator in the family. Alex's mother was invited, but she could not attend for a number of reasons.

The father provided anecdotal information suggesting that he suspected that Alex was exposed to domestic violence between his mother and "stepfather" and that Alex was possibly abused by him. It was evident to me that Alex was struggling in all areas of social interaction. I determined that creating a supportive home environment for him was a top priority before he could begin to process any past trauma. Fortunately, the father was invested in Alex's healing and agreed to frequent conjoint and collateral sessions.

At school, Alex had similar perceptions of his peers as purposely hurting him and of his teacher's failure to attend to his needs. He was observably distressed in sessions as he spoke about his preoccupation with specific incidents in which people would do what he disliked, resulting in his feeling helpless. He would identify "bullies," but when the father spoke with his teacher, no specific peers were identified as being aggressive or mean to him. In fact, the teacher reported that Alex was the one who had difficulties reading social cues and would say rude things that hurt others. In consulting with the teacher, I appreciated her perspective that Alex was rigid in his beliefs about certain people and that his black-and-white thinking had prevented age-appropriate social functioning. She observed that he frequently lacked intuitive understanding of another person's feelings and that he had difficulty taking age-appropriate steps to reciprocate the communication. The teacher also reported that Alex habitually complained about headaches, scrapes, and scratches that she considered to be minor. Although Alex had difficulties listening to others' statements about their feelings, he was able to sustain his attention and could relate to some art expressions, such as a sibling's collage that included a phrase "taking the fun out of summer."

In the absence of a maternal presence in therapy, I was encouraged by his father, who demonstrated a great capacity to love and accept his son. Once the father was free of the active "fixer" role in the family, he was able to access his nurturing nature and become curious about the etiology of the son's early attachment injuries. He supported Alex's recovery from trauma even if it meant witnessing and experiencing his son's aggression toward himself and admitting the need for help with his parenting skills. Alex's father confidently identified himself as the biggest ally to his children, but he was markedly surprised and conflicted when shown the picture of how his son experienced the father (see Figure 3.1).

I offered consultations and coaching to the father on a regular basis to ensure that he remained supportive of his son's open expressions of feelings and thoughts in treatment. Alex's father practiced specific skills to improve the quality of their interactions, including reflective listening and attending to Alex's verbal and nonverbal expressions. Much of the art therapy and parenting support was in preparation for trauma

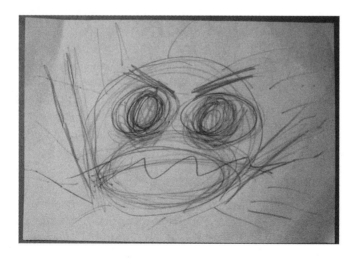

FIGURE 3.1.

processing, so that Alex had a concrete, reliable resource to count on when and if he became distressed. Alex's complaints of what occurred regularly at home and school provided his father with ways to enhance his "listening muscles" and develop an appropriate level of guidance that matched the needs of the son. For example, in one session Alex had dark circles around his eyes because of lack of sleep for several days following his teacher's alleged shaming of him in front of the whole class. The father was able to respond appropriately and promised to speak with the teacher.

Four months into the treatment, Alex disclosed details of how he was physically abused by his "stepfather." Although his father's mixed emotions were visible, he remained calm and supportive of his son and reassured Alex that he was safe now and that it was all over. The father informed Alex that he would not let anyone harm him again, if he could help it. I made the suspected child abuse report in their presence, per Alex's choice, thereby solidifying his assimilation of this new experience in which responsible adults took action on his behalf.

When the father returned the next session, he mentioned the approaching Thanksgiving holiday and that he wanted to see Alex let go of the past and live in the present. The father demonstrated to Alex that he shared the burden of this past, as he himself was affected by the disclosure of the abuse incident. He felt remorseful, but also that he was willing to make peace with his feeling of guilt for not having been there for Alex when the abuse took place. He shared that he knew how hard it was for Alex to live with anger. Alex saw his father's facial and art expressions of his wish for his family's happiness and responded with his own art, expressing the wish to work closely with his father toward this goal. I honored the pace in which the child and parent needed to address and integrate this specific trauma. Once the father was able to be the "container" for Alex's distress and learned to offer collaborative ways to solve problems, Alex was then prepared to explore positive resources, such as drinking sweet tea in my office, and identifying a safe place, such as holding his father's hands (Figure 3.2).

Alex also learned other supportive techniques, including progressive muscle relaxation and asking for specific help from caregivers in an appropriate manner. In addition, he was exposed to experimenting with BLS of different kinds "for fun," including alternating eye movements, ticking sounds to his left and right ears, tapping of his knees, and holding alternately pulsating buzzers in each palm of his hands. This process was facilitated with the intention of instilling positive resources in Alex to strengthen his sense of safety and to enhance his immediate access to something comforting in preparation for the desensitization phase of the treatment.

A target to be processed was established with Alex; approaching cautiously, but immediately, he created the picture of the incident of his being physically assaulted by his "stepfather" (Figure 3.3). Whereas his drawing of the resource (Figure 3.2) included color, he did not use color on this drawing of the disturbing event. In spite of its diminutive size and apparent lack of detail, he stated that the event felt close to him as he looked at it. He gazed at the picture with a grimace that suggested a repugnant response; the picture had a certain quality about it, being half hidden, with only the top portion of the incident showing at the bottom left corner of the paper, as if it could pop up upward anytime like a jack-in-the-box. He made sure to close it up by folding the paper in half once he drew it, but he gave me permission to open it, as needed, to prompt him to think about the incident. All around the two figures were faint but choppy, agitated motion lines, which may be difficult to see in the reproduction.

Through BLS, additional pictures came to mind. Alex remembered that he was unreasonably reprimanded for playing with his mother's cosmetics. It appeared that young Alex, at about the age of 4 or 5, was attempting to be close to his mother when left alone with the "stepfather." He recalled his mother "not doing anything about it" when he

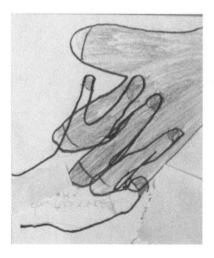 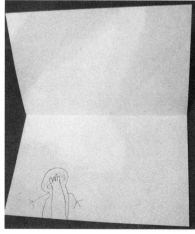

FIGURE 3.2.   **FIGURE 3.3.**

told her about the abuse he endured. The most disturbing part of the picture he identified was his feeling that it was "unfair." He recognized his NC of seeing himself as "unwanted, not lovable" and that he would rather believe (PC) that "I am lovable and cared for." VoC for PC was at 1, completely false, on a scale of 1–7. The emotion that he identified when he looked at the picture was "scared," with the SUDs at 7 on a scale of 0–10, 10 being the highest level of disturbance.

Upon scanning his body, Alex reported that he still felt the pain and "weak in my face. The whole back felt tense." Alex accessed the memory of the sensory disturbance of being smashed against the wall and being pushed down repeatedly with great force. I continued to process with BLS and checked for changes, indicated by new pictures he saw in his mind's eye, to determine if any other disturbing memories emerged. He was able to track with bilateral eye movement and recalled some details of the abuse, mostly his fear response in sensations. His affective state changed from scared to angry to feeling safe in knowing that his father would protect him now. At the end of processing, he accepted that the perpetrator was bad for doing what he did to a little innocent child and that it was not his fault that he was abused.

With some assistance from me implementing a cognitive interweave when he expressed repeated wishes for revenge, Alex successfully created emotional distance as he was desensitized from the incident, and he appeared well regulated. The cognitive interweave I offered prompted Alex to compare the size of the perpetrator to the size of him as a small child. When asked to look again at the original picture he drew of the perpetrator assaulting him, Alex reported it did not bother him because "it was all over." Some of the comforting phrases uttered by his father during the preparation phase were now adapted and internalized by Alex. His cognitive, somatic, and affective responses to the memory were assimilated into the bigger picture and integrated as a memory surrounding the past event, which no longer appeared to have significant bearing on him at the moment. SUDs went down to 0. After a few more sets of BLS installing the PC that he is loved and cared for, he reported VoC of 7, completely true. Finally, the body scan revealed that the original picture (Figure 3.3) no longer activated him somatically. He reported a "light and good feeling" coming down from the top of his head to the rest of his body.

Alex had a few more EMDR sessions when he would report slipping back into negative thoughts, such as when he couldn't find his wallet and thought someone had stolen it and sensed that his father was indifferent about it. His NC was "I am alone and helpless because nobody wants to help me," and his identified emotion was sad and lonely. The PC was "People care about me—I'm not alone." Consequently, he was prompted to recall the first time that he ever felt this way; the original traumatic incident was brought back so that we could then reprocess it with BLS, the same picture (Figure 3.3).

In these follow-up EMDR sessions, Alex recovered at a quicker rate and presented creative resolutions to the problem. His ego strength had visibly increased, as he smiled and explained his thoughts and feelings articulately in his professorial manner, no longer whining to complain about difficult situations that he could not control. His posture was straighter, and he drew images with a steady grip. Although his fine motor skills continued to be challenged, evidenced by his poor penmanship and difficulty in use of certain tools such as scissors, he was mastering his personal expressions through art. One day he reported watching a movie that left a big impression on him. The movie was about a father and son overcoming obstacles together. As he narrated the storyline, he drew a series of pictures of the protagonist who, in spite of adversity, made himself happy. We did slow BLS and installed his positive feelings associated with the movie. It was apparent that Alex had personalized the triumph over his own challenges.

Alex came back to treatment after a holiday and reported that he was getting along better with peers and his family and that he felt happy. With art material available, he opted to cut out a group of human figures and used a split rivet to keep them together. He put his name on the figure at the top, connected to the rest, which fanned out (Figure 3.4).

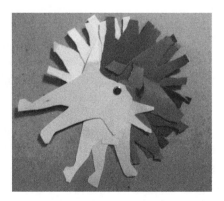

FIGURE 3.4.

This art expression was interpreted as a sign of integration of a layered self as well as integration of himself as part of a bigger social system. It also indicated that he was ready to leave treatment. He had met our 6 months' treatment goal of decreasing problematic behaviors at school and at home as a result of increased affect regulation. His father, seen 5 years later, informed me that Alex was doing "outstanding" in school and that he was very proud of his son.

Ben: Reclaiming Identity

Ben came to see me at the age of 17 after having 6 months of treatment with another clinician, who he described as someone with whom he "did not connect . . . just talking." He was going through a multitude of stresses as he was entering his senior year of high school and at the same time separating from his biological mother who, according to him, was mentally unstable. He had just come out as gay 6 months prior and moved into the home of his other parent, Tori, and her partner. He was the only son of a lesbian couple who had separated when Ben was still very young. When his mother and Tori were together, they conceived Ben through artificial insemination. Ben grew up in an openly gay community with a lesbian godmother and other caregivers who were lesbians. He had just reconnected with his donor father who lived out of state. When I began working with him, he presented with agitated mood, generalized anxiety, and obsessive–compulsiveness. He reported being obsessed over his appearance or what others thought of him and being preoccupied with his own negative thoughts about current events and history. Ben also presented with fear of flying after seeing many TV simulations of the 9/11 terrorist attacks on the World Trade Center over 10 years ago.

He disclosed a history of exposure to his biological mother's repeated emotional outbursts and depressive episodes that resulted in her multiple hospitalizations. Since young childhood he had lived in fear of his mother following through with numerous suicidal threats, and he had witnessed her attempts. He also reported ongoing issues of being bullied by peers and inconsistent support from his mother. His mother was said to have a very high IQ with a low capacity for empathy. She also appeared to have internalized homophobia and projected self-denial on Ben as she called him derogatory names throughout his childhood, despite her own sexual orientation and challenges. His relationships with his current caregivers were said to be "good." He maintained contact with his mother and "still cared for her," but no longer wanted to accommodate her whims. He seemed desperate to establish his autonomy, but worried about his future.

Ben's baseline functioning was fair and he excelled academically. Nonetheless, he typically presented as highly anxious, spoke in pressured speech, averted eye contact when nervous, and exhibited anxiety with social situations that involved people outside of his inner circle of friends and family. He verbalized his wish to not be so anxious and self-conscious. He was very sensitive and artistic. It is likely that he thought of himself as a different kind of creature than others, as indicated in one of his free drawings during assessment (Figure 3.5). Ben considered himself smart, mature, and kind, but his drawing was self-deprecating. He enjoyed doodling and drawing in his spare time and when he made art, he was at his best; he appeared to be at peace with himself, as he was able to stop censoring his own thoughts and was confident in his aesthetic decisions. He began treatment by creating a collage of intricately juxtaposed images that seemed to reflect his multiple ego states (Figure 3.6). What stood out the most to me was the contrast of an image of a crying baby with his eyes cut out and an old bearded man painting intently with others watching, holding a bleeding brush over a broken heart of the baby.

Although Ben's affect was restricted while engaging in art making, he appeared to be relieved each time he completed an artwork. We typically began our sessions with a check-in drawing and discussed issues that came up while he drew, so that he would have this sensory activity to ground him while discussing areas of conflict. Sometimes his concerns compounded his need to fill much of pictorial space with

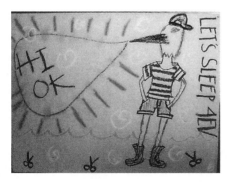

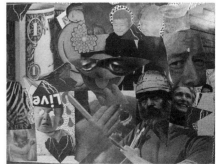

FIGURE 3.5.   **FIGURE 3.6.**

expressions incongruent with his mood (Figure 3.7). In fact, his coping included making a tightly organized bird's-eye view drawing. His drive to control his environment lent itself to the blueprint-like image of his street map (Figure 3.8). Those drawings appeared to have assisted him in compartmentalizing and simplifying visual information as well as other details that inundated him.

His response to stressors fluctuated between underregulating and overregulating his feelings and sensory stimulation, or cognitively shifting from obsession to dissociation. He reported taking hours to ready himself for school in the morning as he had difficulty deciding what to wear. The anxiousness surrounding his identity, his sexual tension, and his concern for his obsessive and disturbing thoughts are shown in his brain drawing (Figure 3.9). I asked Ben to begin exploring his triggers through drawing (Figure 3.10). Ideally with EMDR, the earliest and the most disturbing memory is targeted first in its three-pronged approach of moving from the past, present, and future; if past events should come to a satisfactory resolve, the presently manifesting symptoms are expected to be alleviated (Shapiro, 1995, 2001).

Since Ben's triggers were vague and overwhelming, I felt the need to first attend to his immediate concern to relieve his tension and later utilized a "float back" prompt that asks for the earliest memory in which he experienced a similar level of disturbance. He had difficulty identifying one specific event when he was bullied or hurt because these events were pervasive throughout childhood. He also began taking psychotropic medication around this time to cope better with the compulsivity he experienced. While Ben was adjusting to medications and going through some instability, he preferred to engage in simpler art making

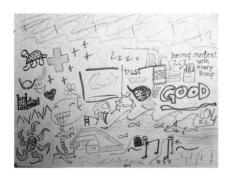

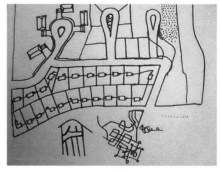

FIGURE 3.7.   **FIGURE 3.8.**

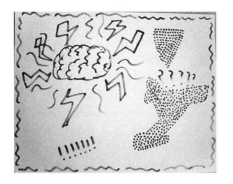 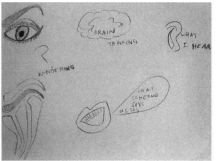

FIGURE 3.9.   **FIGURE 3.10.**

and discussions about interesting quotes, sometimes bringing in his favorite phrases and meditating on them through art making. I provided additional structure and cognitive resources in sessions while continually providing unconditional positive regard and attunement. One day he brought in a quote, in Latin, with which he resonated (Figure 3.11): "*a posse ad esse*," which means "from possibility to reality" or "being able to be," reflecting his high level of motivation for self-actualization. This marked his readiness to take another leap in treatment because he was embracing his own challenge to stretch beyond himself.

EMDR was scary for Ben, but his caregivers encouraged him to test it out with his fear of flying, as a travel arrangement was being made for him to go see his father in a coming month. This was his second visit to his father, and although he looked forward to seeing him, he was concerned about the plane crashing. Ben's earlier artwork was examined for rich metaphors of resources, including the wise self, the nurturing self, and the vulnerable but innocent and beautiful child-self deserving of beautiful things in life (Figure 3.6). Ben also used his favorite season and the favorite time of the day as a safe place to linger (Figure 3.12). Doing an "art review" of all his artwork served to reevaluate his mental status in a global manner and provide a current SUD for the imagined plane crash.

When revisiting older drawings Ben was able to discuss his compulsion to move—move in, out, around, and move on—which led to a discussion of the value of actually completing an action in order to move forward (Figure 3.13). EMDR that was focused on the plane phobia led to his target of feeling unworthy (NC) and therefore feeling doomed to a terrible consequence; it also led to an implicit memory of insecure attachment with his mother. He recalled his mother being glued to

TV after 9/11 and not being available to him while he was scared. The vicarious trauma of 9/11, coupled with ongoing relational trauma and his mother's emotional volatility, exacerbated his anxiety and the belief that the world was not capable of holding him safely.

After he had finished his EMDR treatment he made a poetic observation about a certain period of his life as giving him a sense of four seasons. The most difficult years of his life were labeled as winter. I sensed that Ben had adopted a positive outlook for his future with the understanding that there is a cyclical nature operating in life and that he was deserving of enjoying the fair weather and harvest that were coming his way. With this, his presenting symptoms of generalized anxiety were significantly alleviated along with increased ease of being who he was. He had less concerns for others' expectations of him, and his occasional interpersonal struggles were within normal range of age and culture.

After a year of art therapy with a periodic EMDR booster session, Ben decided to leave treatment. He had graduated from high school, turned 18, engaged in a committed relationship, and made a major decision about his career goal. His choices of personal goals were congruent with his needs, desires, and strengths. His last artwork was the embellished quote from a movie he had enjoyed (Figure 3.14), which reflected his self-acceptance and the PC, "I am worthy." I saw Ben 2 years after his completion of treatment. He informed me of steady advancement toward his career goal with his support system intact. He was no longer nervous about flying. Most importantly, he was less inhibited about showing positive emotions, and he appeared genuinely content with where he was in his life. He continues to "move forward" in the direction of self-determination.

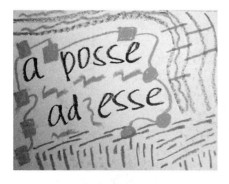

FIGURE 3.11.

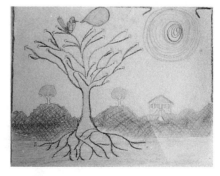

FIGURE 3.12.

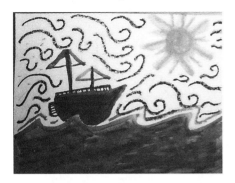 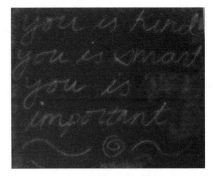

FIGURE 3.13.   **FIGURE 3.14.**

A Group Mural with Children Afflicted by Natural Disaster

In the spring of 2013, I had the honor of visiting one of the elementary schools in Fukushima, Japan, affected by an earthquake and tsunami disaster in 2011. The natural disaster was followed by a dangerous rise in radiation levels in the region due to explosions of two nuclear plants nearby. Those who survived the tsunami had evacuated to temporary housing, away from this beach town, or moved completely out of the area. The principal of the school permitted their school counselor and I to collaborate on making a commemorative mural on an auspicious day of the new school year. The coming of the spring season in Japan is signaled by cherry blossoms and evokes the image of children and youth in new uniforms, walking through the rows of cherry trees with their delicate blossoms falling like confetti. They are indeed blessings from the sky. The cherry blossom's season is short-lived and coveted by adults and children alike. When the tsunami hit the town, the houses of these students as well as the trees were uprooted and destroyed. The school had reopened a year after the disaster, but the trees were not there to welcome the children, who commuted by bus, for over an hour each way, to attend their home school. Enrollment had decreased by one-third, and the school struggled with low morale. Although students were being referred for school-based counseling due to behavioral or emotional disturbances, including peer issues and school refusal, they still possessed the healthy need to play and wished that they had more access to outdoor activities from which they were restricted for health reasons.

A study by Oras, de Ezpeleta, and Ahmad (2004) supports the use of EMDR with refugee children. A group mural was initially proposed for multiple families, but this afternoon event, immediately following the morning ceremony, posed a logistical difficulty for some parents, and so we proceeded with fewer caregivers than students. Specifically, our mural-painting population included 11 students, ranging in age from 5 to 12 years, with six adults directly participating. After a former large-scale earthquake in Japan, local people held ceremonies to plant cherry blossom trees as a memorial (Ohnogi, 2010). I was also aiming to facilitate a culturally sensitive and meaningful activity that serves as a healing ritual for the community. I began with a guided imagery about cherry trees to tap into their positive memories of trees and a global sense of wellness with sensory stimulation. To help children manifest the tree's life force, I modeled the movement of a young growing tree breathing and expanding, with stretched-out branches and its roots firmly anchored in their land. This movement and the image were resourced with BLS in the form of the butterfly hug.

(The butterfly hug was introduced by Lucinda Artigas while she and her colleagues were working with children in Mexico under the EMDR Humanitarian Assistance Program, and it has since been used to aid victims of hurricanes, floods, and other natural disasters. The method of combining butterfly hugs with drawing is now widely known to EMDR clinicians and is found especially suitable for disaster relief settings, where simultaneous accessibility to a large audience is necessary [Artigas, Jarero, Mauer, López Cano, & Alcal, 2000; Gertner, 2008].)

To begin the mural, the volunteers spread out wide on a canvas on the floor to be outlined as trees. The bashful students followed the lead of the school counselor, who modeled the activity, and then they rushed to be the tree themselves. Finger painting was encouraged with the option of using plastic gloves and clear raincoats to encourage mess making (Figure 3.15). The children began exploring the tactile sensations involved in painting with both hands. Some used big fat brushes and painted with huge strokes of dripping paints. I continued to utilize components of EMDR while promoting dual attention to the here and now of the sensory activity by eliciting a recall of their cherry trees every so often.

Over the next 1½ hours, the mural transformed many times. Some students engaged in self-directed, sensory-oriented play with paint. I observed one girl, in particular, who was pouring paint from one hand to another as if she were playing with wet sand at the beach. She seemed to be in a trance. She later painted a series of small "rainbows" in gray and called them to my attention; they appeared to resemble tsunami

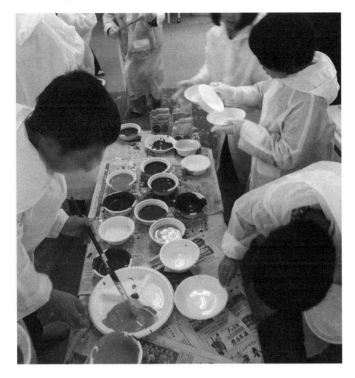

FIGURE 3.15.

water. I acknowledged her work and let her continue with finger painting. Her contribution, probably based on a traumatic memory, became
part of the group mural.

The students were gratified by the process and the resulting art
product. In completing the activity, the group was encouraged to come
up with a title, and the mural was enthusiastically named "Our [XYZ]
school's cherry blossom trees" (Figure 3.16). Giving it a title provided
closure to the activity and containment for the students' excitement.
Silently viewing and appreciating the work together in the end installed
the positive feelings experienced during the activity.

The 11 students from Fukushima who participated in this group
mural project engaged in multimodal reprocessing, first through guided
imagery, followed by the BLS of the butterfly hug to recall positive memories, and finally through active, physical participation in art therapy.
Though all of them impressed me as robust, one female student was particularly notable. She first appeared to have challenges with teamwork,

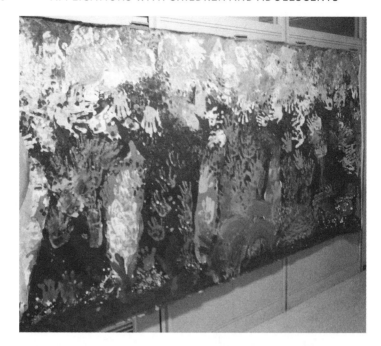

FIGURE 3.16.

displaying the tendency to dominate others or isolate herself in her own art-making process, disregarding others' expressions at times. After participating in the experience of simultaneously attending to the present moment of painting and to the memory of playing at the beach, she became more collaborative with others. Clearly, the parasympathetic nervous system was at work and kept her in the ideal regulated state as she reengaged in the group work to tackle the imagery of cherry trees that implied loss as well as hope for the future.

CONCLUSION

The intent of EMDR is not simply to flood clients with triggers through exposure therapy, but instead to achieve a shift in reality by developing new schemas of life and self-concept through the reorganization of fragmented or distorted memories stored in mind and body. Although its efficiency in rapidly resolving trauma with fewer sessions is unique to EMDR, its standard protocol offers only a basic landscape; the art component provides the roadmap of successful strategies to enhance BLS and facilitate sensory integration. As Steele and Malchiodi (2012) indicate, in trauma-informed practice the focus must remain on the needs of the clients to promote resilience. When working with traumatized children, in particular, judicious delivery of EMDR and art therapy is required.

REFERENCES

Adler-Tapia, R., & Settle, C. (2008). *Treatment manual: EMDR and the art of psychotherapy with children.* New York: Springer.

Ahmad, A. Larsson, B., & Sundelin-Wahlsten, V. (2007). EMDR treatment for children with PTSD: Results of a randomized controlled trial. *Nordic Journal of Psychiatry, 61,* 349–354.

American Psychiatric Association. (2004). *Practice guideline for the treatment of patients with acute stress disorder and posttraumatic stress disorder.* Arlington, VA: Author.

Artigas, L., Jarero, I., Mauer, M., López Cano, T., & Alcal, N. (2000, September). *EMDR and traumatic stress after natural disaster integrative treatment protocol and the butterfly hug.* Poster presented at the EMDRIA Conference, Toronto, Ontario, Canada.

Chemtob, C. M., Tolin, D. F., van der Kolk, B. A., & Pitman, R. K. (2000). Eye movement desensitization and reprocessing. In E. B. Foa, T. M. Keane, & M. J. Friedman (Eds.), *Effective treatments for PTSD: Practice guidelines from the International Society for Traumatic Stress Studies* (pp. 139–155, 333–335). New York: Guilford Press.

Fosha, D. (2003). Dyadic regulation and experiential work with emotion and relatedness in trauma and disorganized attachment. In M. F. Solomon & D. Siegel (Eds.), *Healing trauma: Attachment, mind, body, and brain* (pp. 221–281). New York: Norton.

Gantt, L., & Tinnin, L. W. (2008). Support for a neurobiological view of trauma with implications for art therapy. *Arts in Psychotherapy, 36,* 148–153.

Gertner, K. (2008). *Butterfly hug: An explanation of EMDR for children.* Fort Morgan, CO: Author.

Gomez, A. M. (2007). *Dark, bad day go away.* Phoenix, AZ: Author.

Gomez, A. M. (2011, August). *Repairing the attachment system through the use of EMDR, play, and creativity.* Lecture presented at the EMDRIA conference, Anaheim, CA.

Gomez, A. M. (2013). *EMDR therapy with adjunct approaches with children.* New York: Springer.

Gomez, A. M. (2013, November). *Complex PTSD, attachment, and dissociative symptoms: Treating children with pervasive emotion dysregulation using EMDR therapy* [Webinar]. Phoenix, AZ.

Kemp, M., Drummond, P., & McDermott, B. (2010). A wait-list controlled pilot study of eye movement desensitization and reprocessing (EMDR) for children with post-traumatic stress disorder (PTSD) symptoms from motor vehicle accidents. *Clinical Psychology and Psychiatry, 15,* 5–25.

Korn, D. L. (2011, August). *EMDR and the treatment of complex PTSD.* Workshop presented at the EMDRIA pre-conference, Anaheim, CA.

Korn, D. L., & Leeds, A. M. (2002). Preliminary evidence of efficacy for EMDR resource development and installation in the stabilization phase of treatment of complex posttraumatic stress disorder. *Journal of Clinical Psychology, 58*(12), 1465–1487.

Landgarten, H. B. (1981). *Clinical art therapy: Comprehensive guide.* New York: Routledge.

Levine, P. (1997). *Waking the tiger.* Berkeley, CA: North Atlantic Books.

Levine, P. (2002). *In an unspoken voice: How the body releases trauma and restores goodness.* Berkeley, CA: North Atlantic Books.

Levine, P., & Kline, M. (2007). *Trauma through a child's eyes: Awakening the ordinary miracle of healing—infancy through adolescence.* Berkeley, CA: North Atlantic Books.

Lovette, J. (1999). *Small wonders: Healing childhood trauma with EMDR.* New York: Free Press.

Malchiodi, C. A. (1990). *Breaking the silence: Art therapy with children from violent homes.* New York: Brunner/Mazel.

McNamee, C. (2003). Bilateral art: Facilitating systemic integration and balance. *Art Psychotherapy, 30,* 283–292.

McNamee, C. (2004). Using both sides of the brain: Experiences that integrate art and talk therapy through scribble drawings. *Art Therapy: Journal of the American Art Therapy Association, 21*(3), 136–142.

Ohnogi, A. J. (2010). Using play to support children traumatized by natural disasters: Chuetsu earthquake series in Japan. In A. Kalayjian & D. Eugene (Eds.), *Mass trauma and emotional healing around the world: Rituals and practices for resilience and meaning-making: Vol. 1. Natural disasters* (pp. 37–54). Santa Barbara, CA: Praeger.

Oras, R., de Ezpeleta, S. C., & Ahmad, A. (2004). Treatment of traumatized refugee children with eye movement desensitization and reprocessing in a psychodynamic context. *Nordic Journal of Psychiatry, 58*(3), 199–203.

Parnell, L. (2013). *Attachment-focused EMDR: Healing relational trauma.* New York: Norton.

Parnell, L., & Phillips, M. (2013, August). *Resource-tapping with EMDR.* San Francisco: R. Cassidy Seminars.

Perry, B. D., & Azad, I. (1999). Posttraumatic stress disorders in children and adolescents. *Current Opinion in Pediatrics, 11,* 310–316.

Perry, B. D., & Szalavitz, M. (2006). *The boy who was raised as a dog: And other stories from a child psychiatrist's notebook—what traumatized children can teach us about loss, love, and healing.* New York: Basic Books.

Porges, S. W. (2011). *Neurophysiological foundations of emotions, attachment, communication, and self-regulation.* New York: Norton.

PracticeWise. (2014, Spring). *PracticeWise Evidence Based Services Database.* Satellite Beach, FL: Author. Available online at *www.practicewise.com.* (Restricted site for subscribers only)

Riley, S. (1997). Social constructionism: The narrative approach and clinical art therapy. *Art Therapy: Journal of the American Art Therapy Association, 14*(4), 282–284.

Rothschild, B. (2000). *The body remembers: The psychophysiology of trauma and trauma treatment.* New York: Norton.

Schmidt, S. J. (1999, March). Resource-focused EMDR: Integration of ego state therapy, alternating bilateral stimulation and art therapy. *EMDRIA Newsletter, 4*(1), 8–26.

Schore, A. N. (2000). Attachment and the regulation of the right brain. *Attachment and Human Development, 2*(1), 23–47.

Schore, A. N. (2003). Early relational trauma, disorganized attachment, and the development of a predisposition to violence. In M. F. Solomon & D. Siegel (Eds.), *Healing trauma: Attachment, mind, body, and brain* (pp. 107–167). New York: Norton.

Shapiro, F. (1995). *Eye movement desensitization and reprocessing: Basic principles, protocols, and procedures.* New York: Guilford Press.

Shapiro, F. (2001). *Eye movement desensitization and reprocessing: Basic principles, protocols, and procedures* (2nd ed.). New York: Guilford Press.

Shapiro, F., & Laliotis, D. (2011). EMDR and the adaptive information processing model: Integrative treatment and case conceptualization. *Clinical Social Work Journal, 39,* 191–200.

Siegel, D. J. (1999). *The developing mind: How relationships and the brain interact to shape who we are.* New York: Guilford Press.

Siegel, D. J. (2011, August). *Mindsight and the power of neural integration in healing.* Keynote address presented at the EMDRIA conference, Anaheim, CA.

Steele, W., & Malchiodi, C. A. (2012). *Trauma-informed practices with children and adolescents.* New York: Routledge.

Talwar, S. (2007). Accessing traumatic memory through art making: An art therapy trauma protocol (ATTP). *Arts in Psychotherapy, 34,* 22–35.

Tanaka, M., & Urhausen, M. T. (2012). Drawing and storytelling as psychotherapy with children. In C. A. Malchiodi (Ed.), *Handbook of art therapy* (2nd ed., pp. 147–161). New York: Guilford Press.

Tinker-Wilson, S. A., & Tinker, R. H. (2011, August). *EMDR cases on the cutting edge of neuroscience.* Lecture presented at the EMDRIA conference, Anaheim, CA.

U.S. Department of Veterans Affairs and U.S. Department of Defense. (2010). *VA/DoD clinical practice guideline for the management of post-traumatic stress.* Washington, DC: Authors. Retrieved from *www.oqp.med.va.gov/cpg/PTSD/PTSD_cpg/frameset.htm.*

van der Kolk, B. A. (2008, January). *Trauma, attachment, and the body.* Lecture presented at Meadows conference, Universal City, CA.

Zaghrout-Hodali, M., Ferdoos, A., & Dodgson, P. W. (2008). Building resilience and dismantling fear: EMDR group protocol with children in an area of ongoing trauma. *Journal of EMDR Practice and Research, 2*(2), 106–113.

RESOURCES

EMDRIA (EMDR International Association)
www.emdria.org

AATA (American Art Therapy Association)
www.arttherapy.org

CHAPTER 4

Music and Grief Work
with Children and Adolescents

Russell E. Hilliard

Music has been a source of healing for centuries, and humankind has utilized this powerful medium to develop a sense of connectedness and to express emotions and thoughts. Quite often, words fail to convey the depth and breadth of one's emotions, and the elements of music (melody, harmony, and rhythm) can serve us when verbal expression is too limiting. Grief is one of the most complex emotional experiences because the grieving person often experiences a myriad of emotions, such as sorrow, anger, guilt, anxiety, fear, denial, disappointment, and relief, among others. Grieving adults often struggle through their bereavement, and the experience can be even more complicated for children and adolescents due to their developing understanding of the cycle of life and death (Doka, 2003). Music is a creative tool that can provide a form of emotional expression and assist children in understanding basic death education concepts (Hilliard, 2001; Wheeler, 2015).

Music therapy is an established allied health profession. The American Music Therapy Association (AMTA; *http://musictherapy. org*) defines music therapy as "the clinical and evidence-based use of music interventions to accomplish individualized goals within a therapeutic relationship by a credentialed professional who has completed an approved music therapy program." Although credentialed music thera-pists conduct music therapy, these practitioners are supportive of other professionals using music in their practices with proper education and experience. This use of music is not "music therapy" per se, but coun-selors, social workers, psychologists, and other health care professionals may nevertheless find that music can support their discipline-specific interventions.

Very little is available in the literature regarding counselors' use of music interventions for grieving children and adolescents, but the liter-ature does include the use of music interventions provided by counselors for the terminally ill. In his descriptive article, Brown (1992) claims to have been a health care "troubadour," providing music to the terminally ill for more than 12 years. He states, "Though an associate member of the National Association for Music Therapy, I am by no means a pro-fessional therapist" (p. 13) and "my own working definition of music as therapy is the applied use of music in the context of a nurturing rela-tionship to bring about change" (p. 15). Through case vignettes, Brown illustrates how his singing and guitar playing brought about changes in his clients. He suggests listening to audiotapes as a means of facilitating communication and getting people to open up. He encourages perfor-mance as a means of expression and socialization, imagery with music to increase relaxation, and songwriting to communicate feelings and experiences. Although he identifies the highly specialized training of professional therapists, Brown encourages all caring professionals to use music with their patients and clients.

Lochner and Stevenson (1988) explain how they used music with terminally ill individuals in their professionally trained roles as counsel-ors. Although they admit they are not therapists, the authors make no clear distinction between professionally trained therapists and counsel-ors using music in therapy. They report on music composed by Lochner and how it was used in therapy. Music often opened communication between therapist and client. In one case, the music allowed a 20-year-old man with cancer to begin sharing his feelings about his impending death, after listening to Lochner's song "I Love You, My Friend." In another case, Lochner wrote a song that he felt reflected his patient's feelings about the separation from her family she would soon experi-ence. The patient was a 40-year-old woman with ovarian cancer and had processed her feelings in a verbal therapy session, but she wanted to communicate them to her family. Lochner wrote a song titled "Stay by My Side" and sang it to the family with the patient's permission.

Family members clung to one another and cried as they realized what the patient was feeling. The music provided a way to increase awareness within the family and build a sense of higher cohesion. The authors conclude with a suggested music list for counselors to use when working with terminally or tragically ill individuals.

Music is an important form of creativity for children and adolescents; as such, it has been used therapeutically for a variety of clinical needs. In a study of 19 bereaved children, music therapy significantly reduced grief symptoms and taught participants a variety of healthy coping skills (Hilliard, 2001). It has been used as an alternative form of treatment to traditional verbal therapy for children and adolescents who experienced grief and trauma following the tragedies of September 11, 2001 (Gaffney, 2002). In pediatric health care settings, music therapy has been utilized to provide diversion during routine medical procedures, to convey emotional support, and to address the developmental needs of hospitalized children and adolescents (Robb, 2003). Music therapy has played a vital role in children's hospices to help terminally ill children and their families cope with their feelings of anticipatory grief (Hilliard, 2003; Pavlicevic, 2005). Through case vignettes and sample session plans, this chapter describes the use of music therapy and music-based interventions in grief work with children and adolescents.

MUSIC AND GRIEF WORK

The session format and plans described in this chapter embrace a cognitive-behavioral music therapy model. Cognitive-behavioral music therapy has been used with a variety of client populations and has been demonstrated to be a highly effective and efficient treatment modality (Standley, Johnson, Robb, Brownell, & Kim, 2004). Within this philosophy, "undesirable behaviors and symptoms are modified, beliefs that interfere with healing are re-evaluated, and traumatic reminders are reframed to become normal parts of a child's life, not harbingers of yet another traumatic event" (Gaffney, 2002, p. 58). Cognitive-behavioral music therapy in child and adolescent grief work emphasizes "behavior modification, the identification and expression of emotions, the intellectual understanding of grief, and challenges cognitive distortions while assisting with cognitive reframing and reshaping" (Hilliard, 2001, p. 296).

An essential component of treatment is recognition of the developmental stage of the client. The child's developmental stage plays an important role in understanding and coping with losses. For young children (ages 4–5 years), the idea that the deceased may return is common, as the permanence of death is not yet clearly understood. Children in this age group engage in magical thinking, consider death as punishment for bad behavior, and may have a fear of separation. The elementary school–age child (ages 6–11 years) may feel guilt or regret when a loved one dies, especially if the child disagreed with the deceased. Children in this age group may still engage in magical thinking, are likely to personify death (e.g., see it as a monster), can understand facts, and may have a high degree of death anxiety. Adolescents (ages 12–20 years) may internalize their grief or use unhealthy forms of coping such as experimenting with drugs and alcohol, embrace an adult concept of death, or defy death by engaging in reckless behavior (Doka, 2003). It is essential to utilize music interventions appropriate for the developmental stage of the client.

In addition to the developmental stage of the client, the therapist assesses the client's strengths and problem areas, communication style, learning style, cultural and religious/spiritual background, history with music, and preferred musical styles and genres. In many cases, therapists utilize standardized music therapy assessments, especially in pediatric health care and special education settings (Chase, 2004; DeLoach-Walworth, 2005). Meta-analyses of the medical music therapy literature indicate that the most effective type of music intervention is live music. Recorded music conditions, however, show a more positive effect than do no-music conditions. The type of music shown to have the most positive effect is patient-preferred music. Based on these data, the best types of music interventions are those that utilize patient-preferred, live music (Dileo & Bradt, 2005; Standley, 2000; Standley & Whipple, 2003). Therefore, learning the type of music preferred by the grieving child or adolescent is an important component of the music therapy assessment.

Following the music therapy assessment, the therapist begins the process of treatment planning and the formation of session plans. Much of the work described here was conducted in child and adolescent bereavement support groups under the auspices of a hospice's bereavement center. The format of the sessions remained fairly consistent, regardless of the age of the clients. Each session began with an opening experience designed to help clients motivate themselves to engage in the group and to reduce any feelings of defensiveness or emotional guardedness. These opening group experiences included drumming, singing, or music and movement. Following the opening experience, the therapist facilitated a brief discussion and an emotional check-in for each client, and clients shared how they were feeling at that moment. The central part of the group was the theme of the day. These themes varied, depending on the type of group and age of the clients, but included "the memorial service," "coping with anger (or sorrow)," and "remembering." Because clients often shared intense emotions during the theme-based aspect of the group, the therapist facilitated a closing experience designed to elevate mood and encourage creative musical play. These closing experiences included musical improvisation and the playing of musical games such as Name That Tune or Musicopoly (a music version of Monopoly).

The music and grief work described here has been utilized in bereavement centers associated with hospice programs. Music therapy has been provided for children in a variety of settings: family sessions, individual sessions, time-limited school-based bereavement groups, child and adolescent grief camps, and open bereavement groups at a bereavement center. Family therapy sessions utilizing music therapy have been facilitated prior to the death of the loved one to help children cope with the anticipated death as well as following the death to help them with the mourning process. These sessions are typically held in the home environment and include various family members, such as siblings. Music provides opportunities for the family to engage in intergenerational therapy activities, wherein each person's developmental stage is respected. Individual music therapy sessions for grief and loss can be facilitated, as needed, either in the home or at the bereavement center. These sessions are particularly useful for the child or adolescent who may be nervous or unsure about attending a group setting. Engaging in individual therapy initially may open the door for group participation later. Additionally, individual therapy is essential for clients experiencing complicated mourning or multiple clinical needs.

Time-limited school-based groups are useful in helping maintain continuity and leading a curriculum focused on grief and loss. Children and adolescents attend groups at their schools during the school day for 1-hour sessions once weekly for 8 weeks. The structure of these groups contrasts with the open-group format often facilitated at a bereavement center. In the open groups, clients participate as needed, there is an ebb and flow of clients attending, and the sessions are planned by topic or theme rather than following a systematic curriculum. Child and adolescent grief camps that utilize music have been offered in hospices throughout the country. Clients rotate through many small groups, and music therapy is often offered in these groups. Music is also used in large groups such as memorial services or the closing ceremonies for grief camps.

MUSIC TECHNIQUES

A variety of music therapy techniques is used in grief work. Although most of these techniques employ live music, recorded music can be substituted whenever live music is not possible. The music techniques presented here are easily modified to be appropriate for youngsters of all ages.

Drumming is a popular technique for children and adolescents alike. The important factor to remember when drumming with teenagers is that it is essential to use age-appropriate rhythm instruments. Rhythm instruments such as djembes and bongos can be purchased for a fair price from most local or online music retailers. Paddle drums, hand drums, and tambourines as well as other popular rhythm instruments can be enjoyed by children of all ages. Younger children like drums with bright colors or cartoon characters. There is a variety of ways to facilitate a group drumming experience (Stevens, 2003; Wajler, 2002), such as engaging in a call-and-response pattern wherein the facilitator plays a short rhythm and the group participants play it back. This call-and-response pattern is passed around the group until each member has had an opportunity to play an original rhythm and hear it played back. A short discussion about the experience may follow, with the therapist helping the clients see that the experience resembles a conversation, with times for listening and times for responding.

In addition to call-and-response drumming, the facilitator can encourage improvisation by holding a steady beat while group members play any rhythm, style, and dynamic they wish. By keeping a steady beat, the facilitator grounds the improvisation. One can also divide the group in half and alternate the grounding steady beat with the improvisation, half the group keeping the steady beat at all times. Exploring dynamics (loud/soft) and tempo (fast/slow) and adding movements (marching, playing up high or down low) can also add to the drumming experience. Drumming the rhythm of a group member's name can be a fun and welcoming musical experience, and playing multiple members' names can create a rich polyrhythmic experience. For example, the group can learn to drum, say, Nancy Middleton's name by practicing playing and saying the name in rhythm (i.e., Nan-cy Mid-dle-ton). Once the group can play and say the name together, they can fade out saying the name and just drum. Selecting multiple names to play in small groups creates a richer rhythmic experience. These drumming experiences are useful for opening and closing the group process; they can create a sense of group cohesion, motivate clients who may have depressive symptoms, provide an outlet for hyperactive clients, and foster a sense of working together.

Rhythmic improvisation can be used for the identification and expression of emotions as well. Group members can play what they are feeling, and other group members can guess the emotion. To facilitate this process, it is sometimes necessary to place a variety of instruments on a table or on the floor in the back of the room and have the group members face away from the instruments or close their eyes as the client playing selects the instrument and plays. This method encourages the group members to listen respectfully, decreases off-task behavior, and helps the self-conscious client play expressively and creatively. Free play can also be used with instruments, as the therapist simply responds to the music as the clients make it. In both cases, clients are able to identify and express their emotions—one of the goals of grief work.

Singing well-known songs can assist in developing group cohesion as clients get to know one another through their musical preferences. Songs chosen can also reflect an emotional state when clients choose a song that reflects how they feel when they think of the person who died. To remember the deceased, the clients may also be asked to bring a recording of his or her favorite song to be played in the group. Clients can sing along with a recording of the song, but therapists primarily use live music with guitar or piano accompaniment. Using song lyric sheets helps prompt clients to sing along with the recording or accompaniment.

Combining music and art techniques is useful in fostering creativity among children. There is a variety of ways in which therapists facilitate this type of activity, such as by having clients create a grief collage to music. The therapist brings a recording of short segments of different types of music, and, as the music plays, clients draw freely on a large piece of paper. Each time the music changes, the clients move one seat to the right and begin drawing around the drawing of the client previously seated there. After each musical segment, a short discussion about clients' drawings follows. The end result is a collage of art based on clients' grief experiences. This activity can also be facilitated with live music, with the therapist playing or improvising a variety of musical styles or selections.

Another music and art activity that is well liked by grieving children and adolescents is to create CD covers. The therapist asks the clients to create a series of song titles that reflects their grief experiences. Examples of instructions include "Write a song title about how you felt when you first found out your loved one died," ". . . about how you viewed your relationship with your loved one," ". . . about how you felt at the memorial service (if you attended it)," ". . . about how you feel now when you think about your loved one," and so forth. Clients are instructed to write the song titles on a piece of paper and then decorate it as though it were the cover to a musical recording. During discussion of the song titles, it is useful to have instruments at hand and to ask clients to give a demonstration of how the songs might sound. This type of activity can encourage verbal expression of emotions and help clients engage more easily in verbal counseling.

Music bibliotherapy combines music techniques with story reading and has been used in the field of music therapy to promote academic successes (Register, 2001, 2004) and for counseling after traumatic experiences (Altilio, 2002). Although this technique is primarily used with younger children who enjoy being read stories, it can be used with adolescents as well. Adolescents are encouraged to write their own grief story or poem, to which music is added. For young children, music is added to an existing children's book about grief and loss. There is a variety of such books available; sample titles include *Lifetimes: A Beautiful Way to Explain Death to Children* (Mellonie, 1983), *The Tenth Good Thing about Barney* (Viorst & Blegvad, 1971), and *The Memory String* (Bunting & Rand, 2000). *Grateful: A Song of Giving Thanks* (Bucchino & Hakkarainen, 2006) is useful for helping children cope with grief and the holidays because it deals with being grateful in spite of a loss, and it includes a CD recording of Art Garfunkel's original song for the book.

Therapists who use music bibliotherapy often compose original songs to accompany the story reading. During breaks in the reading of the book, the therapist and clients sing the song, and this singing reinforces the lesson being taught by the book (the therapist can choose a highly rhythmic chant in lieu of an original song composition for a similar effect). The therapist also identifies main characters or actions that are repeated throughout the story. These characters or actions are then assigned a musical instrument (e.g., Barney = maracas; purred =

shakers). Each time the character's name or the action is heard during the reading of the story, the client who has that character or action plays the assigned instrument. This technique helps increase on-task behavior and attention to the story. Books about grief and loss provide opportunities for discussion of group members' experiences and help normalize the grief process. The musical elements assist in the understanding of the lessons learned, provide opportunities for active engagement, and encourage listening skills.

Writing lyrics has been used successfully with children and adolescents in an effort to address a variety of emotional needs (Hilliard, 2001; Keen, 2004). Song or rap lyric writing can be a useful tool in helping children and adolescents express their grief, contract to use healthy coping skills, and remember the person who died. Young children often need structure to help elicit lyrics. The therapist can ask questions about their grief process in a systematic way to develop each line of the song. Questions may include "How did you feel at the memorial service?"; "What are some of the things you remember about the person who died?"; and "How do you express your anger (or sorrow or any other emotion)?" Answers to these questions form the lyrics of the song or rap. Writing a rap is often easy to facilitate because clients readily provide the rhythmic structure. The task of the therapist is to fit the lyrics into the rhythmic structure provided by clients. Sometimes this requires a rewording of the lyrics or a collapsing of ideas into shorter lines. By providing a selection of musical elements such as various keys, tempos, dynamics, and styles, the therapist helps clients compose their own music to fit their song lyrics. Another popular songwriting activity is to provide a musical structure in the style of the blues, for example, and encourage clients to improvise singing over it.

Analyzing song lyrics can facilitate an understanding of death, provide a sense of normalcy, educate clients about grief, and help them identify and express emotions. Therapists often lead a sing-along with guitar or piano accompaniment and then lead a discussion analyzing the song's lyrics. Recorded music can also be used, and there are several children's songs that deal with emotional content such as feeling sad, lonely, or angry and that work well in children's bereavement groups. Peter Alsop has written several songs to help children cope with death, dying, grief, and loss. His videotape *When Kids Say Goodbye* (1996) and audio recording *Songs on Loss and Grief* (1995) contain songs to help children understand their grief emotions and also provide basic death education concepts (e.g., the difference between sleep and death).

Playing either of these provides opportunities for discussion and counseling of the children's needs. Adolescents are often encouraged to bring their own recordings that express their grief emotions and reactions to the group, but it is sometimes necessary for the therapist to require that clients bring edited versions of the recordings to prevent others from becoming offended by the sometimes graphic language. It is useful to have lyric sheets to accompany the songs, and the therapist can point out lines for discussion and opportunities for counseling.

Orff–Schulwerk is an approach to music education created by Carl Orff that embodies the concept that children learn by doing. In this approach, children experience music through playing, singing, and moving as they learn about various musical concepts. Therapists use this approach because the musical elements lend themselves to many therapy goals. A variety of instruments are used in Orff–Schulwerk and may include xylophones, metalophones, glockenspiels, recorders, drums, and other rhythm instruments (Colwell, Achey, Gillmeister, & Woolrich, 2004). A curriculum for grieving children based on the Orff–Schulwerk approach has been developed (Hilliard, 2007) and empirically tested. In this curriculum, children engage in songwriting, improvisation, singing, playing instruments, and moving with music. All of the music is based on issues related to bereavement, and children are able to achieve therapeutic goals through their participation in musical dialogue.

SESSION PLANS

The following session plan is an example of a music-based bereavement group for young children ages 3–6 years. It is the third session in an eight-session format. Either live or recorded music can be utilized in the plan, which is designed for a group of five to eight with a duration of approximately 45 minutes.

Session Theme: Distinguishing Sleep from Death

Purpose

Young children can become confused about the differences between sleep and death, especially if parents or guardians explained the death of the loved one by making statements such as "Grandma is at rest; it's like she's asleep." Sometimes children are unable to distinguish between death and sleep, and they may experience fear or anxiety when they see their living loved ones asleep or when it is time for them to go to bed. The purpose of this session is to help children understand the differences between sleep and death.

Goals

1. Reduce fear/anxiety regarding sleeping situations.
2. Differentiate between sleep and death.
3. Understand basic death education concepts.
4. Learn effective coping skills.

Materials Needed

- A variety of rhythm instruments
- "While I'm Sleepin'" song sheet (music from the *Stayin' Over Songbook*; Alsop, 1994) or a recording of the song by Peter Alsop (from *Songs on Loss and Grief*)
- Guitar or piano for therapist accompaniment or player for recorded music

Procedure

1. Opening experience: Facilitate rhythm and movement experience by passing out rhythm instruments (egg-shaped shakers are good for this age group) and encourage children to shake their instruments while standing in place. Next, have each child take turns adding a movement to the shaking of the rhythm instruments for other children to mirror. Continue this until everyone has a chance to lead. If the children are still quite active, add a popular children's song to the shaker rhythm, such as "Shake My Sillies Out" or "She'll Be Comin' 'Round the Mountain." Begin to slow the music and shaking rhythm and lead the children in sitting on the floor as they play more slowly and softly. Once they are seated in a circle, stop the music. Instruct the children to toss the instruments in the circle for you to collect. This will help reduce off-task behavior.

2. Play the song "While I'm Sleepin'" by Peter Alsop. Lead a sing-along of the chorus: "While I'm sleepin', I'm alive. My heart's beatin', deep inside. I keep breathin', soft and slow. How do I do it? Well, I don't

know." Each verse of the song provides examples of how being asleep is different from being dead and normalizes the fear, anxiety, and confusion about this issue.

3. Lead a short discussion of the song lyrics by asking concrete questions such as "What's the difference between being asleep and being dead?" or "Does a person's heart beat when he or she is asleep? How about when he or she is dead?" Have each child identify a difference between sleep and death. A nice way to end the discussion is to ask, "If you had to explain how being asleep is different from being dead, what would you say?"

4. Pass out the rhythm instruments again and play a variety of rhythms. The call-and-response mode is useful, and adding movement, as needed, helps reduce off-task behavior. Begin to slow and soften the music again to get the children in a seated position. Collect the instruments.

5. Pass around the most interesting instrument (e.g., rain stick or ocean drum). Explain that the instrument is the talking instrument and that when you say "Stop," whoever is holding the instrument gets to talk. Ask questions of each child, such as, "How was it that your special someone died?" or "Who told you about the death?"

6. For a closing exercise, engage the children in singing, rhythmic improvisation, and movement. These activities elevate children's mood and ends the group on an uplifting note.

The following session plan is taken from a music-based bereavement group for adolescents. Using an open format, the group meets twice monthly at the bereavement center, and music sessions are planned for each meeting. This session plan is an example of a typical music-based experience with this type of group.

Session Theme: The Grief Rap

Purpose

Adolescents may struggle with the recognition that grief changes over time and that most grieving people begin to feel better as they process their experiences. It can be useful for clients to see how their grief has changed over time. This activity is designed to help them recognize these changes and honor their own processes.

Goals

1. Identify and express emotions.
2. Recall memories of the deceased.
3. Engage in peer support.
4. Learn effective coping skills.

Materials Needed

- A variety of rhythm instruments
- Client-preferred live or recorded music
- Guitar or piano for therapist accompaniment or player for recorded music
- Grief worksheets and pencils
- Large piece of paper or dry-erase board and markers

Procedure

1. Opening experience: With clients sitting in a circle, play client-preferred music (either live or recorded). Distribute two soft, medium-sized foam balls and have clients toss the balls to each other while the music plays. Stop the music periodically at random and have the two clients holding the balls share how their time has been since the previous group and how they are feeling in their grief process now. Continue the activity until everyone has had an opportunity to share.

2. With music playing quietly in the background, distribute pencils and a prepared worksheet for each client to complete that contains the following questions:

> "What is something your loved one taught you for which you are grateful?"
> "Where were you when you found out your loved one died?"
> "How did you feel when you first found out about the death?"
> "How did you deal with or express that feeling?"
> "When you think of your loved one now, how do you feel?"
> "What is one of the best memories you have of your loved one?"

3. Lead a short discussion of the responses to the questions on the worksheet if clients feel comfortable.

4. Following the discussion, the responses provided on the work-sheet are used to write a rap. Using a drum, play a basic rhythm and ask clients to provide the first line to the rap by choosing one of the responses they wrote on the worksheet. Adolescents easily complete most rap writing, but they sometimes need prompting or suggestions. This guidance can be necessary if clients get off task or become inappropriate with their lyrics.

5. Write the rap on a large piece of paper or dry-erase board. At the end of the group, the rap is written on a smaller piece of paper to be photocopied for each client.

6. For a closing exercise, pass around a bongo drum and ask clients to identify at least one person they trust and with whom they can share their grief emotions until the next group.

CASE VIGNETTES

Jackie, a 4-year-old European American female, was referred to the children's bereavement program after her father died in a tragic accident. On a Saturday afternoon, she was playing in her next-door neighbor's yard when her father arrived home with a new piece of lawn equipment. While he was unloading the equipment from the trailer, he lost control of it and was crushed to death. Jackie witnessed her father's sudden death and experienced an intense state of shock. The child psychologist she was seeing for individual sessions referred her to the bereavement group to give her opportunities to engage with other grieving children.

During the music therapy assessment, Jackie's mother reported that Jackie had problems sleeping at night, displayed an intense level of dependence, had become increasingly inattentive in her preschool, and complained of somatic concerns such as head- and stomachaches. Jackie participated in live music experiences with the therapist during the assessment visit, was creative and engaging, and initiated free musical play with rhythm instruments. When asked about her father, she became withdrawn, looked downward, displayed a sad affect, and would not talk about him. Therapeutic goals for Jackie included increasing her awareness of basic death education concepts (e.g., the finality of death), identifying and expressing emotions, decreasing her problems with sleeping and overdependency on her mother, developing coping skills, and remembering happy times with her father.

Initially, Jackie was quiet, withdrawn, and timid but quite polite and respectful of her peers and the therapist. It took her several weeks before she felt comfortable enough to initiate expression of her own thoughts and feelings, and then she became quite expressive and participatory in the sessions. She was musically motivated, and even before she talked about her experiences, she was readily able to engage in musical dialogue. She enjoyed choosing instruments to play during the rhythmic improvisation and Orff-based musical experiences. While playing, she smiled, giggled, and was able to share with her peers. These experiences seemed important for her, as they helped her develop therapeutic rapport with the therapist and the other children in the group.

Over time, Jackie began to share her grief experiences. Following a musical improvisation, she expressed feeling sad about her father's death. One of the other children asked her how he died, and, without hesitation, she told the group what had happened to him. This was the first time she had acknowledged the actual event. She said, "I thought it was a bad dream, but he's not coming home." Immediately afterward, she began improvising a melancholic melody on the xylophone that was in front of her. Jackie displayed an awareness of her father's death, and she was able to recognize that he was not going to return. The music helped her cope with her grief emotions after verbally sharing with the group, and it seemed as though her engagement in the musical dialogue helped her feel comfortable enough to share her thoughts and feelings verbally with the group.

In subsequent music therapy sessions, Jackie became increasingly expressive and talked openly about her father's death, her memories of him, her family's spiritual beliefs, and her reactions to her mother's grief (she became nervous when she witnessed her mother crying). She often initiated musical experiences by making requests or leading musical improvisation experiences. Jackie's mother reported that Jackie's symptoms (sadness, sleep disturbance, overdependency, somatic concerns) continued to improve, although she remained unable to sleep through the entire night. With a curious affect, her mother reported that Jackie enjoyed coming to group and would often ask, "Is this group night?" This is a common reaction among group participants, who apparently feel supported and affirmed in the group and are able to make friends with one another; even though the topic of the group can be emotionally heavy, the music experiences seem to offer a sense of lightness and provide opportunities for mood elevation and even joy.

Tyrone, a 13-year-old African American male, was participating in music therapy sessions prior to his mother's death. His mother, diagnosed with HIV/AIDS, received home care hospice services, and, as part of the interdisciplinary team, the therapist visited the patient and family prior to the patient's death. Tyrone was present for and participated in several of his mother's music therapy sessions. At times, the therapist and Tyrone met together without his mother, and these sessions were important in helping Tyrone deal with her impending death. Tyrone wanted to learn how to play the guitar, and the therapist taught him several basic chord progressions. Tyrone's music therapy treatment was part of the overall interdisciplinary care plan for his mother. Goals for Tyrone included engaging in meaningful experiences with his mother, identifying and expressing emotions, and learning healthy coping skills.

His mother's symptoms became difficult to manage at home, and she was admitted to the hospice's freestanding inpatient unit. When Tyrone's mother died, he went to the therapist's office in the inpatient unit and informed the therapist of her death. Tyrone's affect was flat, his eyes were vacant, and he was not crying; he appeared to be numb. He picked up the guitar in the corner and began playing a D chord repeatedly while improvising a song about his mother. While vocalizing and playing, he became tearful, and these tears quickly led to intense sobbing. With his eyes closed, he sobbed as he sang and played in an apparently cathartic experience. As his sobs lessened, he stopped vocalizing and eventually stopped playing the guitar. After the music and cathartic expression, he appeared tired and was able to begin talking about his mother's life and death.

Tyrone continued participating in individual music therapy sessions and eventually agreed to attend an adolescent bereavement group. In the group, he openly engaged with his peers and continued to prefer expressing his emotions nonverbally through his participation in live musical dialogue. Music helped Tyrone engage in meaningful experiences with his mother prior to her death, and he often shared memories of these experiences with his peers in the bereavement group. Typically resisting verbal discussion of his emotions, he used the music experiences as a means of expressing them. In his time outside of the therapy sessions, Tyrone used music to alter his mood and help him cope with his grief. He rarely left his home without his MP3 player, and he often brought his favorite recordings to the group to share with his peers.

CONCLUSION

Music therapy has been used effectively in helping children and adolescents cope with traumatic experiences and subsequent feelings of grief and loss. Research documenting music therapy's effects on mood and behavior of grieving children supports music therapy as a viable treatment option for significantly reducing the symptoms associated with bereavement (Hilliard, 2001). It has also been used to help children and adolescents cope with the aftermath of the September 11, 2001, tragedies (Altilio, 2002). Although music therapy is conducted most effectively by a board-certified therapist, other mental health professionals may find that the use of music in their practice can support their therapeutic interventions. By using recorded music in lieu of live music, counselors can explore new and creative ways to help children and adolescents in the counseling process. A variety of musical techniques used by therapists can lend themselves to verbal therapy sessions. Such techniques include lyrical analyses and using background music combined with art activities. When counselors and therapists work together, clients benefit from the expertise provided by both disciplines. Sharing information is essential for children and adolescents to have better access to treatment in a world they understand—the world of creativity and play.

REFERENCES

Alsop, P. (1994). *Stayin' over songbook for kids, parents and teachers.* Minneapolis, MN: Moose School.

Alsop, P. (1995). *Songs on loss and grief.* Minneapolis, MN: Moose School.

Alsop, P. (1996). *When kids say goodbye: Helping kids with sad feelings.* Minneapolis, MN: Moose School.

Altilio, T. (2002). Helping children, helping ourselves: An overview of children's literature. In J. Loewy & A. Hara (Eds.), *Caring for the caregiver: The use of music and music therapy in grief and trauma* (pp. 138–147). Silver Spring, MD: American Music Therapy Association.

Brown, J. (1992). When words fail, music speaks. *American Journal of Hospice and Palliative Care, 9*(2), 13–17.

Bucchino, J., & Hakkarainen, A. (2006). *Grateful: A song of giving thanks.* New York: HarperCollins.

Bunting, E., & Rand, T. (2000). *The memory string.* London: Clarion Books.

Chase, K. M. (2004). Music therapy assessment for children with developmental disabilities: A survey study. *Journal of Music Therapy, 41*(1), 28–54.

Colwell, C. M., Achey, C., Gillmeister, G., & Woolrich, J. (2004). The Orff approach to music therapy. In A. Darrow (Ed.), *Introduction to approaches in music therapy* (pp. 103–124). Silver Spring, MD: American Music Therapy Association.

DeLoach-Walworth, D. (2005). Procedural support for music therapy in the healthcare setting: A cost-effectiveness analysis. *Journal of Pediatric Nursing, 20*(4), 276–284.

Dileo, C., & Bradt, J. (2005). *Medical music therapy: A meta-analysis and agenda for future research.* Cherry Hill, NJ: Jeffrey Books.

Doka, K. (2003). *Living with grief: Children, adolescents, and loss.* Washington, DC: Hospice Foundation of America.

Gaffney, D. (2002). Seasons of grief: Helping children grow through loss. In J. Loewy & A. Hara (Eds.), *Caring for the caregiver: The use of music and music therapy in grief and trauma* (pp. 54–62). Silver Spring, MD: American Music Therapy Association.

Hilliard, R. E. (2001). The effects of music therapy-based bereavement groups on mood and behavior of grieving children: A pilot study. *Journal of Music Therapy, 38*(4), 291–306.

Hilliard, R. E. (2003). Music therapy in pediatric palliative care: A complementary approach. *Journal of Palliative Care, 19*(2), 127–132.

Hilliard, R. E. (2007). The effects of Orff-based music therapy and social work groups on grieving children. *Journal of Music Therapy, 44*(2), 123–138.

Keen, A. W. (2004). Using music as a therapy tool to motivate troubled adolescents. *Social Work in Health Care, 39*(3–4) 361–373.

Lochner, S. W., & Stevenson, R. G. (1988). Music as a bridge to wholeness. *Death Studies, 12,* 173–180.

Mellonie, B. (1983). *Lifetimes: A beautiful way to explain death to children.* London: Banton.

Pavlicevic, M. (2005). *Music therapy in children's hospices.* London: Jessica Kingsley.

Register, D. (2001). The effects of an early intervention music curriculum on prereading/writing. *Journal of Music Therapy, 38*(3), 239–248.

Register, D. (2004). The effects of live music groups versus an educational children's television program on the emergent literacy of young children. *Journal of Music Therapy, 41*(1), 2–27.

Robb, S. L. (2003). *Music therapy in pediatric healthcare: Research and evidence-based practice.* Silver Spring, MD: American Music Therapy Association.

Standley, J. M. (2000). Music research in medical treatment. In D. Smith (Ed.), *Effectiveness of music therapy procedures: Documentation of research and clinical practice* (3rd ed., pp. 1–64). Silver Spring, MD: American Music Therapy Association.

Standley, J. M., Johnson, C. M., Robb, S. L., Brownell, M. D., & Kim, S. (2004). Behavioral approach to music therapy. In A. Darrow (Ed.), *Introduction to approaches in music therapy* (pp. 103–124). Silver Spring, MD: American Music Therapy Association.

Standley, J. M., & Whipple, J. (2003). Music therapy in pediatric palliative care: A meta-analysis. In S. Robb (Ed.), *Music therapy in pediatric healthcare: Research and evidence-based practice* (pp. 1–18). Silver Spring, MD: American Music Therapy Association.

Stevens, C. (2003). *The art and heart of drum circles.* Milwaukee, WI: Hal Leonard.

Viorst, J., & Blegvad, E. (1971). *The tenth good thing about Barney.* New York: Atheneum.

Wajler, Z. (2002). *World beat fun: Multicultural and contemporary rhythms for K–8 classrooms.* Miami, FL: Warner Brothers.

Wheeler, B. L. (Ed.). (2015). *Music therapy handbook.* New York: Guilford Press.

CHAPTER 5

Art Therapy as an Intervention for Mass Terrorism and Violence

Laura V. Loumeau-May
Ellie Seibel-Nicol
Mary Pellicci Hamilton
Cathy A. Malchiodi

This chapter focuses on the impact of mass violence on children and the use of art therapy to help those children impacted by traumatic grief to develop coping skills and resiliency. Mass violence comprises political violence (including terrorist acts), ongoing exposure to street violence, and mass single-incident shootings. Although mass trauma can result from natural disasters, this chapter concentrates on mass trauma inflicted by humans, notably mass terrorism and nonterroristic mass violence. Two powerful single-incident examples of mass violence—the September 11, 2001 (9/11), terrorist attacks and the December 14, 2012 (12/14), school shooting in Newtown, Connecticut—are highlighted with case examples to demonstrate the therapeutic needs of the children affected and how clinical interventions are structured to address these needs. This chapter validates how art therapy interventions support the role of creativity in trauma recovery from mass terrorism and violence.

MASS TERRORISM AND MASS VIOLENCE

Terrorism has an impact on children that exceeds the loss of life and property; their lives and outlooks are dramatically changed. On 9/11, 3,051 children and teens lost parents in the worst mass terrorist attack on the United States in history. Even those children who did not lose a parent were affected. Thousands witnessed the terror firsthand from their homes and schools, and millions more saw the destruction of New York City's World Trade Center on television.

Mass shooting is defined as four or more people being shot during the same incident or time period. Twenty-six people, including 20 children and 6 adults, were shot and killed at Sandy Hook Elementary School on December 14, 2012. As a result of this act of violence, children lost their lives or were directly impacted by trauma, narrowly escaping themselves while witnessing their friends or teachers be killed. People affected by mass violence may identify themselves as part of a targeted group, such as the Sandy Hook Elementary School, Columbine High School, or Virginia Tech mass shootings, the Boston Marathon bombing, or 9/11, or cases of disgruntled employees returning to places of past employment. At other times, the shooting is perceived as random; survivors may feel that they were in the wrong place at the wrong time, as was the case in the movie theater shooting in Aurora, Colorado, in July 2011.

The trauma of mass terrorism is inflicted upon a large group such as a community or nation and differs from other forms of mass trauma in scope, cause, and intent. Terrorism is purposeful and intersocietal rather than interpersonal, as is the case in familial abuse or even random violence. The end goals exceed physical and economic destruction; they are psychological, with the aim of demoralizing the targeted population. Mass terrorism is also characterized by the scale of human and property loss. Targets are often large symbolic public sites thought to be invulnerable, so that their destruction creates widespread panic. The ripple effects of consequences impact the larger society and create a massive diversion of resources to control and repair the damage (Doka, 2003), such the events of 9/11 in the United States. For example, the perception of the country being under attack lasted for months after the events, and trauma-induced fear had spread throughout society.

In contrast, terrorist acts consisting of repeated incidents on a small scale are experienced differently than mass terrorism. People living in communities where isolated car, subway, and suicide bombings occur at intermittent frequency experience a state of constant hypervigilance (McGeehan, 2005). The occurrences are generally limited in scale and the targets arbitrary. No one knows when or where the next incident will occur. According to Kalmanowitz and Lloyd (2005), "When violence is ongoing, pervasive and unremitting, it may form an integral part of each individual's internal world, identity, values, beliefs and history and not only affect a part of their present, but also inform who each person will become. It will invariably inform the community itself" (p. 15). Political violence affects the cultural memory of a society when the artifacts or symbolic structures of a community that represent its identity are destroyed. This was true of the World Trade Center's Twin Towers, which were symbols of Western economic might, free trade, and power.

Many inner-city neighborhoods are besieged by recurrent street violence, similar to sporadic terrorism. Children and teens living under such conditions experience violence inflicted by others on a regular basis, with danger to themselves, their peers, and their loved ones. Their internal responses are similar to those of people who experience ongoing unpredictable terroristic activity, as noted by McGeehan (2005). Additionally, domestic violence can be similarly perceived because it often occurs sporadically or with little warning and involves danger to self and caregivers (Malchiodi, 2012).

Finally, media coverage of incidents of mass terrorism and mass violence is extensive and pervasive, complicating short- and long-term interventions. Coverage of the actual attacks and repercussions of September 11th was unprecedented and has been linked to acute stress reactions (Silver et al., 2013). Allen, Tucker, and Pfefferbaum (2006) note the same phenomena in Oklahoma City in 1995. In the case of 9/11, grieving families were reexposed to the images of the planes hitting the Twin Towers and the Pentagon—the murder of their loved ones—every day. This repeated display of the traumatic event was experienced as intrusive and potentially retraumatizing, and many people responded by turning off their televisions and stopping news deliveries (Rathkey, 2004).

CHILDREN'S AND ADOLESCENTS' RESPONSES TO MASS TRAUMA AND VIOLENCE

Children and youth experience psychological stress after traumatic events, including those involving mass trauma and violence. Disasters may leave them with harmful, long-lasting effects; even when children only see a large-scale traumatic event on television or overhear parents or friends discussing it, they may feel scared, confused, or anxious. They also may react to trauma differently than adults; some may react immediately, whereas others may show signs that they are having a difficult time weeks and months later. This variability can make relief efforts difficult in some cases.

The reactions noted below are normal when children and teens are experiencing stress right after an event. If any of these behaviors lasts for more than 2–4 weeks, or if they suddenly appear later on, it may indicate that intervention is needed to support coping and relieve symptoms. The following information is summarized from the National Child Traumatic Stress Network (NCTSN; 2014).

Preschool Age: 0–5 Years Old

Very young children may regress to behaviors such as wetting the bed at night after a mass trauma. They may fear strangers, darkness, or monsters or to want to stay in a place where they feel safe. They may depict the trauma repeatedly in their play or drawings or become hyperaroused when telling stories about what happened. Eating and sleeping habits may change, and some children may complain of aches and pains that cannot be explained. There may be aggressive or dissociative behavior, hyperactivity, speech difficulties, and disobedience. Infants and those children younger than 2 years cannot understand that a trauma is happening, but they know when their caregiver is upset. They may mimic the same emotions as their caregivers or cry for no reason, withdraw from people, and not play with their toys. Preschool children, ages 3–5 years old, may have problems adjusting to change and loss and may become more dependent on adults.

Childhood to Adolescence: 6–18 Years Old

Children and teens may have some of the same reactions to trauma as younger children. Often younger children want much more attention from parents or caregivers and may stop doing their schoolwork. Children may fear going to school and stop spending time with friends. They may not be able to pay attention and do poorly in school overall. Some may become aggressive for no clear reason. Or they may act younger than their age by asking to be fed or dressed by their parent or caregiver.

Because adolescents, 11–19 years old, go through a lot of physical and emotional changes due to their developmental stage, it may be even harder for them to cope with trauma. Older teens may deny their reactions to themselves and their caregivers. Older children and teens may feel helpless and guilty because they cannot take on adult roles to respond to a trauma or disaster. They may respond with a routine "I'm okay" or even silence when they are upset. Or they may complain about physical aches or pains because they cannot identify what is really bothering them emotionally. Some may start arguments at home and/or at school, resisting any structure or authority. They also may engage in risky behaviors such as using alcohol or drugs.

CHILDHOOD TRAUMATIC GRIEF

Childhood traumatic grief may occur following the death of someone important to the child when the child perceives the experience as traumatic. The death may have been sudden and unexpected (e.g., through violence or an accident) or anticipated (e.g., from illness or other causes) (NCTSN, 2014). The distinguishing feature of childhood traumatic grief is that the trauma symptoms interfere with the child's ability to go through the typical process of bereavement. The child experiences a combination of trauma and grief symptoms so severe that any thoughts or reminders—even happy ones—about the person who died can lead to frightening thoughts, images, and/or memories of how the person died.

The term *complex traumatic grief* is used to describe children's exposure to multiple traumatic events that are pervasive and include wide-ranging, long-term exposure (NCTSN, 2014). Complex traumatic grief can develop in children who lost a loved one under sudden, horrifying circumstances or under expected medical conditions if the child's perceptions of the death were that it was shocking, unexpected, or terrifying (Epstein, 2013). Although this term often refers to contexts involving interpersonal violence, past and persistent traumatic events in children's lives may compound their reactions to mass terrorism or violence. In particular, chronic abuse or neglect affects children's relationships with caregivers, who may be perceived as unavailable or undependable during crises and as unable to provide the social support and security necessary to foster resilience in children.

Traumatic factors can complicate bereavement (Rando, 2003). When the experience of grief is coupled with trauma, addressing trauma goals and needs, such as safety and affect regulation, must take priority over grief work. This is true for children who have experienced acute, violent loss, such as the Oklahoma City or Boston Marathon bombings, children of 9/11 victims, and survivors of community violence and school shootings/bombings, such as those at Columbine High School in Colorado or Sandy Hook in Connecticut or at the Boston marathon; there were varying degrees of trauma exposure within these events. In Sandy Hook, some children witnessed the deaths of their teachers and friends. Others were witnesses through sound and the experience of being in a school lockdown, followed by the evacuation to the firehouse and seeing fear and panic in their parents' faces. In contrast, children of 9/11 victims experienced the loss of safety in a different form; they lost a primary caregiver, and there was a sense of impending danger to the entire country. Images and televised replays of the towers collapsing reinforced a sense of danger and the experience that they were seeing their parents killed over and over again.

ART THERAPY, MASS TRAUMA, AND MASS VIOLENCE

Creative expression plays an important role in healing in the aftermath of a public tragedy (Bertman, 2003). Art helps a society to cope and provides comfort; it helps to resist and protest what has occurred; and it consoles and gives voice to the philosophical, political, and spiritual questions. Spontaneous public and private art making have helped start the recovery process for single incidents of mass violence such as 9/11, the Oklahoma City bombing, the Boston Marathon bombing, and the shootings at Columbine and Sandy Hook. Almost immediately after the 9/11 attacks a number of ad hoc altars, walls plastered with pictures and tokens of love and memory, firehouses, and an armory filled with gifts of children's artwork appeared around New York City. Ad hoc altars were also created in quick response to the Sandy Hook Elementary School shootings in 2012. Public ceremonies following these events addressed the need for healing, not only for the loved ones of the victims, but also for the collective soul of the society (Benke, 2003).

In terms of art therapy treatment models for mass terrorism and violence, there are relatively few studies to date that provide guidelines for art-based intervention. There is also no one art therapy theory used to address children's needs after human-inflicted disaster. Carr and

Vandiver (2003) underscore that semistructured activities and limiting art materials may be preferable when working with children in emergency shelters postdisaster. In trauma-informed practice, art-based approaches that support resiliency and strengths through increasing a sense of safety and connection are effective during large-scale crises (Malchiodi, 2012). Others report that an increasing number of pediatric disaster survivors are being treated with art therapy (Goodman, 2014; Hussain, 2010).

In general, art making is believed to be a way for children to distance themselves from the effects of mass disaster and to encourage adaptive coping skills and self-empowerment through creative expression. As described in other chapters of this book, art therapy helps children bridge thinking and feeling; channels energy in positive, pleasurable activities; and capitalizes on the self-soothing qualities of art materials and creative expression. Creating art after events involving mass terrorism, violence, or loss provides a way for children to make sense of their experiences, to express grief, and to become active participants in their own process of healing. In essence, art therapy offers a way for children to see themselves as survivors and eventually as "thrivers" (Malchiodi, 2012).

INTEGRATING ART THERAPY AND CURRENT BEST PRACTICES IN TRAUMA INTERVENTION

The following case examples illustrate how we use art therapy to address mass terrorism and violence with children, applying best practices in the fields of art therapy, trauma intervention, and bereavement therapy. Examples include early intervention and individual and group interventions provided to Sandy Hook Elementary School child survivors and to children who lost parents as a result of the events of 9/11.

Early Intervention Using Art Therapy with Sandy Hook Elementary School Students (Ellie Seibel-Nicol)

An acute posttraumatic reaction generally occurs in the first 5 weeks after a mass trauma; chronic posttraumatic stress and related disorders are diagnosed 2–3 months after a trauma. In the acute or "peritraumatic" phase, therapists assess for symptoms, provide psychoeducation, introduce coping strategies to reduce trauma-related symptoms, and monitor the status of symptoms (Marans & Epstein, 2013). During this phase almost any change in behavior can be viewed as a response to the trauma.

In the acute phase following a trauma, treatment focuses on reestablishing sensory safety and normalizing feelings to increase self-regulation. In response to the Sandy Hook Elementary School Shooting, an art therapy group was offered to address these needs. Many trauma specialists and protocols advise against group work when treating trauma survivors. The concern is that one group member may inadvertently cause an emotional response in another group member. The ability of the therapist to facilitate any group of traumatized individuals with a trauma-informed approach is very important. However, group work can be essential for survivors of mass violence because participants have the ability to identify with others' experiences and therefore not feel so isolated. Group members have a high degree of empathy for one another, can learn effective coping strategies from one another, and have the opportunity to share with others what is helpful to them. For many, being able to help others builds resilience and fosters growth.

In facilitating a group for child survivors of the Sandy Hook shooting, it was important to recognize the specific stimuli to which each child was exposed. For example, the public address system was on and everyone in the school heard screams and gunshots; some survivors believed a wild animal was in the building or thought they heard hammering sounds. Others were able to identify gunshot sounds; some individuals witnessed the massacre in its entirety.

The group began approximately 3 weeks after the shooting and continued on a weekly basis for about 3 months. Participants were presented with a very clear statement about why the group was created. The goals for treatment included creating a safe environment for the children to express and explore their feelings about their experiences while increasing a sense of control over, and tolerance for, those feelings. Some of the children wanted to talk about the shooting, the stories that they heard about it, and many of the misconceptions that had circulated throughout the community. I thanked them for their willingness to talk and asked them to wait because we had other group tasks to do before we could get into those stories.

Although these children were screened before entering this group, I needed to make sure that a child would not be affected by hearing another's story. I engaged the children in creating group rules; these included no hitting, no teasing, and mutual respect. The last rule concerned talking about the shooting. This rule established that group members would never be forced to talk about the incident if they did not want to, and if hearing another group member talk about the incident became too upsetting, children could use a key word to interrupt the discussion. Each member then came up with a key word, and the group voted on one. These simple steps and directives established the purpose of the group and rules for safety; additionally, all participants were empowered to control the pace of the session and to self-regulate.

I set up several sensory-oriented rituals for the beginning and ending of each group. For instance, to begin subsequent groups each child was given a piece of modeling clay. The instruction was to hold it behind their backs and model it into something without looking at it. We then passed it to the person on the right without looking at the piece. Each group member then guessed what had been passed to him or her. The soft and smooth texture of the modeling clay (in this case, Model Magic) is soothing to touch, and its flexibility serves as an effective stress reliever. It functioned as a mindful activity that grounded the group in a common task, promoted calm, and set the stage to get into the deeper group work.

A couple of the children reported that they liked the group because they were not talking about the shooting in school and they did not want to talk about it at home. This particular group provided a safe place to process their experiences and express their thoughts and feelings about the events, and then relinquish them until the next group. The group essentially became a sacred holding space; the children felt like it was their own special "private club."

Art Therapy Group Intervention with Sandy Hook Elementary School Students (Mary Pellicci Hamilton)

The Rainbow Fish Project

When working with groups of children exposed to trauma, it is important to expand beyond cookie-cutter methods and blanket directives such as "Draw a safe place." Interventions should be designed to facilitate and provide safety and security through symbolic, sensory, and metaphorical content. In most cases, traumatized children may not have the capacity to conceptualize any physical surrounding as safe. Therapists must help child clients identify sensory elements that increase children's secure feelings and allow them to feel the safest possible. This process helps normalize feelings of vulnerability and fear by encouraging empowerment.

The Rainbow Fish Project included a reading program and creative arts therapy session for children of Newtown, ages 4–7 years. Even though in the early aftermath of the tragedy, many families avoided the bombardment of outside reminders by remaining in their homes, this program was well attended, with preregistration of 26 families and later walk-ins. The program began with several storytelling sessions, including a reading of *The Rainbow Fish* (Pfister, 1992) by co-organizer Amber Kemp-Gerstel, PhD.

The Rainbow Fish is a child's tale centered around the discovery of magnificent support and friendship through giving. The tale was chosen for this specialized program and adapted for its creative metaphorical and symbolic content, so appropriate during the early phase of trauma exposure. A therapeutic art activity based on the tale followed the reading. The children were directed to create their own rainbow fish by applying layers of metallic scales onto a paper template. Since this group was held 3 weeks after the shooting, it was focused on communicating protection and containment. Instead of bringing up the traumatic events, children were invited to use creative metaphor and group discussion centered around the protective function of fish scales. One participant created a flounder fish with a decoy eye as a defense mechanism against predators (see Figure 5.1). He explained that the flounder fish avoids predators by hiding at the bottom of the sea; it also possesses inherent decoy and survival qualities. The art-making process for most children consisted of creating a heavy overlay of appliqué scales made from metallic cutouts. Scales adorned not only the main body of the fish, but were stuck to fins and tails like weighted armor. Other children gravitated toward colored magic markers or a combination of both marker and appliqué cutouts.

As a metaphorical crossover from the storyline, participants were encouraged to give one of their radiant fish scales to a fellow participant to increase a sense of social support among group members and as a gesture representing shared strength and community. To convey personal control, the option was then given to participants to attach their fish to an ocean wall mural, which many thoughtfully did. Much care and thought were involved with choosing the personal location and placement of the fish onto the mural. Some were grouped together in circular schools, whereas others floated atop as if to survey the environment. Interestingly, each fish was placed in the same swimming pattern (left

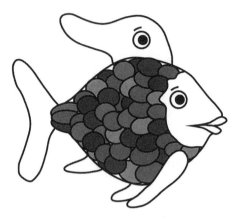

FIGURE 5.1. It was essential for this 7-year-old male participant to incorporate safety mechanisms in his rainbow fish by adding a decoy eye. Predators were avoided by "hiding at the bottom of the sea." Fish image reprinted with permission from Marcus Pfister.

to right), perhaps as an unconscious collective understanding of community resilience and hope.

At session end, some children chose to allow their fish to remain on the group mural, whereas others opted to take their artwork home. Giving children the option to leave their artwork in the therapist's safekeeping is an important practice intervention because it underscores the fact that an extension of them—through their artwork—is being held in the therapist's protective space. Many times, child trauma survivors prefer to leave their art creations in the therapy office as a place of reassurance and containment, which they trust. This choice to leave the artwork most often occurs when the artwork provokes feelings of vulnerability associated with the traumatic event, which the child unconsciously wants the transference relationship to hold, manage, and regulate. During therapeutic growth periods, clients may wish to take ownership of their art piece and transition it to their home living space. This part of the healing process can be guided and interpreted to the client as a measure of posttraumatic recovery.

The art therapy directives in the Rainbow Fish Project communicated safety and protection to the children of Newtown by allowing them to work with their parents and siblings. The session supported a secure physical environment, personal expression, and reinforced community and parent involvement.

Kids Share Newtown

A group of Sandy Hook Elementary School children participated in a 2-week creative writing and art therapy program through Kids Share Workshops (2013). Creative and therapeutic writing themes were developed for a bookmaking workshop to reinforce and communicate safety, self-expression, and community. Multilayered and symbolic themes included time-travel superheroes, an island treasure hunt, and a royal kingdom to provide an increased sense of safety, empowerment, triumph, and discovery. The Sandy Hook students explored their fears, wishes, and conflicts through the use of these metaphors and symbolic themes. Through the creation of paper art illustration, the children experienced their own self-transformation within the art-making process. The workshop provided the children with a secure and structured environment and creative experiences to help them give artistic and written expression to their feelings 4 months after the Sandy Hook event.

A group of first and second graders from Sandy Hook Elementary School created "The Kingdom of Kindness" (Figure 5.2). Some of these children had witnessed the full aftermath of the shooting as they were escorted out of their school by first responders. One child suffered vicarious traumatization through her siblings' and mother's direct exposure and her own exposure to sounds and smells. The children's writing and artwork revealed symbolic imagery that included a number of themes: power (king/queen/money/gold/chocolate coins); protective boundaries (doorbell/castle surrounded by flowers/fish/teachers); security and control over their environment (remote castles/moat with alligators/shields) (Figure 5.3); escape through rich, enchanted fantasy (talking animals/pink-winged lion/unicorns/royal bunnies/magical garden); absence of death (special medicine/everyone lives forever); and happiness (canary/thrones of rainbows and sunshine/sparkles/National Happy Day). This is an excerpt from the writing of one of the Sandy Hook Elementary School students who was exposed to the aftermath of the shooting: "The Kingdom of Kindness is the best place to live because everyone is happy and safe! This is because of our protective shield. The shield keeps all bad things out of the kingdom. In the Kingdom of Kindness, everyone drinks a special medicine that keeps them from getting old. Everyone lives forever in the Kingdom of Kindness. In other words, everyone lives happily ever after."

During a group activity to develop writing ideas, the children picked a hidden object from a box of various concealed objects. A common

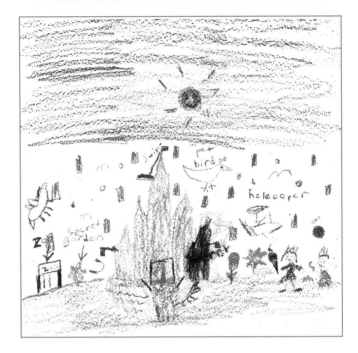

FIGURE 5.2. In the Kingdom of Kindness, created by first and second graders at Sandy Hook Elementary School, several themes emerged, including power and control, safety and security, everlasting life, enchanted fantasy, and blissful happiness.

chalkboard eraser was selected. As discussion unfolded, fears and wishes of undoing emerged to "erase scary and bad memories." Together the group members agreed that they "would erase the bad man. Whenever enemies come to our kingdom, we can erase them." The children creatively utilized a randomly selected object to gain empowerment and victory over their fears and vulnerabilities.

Art Therapy Intervention and Trauma-Focused Cognitive-Behavioral Therapy with Sandy Hook Elementary School Students (Ellie Seibel-Nicol)

Two days *before* the Sandy Hook Elementary School shooting, a mother brought two of her three sons in for treatment to work with me. The oldest son had a long history of emotional disturbance and therapeutic intervention. The youngest was beginning to display behaviors that

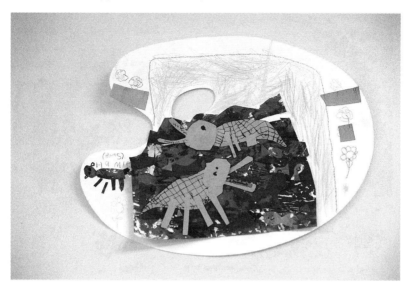

FIGURE 5.3. Multiple layers of protection were applied to guard the castle, including giant-sized alligators and fish surrounding the castle moat.

concerned the mother. She inquired about a social skills group for her youngest son, Owen, who was in first grade at Sandy Hook Elementary School.

On the day of the shooting, Owen was in a classroom where half of the children and his teacher were shot and killed. The gun was pointed at Owen's head when it jammed. Another child yelled "Run!" and Owen ran along with the other children, out of the classroom, past the dead principal, and out the front door. They ran down the street until another mother, who was coming to school for gingerbread-making day, stopped them, asked what had happened, called the police, and drove them to the police station.

Two hours later, Owen's mother was reunited with him at the police station and then she called to schedule a session; to this day she still doesn't remember making that call. Owen's initial drawings, made during this session, were impulsively drawn and chaotic in appearance. Many of his drawings were riddled with dot marks (Figure 5.4). He talked about the bad man that came to his school and killed his teacher, his principal, his friends, and most importantly, his girlfriend. He drew the broken glass from the front entry of the school and a gingerbread man strewn with dots that looked like bullet holes.

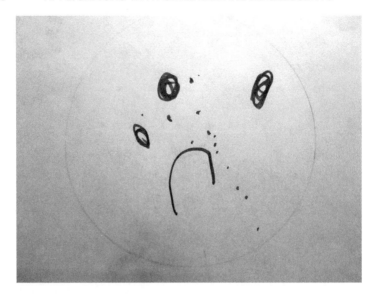

FIGURE 5.4. One of Owen's pictures, titled "Gingerbread Man," was riddled with dots.

Mom described Owen as a silly, happy, mischievous, and occasionally demanding young boy prior to the shooting. He ate well and could play alone. After the shooting, she reported that he became irritable and increasingly demanding at times, had a decreased appetite, needed to sleep with her or his (middle) brother, and was reactive to loud bangs and slamming doors. He stiffened up when asked about the day of the shooting, but he talked about the event constantly and in a graphic way. These symptoms continued for many months.

After Owen attended the first art therapy group, it was determined that group was not an appropriate option for him; his behavior might also adversely affect others in the group. He began individual art therapy on a weekly basis. Owen remained in a hyperaroused state during his art and play, where he reenacted the traumatic day of the shooting. One day, when Owen was using a box of magic markers, he repeatedly stood up two markers and then used another marker to knock them down. He said that the standing markers were the bad guy's legs and by knocking them down, he was knocking down the bad guy. As a child in the classroom the day of the shooting, the "bad guy's legs" were what he saw at eye level. Owen was playing out rescue fantasies, perhaps also driven by survivor guilt. When he was told it was getting close to the time to end the session, Owen picked up the markers and said, as he put them back in the box, "I'm putting the bad guy in jail now." Owen continued to reenact the day of the shooting through drawings and modeling clay, including images of destruction and chaos.

Trauma-focused cognitive-behavioral therapy (TF-CBT; Cohen, Mannarino, & Deblinger, 2012) was implemented in conjunction with art therapy to increase the structure of the sessions. TF-CBT is a protocol that integrates trauma-sensitive interventions with cognitive-behavioral strategies. It is used with children who have been abused, have witnessed something traumatic, or have been involved in mass traumas such as school shootings. TF-CBT integrates attachment theory, developmental neurobiology, family therapy, empowerment therapy, and humanistic therapy (Epstein, 2013). Its goals include reducing children's negative emotional and behavioral responses to trauma, correcting cognitive distortions related to the abuse or trauma, and providing caregivers with support and the skills to respond optimally to children.

The initial phases of psychoeducation, relaxation training, and affect regulation are all about skill development and gradual exposure. Addressing the specific trauma on a more personal level comes later. During the affect regulation phase, Owen learned how to identify, tolerate, modulate, and integrate his feelings.

One way in which Owen learned how to identify his feelings was through a game in which he was given index-card-size pieces of paper and markers and asked to identify as many feelings as he could by drawing a face on each piece of paper expressing that feeling. He was then asked to write the matching word under the face. Owen and I spread out the drawings on a table. The game is to tell a true story, and every time the storyteller comes to a feeling that was experienced during the story a "feelings chip" (poker chip) is placed on that paper. To convey the strength of that feeling, more than one chip can be placed at a time. The therapist goes first to show the child how the game is played. If needed, the therapist can tell a true story about the child. The child then tells a true story, using the chips to identify and rate each feeling. This story is not necessarily the trauma story. However, after playing this game, children like Owen are able to identify how a child might feel if he or she had experienced a trauma like the one he did, how strongly the child might feel it, and how the child could manage or regulate that feeling. This is part of the gradual exposure component of TF-CBT.

Sally was also a Sandy Hook Elementary School student who was in first grade the day of the shooting. She heard the gunshots, and the sound made her think of bombs. TF-CBT and art therapy were implemented individually. Sally lost many of her Daisy troop friends in the shooting and a boy who was a close friend; she was likely to experience complex traumatic grief. After she completed the first few modules of psychoeducation, relaxation training, and affect regulation, Sally started bringing in photographs of a family dog that had died a year or so before the shooting. She asked if she could draw pictures of him (Figure 5.5). Sally's grief related to the shooting was being displaced. It was safer for her to talk about and remember her dog than it was to grieve her friends. Understandably, she was not ready to grieve her friends because thoughts of them were still arousing trauma responses.

With the psychoeducation and the relaxation skills in place, Sally drew a picture showing how she felt the day of the shooting (Figure 5.6). In this picture she is screaming, her heart is beating fast, and she has a tummy ache; there a picture of her dog is in her head and she has lines drawn in her arms and legs that she described as her stiff bones. With reminders of how to use soothing activities such as art and relaxation techniques, Sally became more able to tolerate and manage these

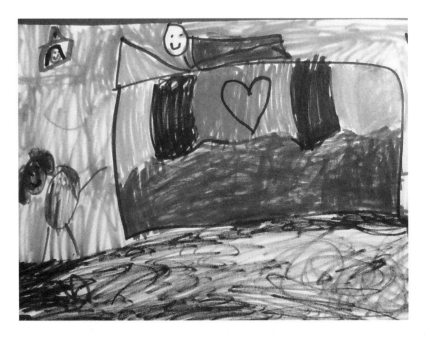

FIGURE 5.5. Sally drew herself safe and smiling in her bed, high above ground level, with her dog happily standing beside her, yet out of reach.

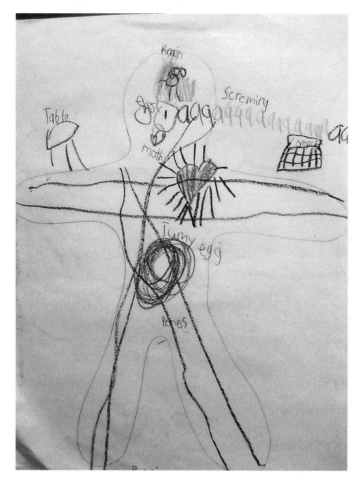

FIGURE 5.6. Sally's depiction of what she felt in her body on 12/14.

extreme feelings. By the time complex traumatic grief was addressed, Sally was able to draw a picture of a close friend she had lost in the shooting (Figure 5.7).

Traumatic Grief Work with Bereaved Children after the 9/11 Attacks (Laura Loumeau-May)

Although families of 9/11 victims did not experience trauma directly, the vicarious experience of trauma was intensified by vivid and constant media coverage of a horrifying event. The knowing and not-knowing of

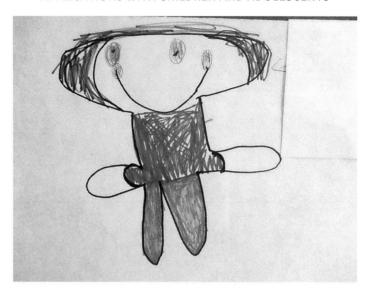

FIGURE 5.7. Sally's picture of the close friend she lost on 12/14.

what their loved ones had suffered was reinforced by the absence of (or partial) human remains and contributed to their imagination of the event. At the same time, the nation responded to its own trauma with hypervigilance, which heightened the sense of traumatization for grieving families of the victims.

Through the Journeys Program of Valley Home Care in Paramus, New Jersey, I worked with children, over the course of 4 years, from most of the 31 9/11 bereaved families served by this agency. Included in the services offered were community workshops, family memorial events on the first two anniversaries, individual art therapy, and ongoing age-appropriate groups. Focus shifted from goals related to trauma during the initial phases of treatment to the processing of grief.

Initial Goals: Coming to Terms with the Trauma

Children who entered the art therapy program in the first months following the terrorist attacks displayed a need to release and share fearful images combined with a need to defend against these overwhelming thoughts. During the first phase of treatment psychological stability and structure were provided to increase opportunities for safety and mastery in art expression. We created an open, supportive atmosphere that was receptive to catharsis while monitoring children's tolerance for emerging affect. Kalmanowitz and Lloyd (2005) discuss the importance of remembering and forgetting in the amelioration of trauma. Remembering and being able to speak about the traumatic experience is validating and healing, but remembering too much too soon can also overwhelm the mind. Therefore, caution must be practiced. Even for a skilled therapist, it is not always possible to modulate when and how memories emerge. It is important, therefore, when guiding expression, to respect defenses and recognize the vulnerability of clients before encouraging them to narrate too soon. Thoughtfully selected art materials, as well as directives, can simultaneously provide the structure to contain and the stimulation to express.

Once a safe "holding environment" was established, trauma-related goals (Rando, 1996) included (1) teaching children ways to self-soothe and regulate, (2) helping them to understand and express emotions, (3) identifying and developing healthy defenses, (4) achieving mastery to counteract helplessness, (5) recalling and narrating trauma witnessed or imagined, and (6) managing anxiety related to memory or present fears. Techniques such as guided imagery and music and the creation of safety boxes (Cohen, Barnes, & Rankin, 1995) provided containment and comfort. Painting, clay work, multimedia collage, and scratchboard released energy for the expression of more difficult emotions such as anger. The use of storyboards, puppetry, and sandplay encouraged literal and symbolic narratives.

Personally created stories afforded the children some control; many provided symbolic versions of the trauma. In her storyboard, one 10-year-old girl created the tale of a "little blue man" who built his house on the shore (Loumeau-May, 2008). In the story, his house was swept out to sea by a gigantic tidal wave and destroyed. Two years later, alone on an island, the little blue man, situated between two palm trees, was still yelling "Help!" as loud as he could. The blue in this story may be a verbal metaphor for sadness, death as in lack of oxygen, or the process of vaporizing into air. The tale told was of an isolated person overwhelmed by a catastrophic event. The tidal wave may have symbolized the suddenness of the attack that killed her father as well as the experience of being overcome by a deluge of tears. The "home" may have represented both a building and her home life as she had known it prior to the attacks. The choice of 2 years may have represented both the towers and the anticipated duration of grief. Through the rich metaphor of her story, this child was able to discuss her psychic process without direct confrontation.

Gradually introduced, creative approaches were used to help children and teens release blocked emotions. One multimedia experience utilized Wallace's (1990) tissue paper collage technique in conjunction with listening to New Age music and the reading of Pablo Neruda's poem "Loneliness" (1970). Printed phrases from the poem were provided to be included in the collage. The goal of this directive was to use the aggressive tearing of the tissue paper, augmented by discordant music and Neruda's lament to tap into and provide release for emotions that were still guarded, apprehensive, and superficial. Ambiguous music intermingled with the soothing process of brushing glue over the tissue paper and seeing the brilliance of the emerging colors, provided an opportunity for both the expression of pain and the containment of it. A collage created by "Bob" (Figure 5.8), intended to depict fire trucks rushing to the scene of the attack, is characterized by the fragmentation of apparently exploding objects. Bob glued many of the poetry phrases onto his collage, indicating his shock and confusion: "on that day," "so

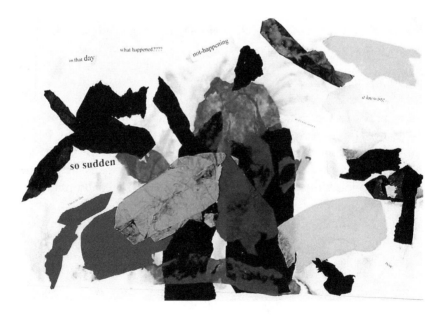

FIGURE 5.8. A multimedia approach, combining tissue paper collage with New Age music and poetry, helped Bob release blocked feelings.

sudden," "not happening," "not knowing," and "I have no idea." The effect of the "bleeding" tissue paper colors vividly conveys yellow-orange flames emanating from a burning building. The collage itself is a visual catharsis of shock, pain, destruction, and confusion.

Periodically, over the course of treatment, metaphorical directives such as "The Road of Grief" or "Before and After" drawings were offered to measure change, ascertain how each child perceived the event, and to see how their coping skills had improved. Toward the end of June 2002, children were encouraged to draw "Before and After" images that reflected what they remembered as the most difficult part of 9/11 itself and what was the most difficult thing now. Several drew the familiar image of the attack itself as the memory of the event and changes in the family as their current challenge (Figure 5.9). One 8-year-old girl drew herself in her classroom on September 11, when her teacher informed the class about the attacks, thinking of her father. On the other half of

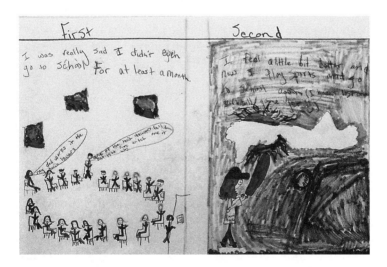

FIGURE 5.9. An 8-year-old girl was unaware that the cloud shape she drew to emphasize her successful hit in a softball game resembled a plane. Similarly to Owen's drawings, where the imagery of bullet holes unconsciously appeared in his pictures, images of planes and structures being penetrated or severed persisted in the artwork of children affected by 9/11. This image illustrates both resiliency through content (portrayed herself as active and empowered) and formal elements (developmentally more mature and larger depiction of human figure in second image as well as fuller use of space and color) and the lingering effects of traumatic memory.

the paper, she drew a picture of herself playing softball 9 months later, saying her father would be proud of how well she was doing now. In the drawing, a large cloud superimposed against an explosion-like burst where the bat has made contact with the ball resembles an enormous plane silhouetted against the blue sky. This drawing simultaneously reflects her coping skills and the lingering traumatic memory, which she was not yet ready to deal with directly. Similar images of penetration or rupture reminiscent of the attack appeared in many children's artwork throughout their time in the program.

Bereavement Goals: Experiencing the Reality of Death

One of the characteristics of early grief in response to trauma is numbness, a feeling that the loss is only a terrible dream. When that passes, the reality of the loss can be devastating. In the second year following the attacks, the children slowly began to deal more directly with the traumatic aspects of their parents' deaths. The younger children were just becoming fully cognizant of what had actually happened. Many began to explore specific questions about the attack and death. The children and teens in the program wanted to hold on to positive memories to ward off the frightful ones. However, that was becoming harder to do. Art therapy interventions concentrated on examining changes, providing continued structured review of the deaths, fuller acceptance of uncomfortable emotions, memory work, and life review.

Following a warm-up technique of looking at, touching, and examining nature objects such as driftwood, shark teeth, bone, amber, and petrified wood, as a lead-in to a discussion about the life cycle, a lively interchange stopped short when one child, remembering the movie *Jurassic Park* (Kennedy & Molen, 1993), excitedly proclaimed that the amber might have some DNA in it. This triggered a memory for another child, "Anna," whose mother had died in the towers. She told the group that her father had to take her mother's hairbrush into Manhattan "to give her mother's DNA." Rescue workers had later found a part of her mother. The group started to compare notes on whose parents had been found and whose had not been. They wanted to know why there had only been "parts" found. The group started to share what they remembered: the planes, the fire, the collapse, and how everyone was trapped inside.

The children, who had avoided the topic up until now, were interrupting each other to tell what they knew and what they thought.

Suddenly they needed a way to share the awful facts they had heard and to find out if the others harbored similar scary thoughts and unpleasant memories. Each child now filled in the blanks of their knowledge with imagination. In the drawings they later produced, they replayed the impact of the terrorist attack—not merely what they may have seen on television, but what they imagined their parents may have experienced during the attacks. They all knew what had happened to the towers, but no one could know what had happened to each of their parents. They wondered if their parents had jumped. They wondered how their parents had died or what they had been thinking and feeling at the end. Offered art materials, they were encouraged to either draw what they thought happened or something that would make them feel good, or both. All drew the outlines of towers; inside several showed staircases with flames rising up through the center of the building and tiny stick figures of people trapped inside. All of the children said they had thought about these images before, but tried not to; they did not like talking about it at home because it was too scary and it upset their remaining parent. Steele (2003) suggests that adults are so fearful that their children will be overwhelmed by trauma that they encourage them to avoid thinking about it.

Traumatized children need to be allowed to tell their story when they are ready and to have their internal experiences witnessed. It took over a year for these girls, who had been 6–8 at the time of the attacks, to externalize their images and have the courage to ask unanswerable questions. In addition to facing the trauma, this group had started to tackle two important aspects of bereavement: their cognitive under-standing of death and empathy for the plight of their parents.

Many children of the victims revealed that the defining moment for them of the loss was not the attack itself, but the arrival at their homes of policemen to inform them that the body of their father or mother had been identified (Freeman, 2005). For example, the shock that Bob had so vividly portrayed in a collage during the first year was contrasted by the loneliness he depicted 2 years later in a drawing about when he acknowledged the death. Choosing black paper and oil pastels, this boy drew himself sitting alone on the edge of his bed in his room. In the picture, the large bed, onto which he is bracing his arms, makes him look small. The emptiness of the room is broken only by the two open windows behind him, a calendar on the wall, and the light fixture on the ceiling. He described looking out his window and seeing the police car pull up to his house as the officers arrived, but remaining in his room because he knew why they were there. Like others whose loved ones' bodies had been found, Bob admitted that up until the point when the police came, he held out hope that maybe his father was trapped and surviving on water and food found in the rubble. It was not until he saw the police car that he admitted to himself that his father was dead. The reality of the loss swept over him as he sat alone in his room; he did not need to hear the words.

People who have experienced trauma or bereavement are prone to sleep disturbances. Another youth had a dream in which he and his father were in one of the towers as it was attacked (Figure 5.10). Both managed to get out safely, but his father went back in to save someone, as he had actually done in a previous 1993 terrorist attack on the World Trade Center. "Donald" was safe outside as the building collapsed with his father inside. Donald told the story of his dream, which he later painted, with much hesitation and difficulty. In his

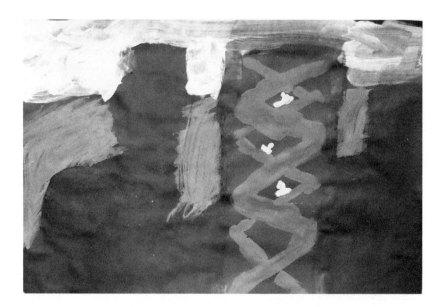

FIGURE 5.10. Many children and adolescents created images of what they imagined their parents experienced being trapped inside the towers. In this painting, based on a dream in which he replayed and tried to change the ending unsuccessfully, Donald re-created the horror of his father's death. Two years after the 9/11 attacks, through externalizing the frightening image and processing his dream, Donald was able to emotionally face the trauma. This enabled him to subsequently engage more deeply in his grief work.

painting, the black skyline is silhouetted against a purple sky. A fiery red, crisscrossing stairwell dominates the interior of one tower. On the way down the burning stairs are three small yellow figures, which look like flickering flames against the red and black. The sky above is also fiery yellow. Donald had painted himself back in the building. He spoke of his father's bravery. He was reassured that it takes courage to enter a burning building, even in one's imagination; he had allowed himself to experience what he felt his father had. Out of love for his father, he had faced the imagined horror of being trapped inside the building. Not only "survivor's guilt" but also his longing to be united with his father took him back into that building. But even in his imagination, he could not change what had happened. He could not effect a rescue as his father had so many years earlier. The sense of helplessness, of not being able to change that reality, was palpable. Donald, as Bob, and the younger children discussing DNA, had faced the trauma of his father's death and had begun a deeper and more conscious exploration of his grief.

Final Goals: Preserving the Connection

By the end of the third year, many children were grieving less intensely and had come to identify themselves as members of an exclusive group who shared experiences that no one else could understand. They wanted to "normalize" their lives. Their perspectives were changing. Art directives at this point concentrated on revised world outlooks, review of the previous relationships with their deceased parents, and ways of memorializing and internalizing their parents.

In the spring of 2004, the first selection of controversial plans to replace the Twin Towers were being formulated and made public. Some children and teens were in favor of the plans; some opposed them. Anna said, "Our parents died there; it is sacred ground." This concept of sacred ground provided the theme for an appropriate project; they created and constructed their own memorial designs (Loumeau-May, 2008). A group quilt (Figure 5.11), onto which the children and therapists contributed panel designs, also offered a way to memorialize and look toward the future. Anna proudly depicted herself growing from a child to a teen to an adult.

The power of memory is important in processing both trauma and loss. In the bereavement process memory is a symbolic way to hold onto the deceased. It attests to the endurance of love and relationship; it is

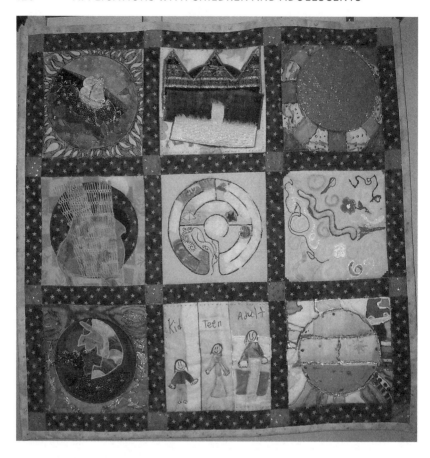

FIGURE 5.11. Memorial Quilt, organized by art therapy intern Tamara Bogdanova, in which Anna optimistically visualizes her growth from child to teen to adult.

not merely the physical presence of the loved one that constitutes the connection, but what the lost person has been to the bereaved and all that has transpired between them. Grief work is a dance between holding on and letting go. Native American wisdom reminds us: "A person is alive as long as someone can tell their story." Young children, because of their developmental stage, will forget much. One young child was poignantly aware of this: "I'm scared . . . because sometimes I think . . . when I grow up I won't remember him" (Payson, 2002). In the earliest stages of trauma, images of their parents' violent death interfered with children's ability to remember their parents as whole and healthy—as illustrated by an early collage Donald had created, using reflective metallic cardboard cut into a silhouette to depict a faceless image that he reported could be either himself or his father; he stated that for a while after the attacks, he could not recall how his father had looked just prior to his death (Loumeau-May, 2011). As children of the victims continued to process and work through the traumatic aspects of their grief, they were encouraged to use photographs of their parents to do portraits of them. Studying and reproducing images of their parents' faces as they painted them deepened an emotional presence with the work that both tolerated sorrow and reestablished joy.

Even when life and grief reviews indicated that the youth remaining in the program had reinvested and found new foci in their lives, letting go of active mourning as a way to maintain attachment to their parents provided a final challenge. Self-portraits in which they represented incorporated aspects of their parents helped reveal internalized strengths. Much of Donald's artwork prior to the depiction of his dream had been reminiscent and idealized. It took a brave leap for him to let go of his facade of strength and allow himself to feel the full pain and sorrow of separation, which he had finally done. It was necessary for him to fully experience the separation before he could reconnect with his father on a deeper level. Now he had processed both his trauma and his loss and was able to create a very different self–father portrait.

Donald's project was a combined self-portrait, inspired by a directive I based on a scene from *The Lion King* (McArthur & Schumacher, 1994), when Rafiki tells Simba to look into his own reflection to find his father, who "lives in" him. In order to represent how his father continued "to live in him," Donald divided his portrait in half. He drew his father's face on one side and his own on the other. He surrounded the portrait with a series of stripes symbolizing the various sports teams they both enjoyed (Freeman, 2005). Even as he had been struggling in adjusting to life without his father, Donald had also been noting many areas of identification with his father, which included his physical appearance as he grew older, his interests, and the development of similar academic strengths to his father, such as math. He began to realize, on a deeper level, that his father resided in him, not just by the memories he tried to preserve, not just by their same names and similar physiques, but on a deep level by the way they had connected, what he had learned from him, and who he was growing up to be. This growth occurred as a result of the solid foundation his father had taught him and the strength he had developed in coping with his father's death.

CONCLUSION

In discussing their work with traumatized families, Abu Sway, Nashashibi, Salah, and Shweiki (2005) say, "The power of the arts as a means of self-expression is that it brings out the deep-rooted pain in the self without posing a threat to it" (p. 159). The arts provide a safe transitional space that allows the child to experiment until attaining integrity and control. The use of art in treating trauma and grief has been recognized in work with children who have survived mass violence—directly in the Sandy Hook event and indirectly with children who lost parents in 9/11. The healing work involved the double challenge of helping children deal with both the trauma of the attacks and personal loss. The use of drawing and other art modalities actively engaged children in their own healing (Steele & Raider, 2001). Art therapy continually provided a safe vehicle through which full self-expression was possible.

The cases described in this chapter provide examples of how clinically focused art therapy promotes resilience and recovery in children affected by mass trauma and violence. Practitioners using this material as a resource must remember to evaluate the unique aspects of the particular trauma to which children are reacting and make adjustments according to specific needs. Additionally, sensitivity to a child's trauma history, clinical presentation, coping mechanisms, and sources of support is essential to meet the needs of the individual child. Establishing safety and instilling the inner strength to modify overwhelming emotions and memories produced by trauma is necessary before grief work can begin. Short-term trauma-related goals demonstrated in the clinical examples above also include self-regulation, metaphorical exploration of the trauma narrative, and attention to adaptive coping skills. Long-term bereavement goals helped children affected by 9/11 deal with recognizing and adjusting to external and internal life changes, evaluating self-growth, experiencing the fullness of grief, internalizing aspects of the parent, and creating memorials to them. Vital to grief and trauma work is the role of the therapist in witnessing and providing an open and supportive environment. Any therapist working with traumatized children must be fully present and able to tolerate their pain, and must work with them to help decrease their feelings of isolation, validate their experiences, and enhance a sense of courage and resilience.

Finally, the role of society in healing from these events must be honored and included in treatment. Meaning can be found in taking action; action in thought, choice, attitude, and behavior transforms tragedy into will and meaning and is empowering. We have witnessed this through acts of philanthropy, volunteerism, advocacy, dedications and memorials of parks and programs, marches, and legislative mediation. For example, in Manhattan, the 9/11 memorial features symbolic reflective pools that honor lost loved ones by their position in the footprints of the Twin Towers. The "Sandy Hook Promise" to "Choose Love" slogan, chosen early in the recovery process, demonstrates the intention of the Newtown community to lead purposeful and meaning-centered lives and the conscious choice to possess and empower thoughts and attitudes with "love, belief, and hope instead of anger" (Make the Sandy Hook Promise, 2012).

Through actions and memorials, individuals and groups can sublimate their suffering and find meaning and hope. According to Seligman, Reivich, Jaycox, and Gillham (1995), supporting a cause larger than oneself through philanthropic acts promotes positivity. The search to create meaning from suffering is seen repeatedly in society's response to mass violence such as the events discussed in this chapter.

REFERENCES

Abu Sway, R., Nashashibi, R., Salah, R., & Shweiki, R. (2005). Expressive arts therapy healing the traumatized: The Palestinian experience. In D. Kalmanowitz & B. Lloyd (Eds.), *Art therapy and political violence* (pp. 154–171). London: Routledge.

Allen, J. R., Tucker, P., & Pfefferbaum, B. (2006). Community outreach following a terrorist act: Violent death and the Oklahoma City experience. In E. K. Rynearson (Ed.), *Violent death, resilience and intervention beyond the crisis* (pp. 311–334). New York: Routledge/Taylor & Francis.

Benke, D. (2003). A healing ritual at Yankee Stadium. In M. Lattanzi-Licht & K. Doka (Eds.), *Living with grief: Coping with public tragedy* (pp. 191–201). Washington, DC: Hospice Foundation of America.

Bertman, S. (2003). Public tragedy and the arts. In M. Lattanzi-Licht & K. Doka (Eds.), *Living with grief: Coping with public tragedy* (pp. 203–217). Washington, DC: Hospice Foundation of America.

Carr, M., & Vandiver, T. (2003). Effects of instructional art projects on children's behavioral responses and creativity within an emergency shelter. *Art Therapy: Journal of the American Art Therapy Association, 20*(3), 157–162.

Cohen, B., Barnes, M., & Rankin, A. (1995). *Managing traumatic stress through art: Drawing from the center.* Baltimore: Sidran Press.

Cohen, J. A., Mannarino, A. P., & Deblinger, E. (2012). *Trauma-focused CBT for children and adolescents: Treatment applications.* New York: Guilford Press.

Doka, K. (2003). What makes a tragedy public? In M. Lattanzi-Licht & K. Doka (Eds.), *Living with grief: Coping with public tragedy* (pp. 3–13). Washington, DC: Hospice Foundation of America.

Epstein, C. (2013). *Child and parent trauma-focused cognitive-behavioral therapy.* New Haven, CT: Yale Childhood Violent Trauma Center, Yale Child Study Center, Yale University School of Medicine.

Freeman, V. (2005, October). Between trauma and transformation: The alchemy of art therapy. *Alternative Medicine,* pp. 43–48.

Goodman, R. F. (2014). Talking to kids about their art. Retrieved January 20, 2014, from *www.aboutourkids.org/articles/talking_kids_about_their_art.*

Hussain, S. (2010). Images of healing and learning: Art therapy for children who have survived disaster. *American Medical Association Journal, 12*(9), 750–753.

Kalmanowitz, D., & Lloyd, B. (2005). Art therapy and political violence. In D. Kalmanowitz & B. Lloyd (Eds.), *Art therapy and political violence* (pp. 14–34). London: Routledge.

Kennedy, K., & Molen, G. (Producers), Crichton, M. (Writer), & Spielberg, S. (Director). (1993). *Jurassic Park* [Motion picture]. Universal City, CA: Universal Pictures.

Kids Share Workshops. (2013). BerylMartin, IN: Kids Share Workshops and Publishing.

Loumeau-May, L. V. (2008). Grieving in the public eye: Art therapy with children who lost parents in the World Trade Center attacks. In C. A. Malchiodi (Ed.), *Creative interventions with traumatized children* (pp. 81–111). New York: Guilford Press.

Loumeau-May, L. V. (2011). Art therapy with traumatically bereaved children. In S. Ringel & J. Brandell (Eds.), *Trauma: Contemporary directions in theory, practice and research* (pp. 98–129). Thousand Oaks, CA: Sage.

Make the Sandy Hook Promise. (2012, December). Sandy Hook Promise. Retrieved May 29, 2014, from *www2.sandyhookpromise.org/the_promise.*

Marans, S., & Epstein, C. (2013). *Trauma-focused symptom screening and assessment and early trauma-focused mental health intervention strategies.* New Haven, CT: Yale University School of Medicine.

McArthur, S., & Schumacher, T. (Executive Producers), Mecchi, I., Roberts, J., & Woolverton, L. (Writers), & Allers, R., & Minkoff, R. (Directors). (1994). *The lion king* [Motion picture]. Burbank, CA: Walt Disney Studios.

McGeehan, I. (2005). Creativity from chaos: An art therapist's account of art work produced in the aftermath of a bombing in her community, Omagh, Northern Ireland. In D. Kalmanowitz & B. Lloyd (Eds.), *Art therapy and political violence* (pp. 126–141). London: Routledge.

National Child Traumatic Stress Network. (2014). Types of traumatic stress. Retrieved on January 4, 2014, from *www.nctsn.org/trauma-types*.

Neruda, P. (1970). *Selected poems*. New York: Delta.

Payson, J. (Executive Producer). (2002, March 7). *Primetime Thursday: Tender hearts—art helps children of 9/11 express emotions and heal* [Television broadcast]. New York: American Broadcasting System. In J. Rubin (2004), *Art therapy has many faces* [DVD]. Pittsburgh, PA: Expressive Media.

Pfister, M. (1992). *The rainbow fish*. New York: North–South Books.

Rando, T. (1996). Complications in mourning traumatic death. In K. Doka (Ed.), *Living with grief after sudden loss* (pp. 139–159). Washington, DC: Hospice Foundation of America.

Rando, T. (2003). Public tragedy and complicated mourning. In M. Lattanzi-Licht & K. Doka (Eds.), *Living with grief: Coping with public tragedy* (pp. 263–274). Washington, DC: Hospice Foundation of America.

Rathkey, J. (2004). *What children need when they grieve*. New York: Three Rivers Press.

Seligman, M. E. P., Reivich, K., Jaycox, L., & Gillham, J. (1995). *The optimistic child*. Boston: Houghton Mifflin.

Silver, R. C., Holman, E. A., Andersen, J. P., Poulin, M., McIntosh, D. N., & Gil-Rivas, V. (2013). Mental- and physical-health effects of acute exposure to media images of the September 11, 2001, attacks and the Iraq war. *Psychological Science, 24*(9) 1623–1634.

Steele, W. (2003). Using drawing in short-term trauma resolution. In C. A. Malchiodi (Ed.), *Handbook of art therapy* (pp. 139–151). New York: Guilford Press.

Steele, W., & Raider, M. (2001). *Structured sensory intervention for traumatized children, adolescents and parents: Strategies to alleviate trauma*. Lewiston, NY: Edward Mellen Press.

Wallace, E. (1990). *A queen's quest: Pilgrimage for individuation*. Santa Fe, NM: Moon Bear Press.

CHAPTER 6

Treating Dissociation in Traumatized Children with Body Maps

Bart Santen

Dissociation is an adaptive coping reaction that is used by people of all ages to manage overwhelming distress. Dissociation occurs when the individual compartmentalizes traumatic events in order to keep from feeling psychological and/or physical pain. Children who are dissociative may experience trance states in which they have lapses in attention; they may forget parts of their lives or what was happening minutes before; or they may stare blankly, seemingly inattentive. They may have dramatic changes in mood or personality or insist on being called by another name. It is believed that these reactions reflect these children's capacity to separate parts of themselves, also known as *fragments* or *fragmentation*. Children who have episodes of problematic dissociation may display reactions that can be attributed to other emotional or cognitive problems.

Children who have experienced traumatic events are often depressed or have suicidal ideations (Hornstein, 1998), and they may dissociate to escape their unbearable experiences. Since hurt caused by trauma captures their feeling process, they survive through living in a trance. Their free-floating anxiety warns us to keep our "fingers away from what the fear is hiding!" (O. Fenichel, as cited in Rohde-Dachser, 1979, p. 126), but underneath we can often sense their cry for help. The prize of encapsulation may be too high. As Emily, a 16-year-old girl, verbalized in her recovery (Santen, 2014), "You suppress the experience, and this transforms into a voice, to a person in your head. In that way you don't have to deal with it directly, but in the end you have to after all, because that voice directs you towards insanity and destruction" (p. 79).

Dissociated children need a helping hand when they try to leave the defensive cage that they have created. But vehicles for escape may be hard to find because of fierce inner resistance. When explicit (narrative) memory is locked inside, interventions that operate at a lower level of consciousness are needed to enable these children to reconnect.

This chapter introduces *experiential body mapping* (Santen, 2007, 2014), a focusing-oriented technique (Gendlin, 1996, 2003) developed to enable children to get closer to their well-guarded hurt at a level that they can bear and that protects them against self-destruction. This approach helps these children to visualize their subconscious survival strategy after a traumatic experience, by picturing the inner landscape that emerged as a way to cope. Doing so can help them reconnect with "felt experience" as a starting point for processing trauma.

I also introduce characteristics of structural dissociation, followed by an introduction to experiential body mapping, which is illustrated by a case example of a boy who had walled off his "bodily knowledge" about his painful history with physical violence. The case demonstrates how body mapping helped him recall the memory and integrate the trauma.

CHARACTERISTICS OF STRUCTURAL DISSOCIATION

The notion of *structural dissociation* is a currently accepted theory of dissociation. The central concept underscores that parts of the personality are not integrated in childhood due to excessive exposure to traumatic events. Children who live in such dissociative states need a special therapeutic strategy.

In focusing-oriented child psychotherapy (Santen, 1993, 1999) it is important to listen unconditionally and provide children with a safe and steady environment. These conditions give them the opportunity to engage in playing and/or in focusing-oriented art therapy (Rappaport, 2009, 2010) to facilitate their focusing ability (also see Rappaport, Chapter 14, this volume, for more information on focusing-oriented art therapy). Children who are experiencing structural dissociation, however, may be consumed by fear so pervasively that they need additional intervention techniques. A "slumber fear" is generated to prevent access to traumatic memories and emotions (Santen, 2014). This response system is continuously active and, as a result, these children have no peace. Their need-to-reconnect clashes with their need-to-keep-deleted in a predominantly subconscious struggle that causes arrest. Many of these children talk about a "something" inside that "explodes, expands, and gets worse and starts all over again." That "something" knocks on the door, but seems too hurtful to be addressed. According to Ogden, Minton, and Pain (2006), "An uncontrollable cascade of strong emotions and physical sensations, triggered by reminders of the trauma, replays endlessly in the body" (p. xviii).

Children who generally score high on the Child Dissociative Checklist (Putnam, 1997) are stuck in what is referred to as *inner fragmentation* (van der Hart, Nijenhuis, & Steele, 2006). They have created a hierarchy of alters—self-fragments that hold traumatic memories and emotions. These "internal voices tend to be menacing toward the child or others" (Wieland, 2011, p. 8). Many of these children report that they perceive their primary alter as a disturbing "inner voice" that puts them down with degrading comments and frequently advocates suicide. During therapy sessions, this voice can block the child's memory of what has been achieved and express itself in distracting ways.

Who is the one who distracts? Who is it that misleads? "To debate the reality or unreality of alters, voices, or parts of the mind is to miss the point—that this metaphor resonates powerfully with how these children feel about themselves" (Waters & Silberg, 1998, p. 136). The dissociated child is "one, but also two" (Santen, 2014, p. 88). The child and the primary alter perceive themselves as united, but also split in a collusion that reflects the child's deeply hidden ambivalence about a freeze response versus disclosure. Elsewhere (Santen, 1993) I have described how 13-year-old Rachel painted herself as such a desperate, colluded pair:

> Two identical females . . . were tied together. Their backs were sticking in a pie. Handcuffs chained them to themselves as well as to each other. They were facing us without a face to look. We could look straight into their heads. Their thoughts merged continuously. . . . Rachel explained that they hated each other. "They both don't know what to do. Sometimes there is some space between them, but they are absolutely stuck." (p. 51)

When Emily (described in the beginning of this chapter) allowed me to consult her primary alter, named Alice, this self-fragment verbalized the confusing deadlock from her own point of view. I put together what she told me in bits and pieces:

> "I told Emily that I didn't want to talk. At first instance, she says that I must talk anyway. And then she says that I betray her by telling more about the secret. Then it becomes a mess. If you ask Emily what the secret is she doesn't know, but in spite of that she feels that it cannot be told. She stops it, so that I am present, but the part in me that knows the secret isn't. It is as if she has taken my position now. We change positions. When she talks I keep the secret, and now that I talk she suddenly keeps it. So then I say something, or she says something, and in the end you hardly know who said it anyway, because in fact you are one, but also two. We really don't know how this can be solved. Defending something is easier than letting go." (Santen, 2014, p. 88)

Verbal therapy is not helpful in such a state of alienation. Other interventions are needed to give these children the chance to redefine the relationship between their "person underneath" and their defensive creations.

BODY OUTLINE DRAWING, BODY DIAGRAMMING, AND BODY MAPPING

Creative interventions that foster externalization of traumatic material have potential to help the traumatized child (Malchiodi, 2008). If successful, such interventions establish more space between the child's core self and his or her defensive system and can help to create a vantage point that allows the core self to reconnect with the body and its wisdom. Experiential body mapping adds to that potential. What the different parts of the child's defensive system ("inner voices") say during therapy, they do themselves. However, the child can only successfully draw the various parts of the defensive system from the position of a core self. Because visualization of the child's defensive strategy explicitly requires that that child is capable and willing to detach from that strategy, it is an actual first step in dismantling that emergency state. "You cannot break your chains when they are not visible" (Kafka, as cited in Janouch, 1965, p. 51); when the child visualizes those chains, that process actually starts to break them. Not surprisingly, the inner network's initial response to this "betrayal" is one of confusion and uproar. Detecting and visualizing this defensive system through experiential body mapping takes courage and self-conquest.

Several clinicians provide guidance and approaches that are related to experiential body mapping. Steinhardt (1985) introduced the use of body outlines as a therapeutic tool for 6- to 13-year-old children with a variety of emotional problems. She placed each of these children on the floor (or up against the wall) on/against a piece of paper large enough to accommodate their bodies, and then let them draw their body outlines. They could fill their outline up in any way they chose, to "depict their external perception of their body, which also reflected their inner perception and reveals emotional content" (p. 25). Mendel, a focusing-oriented South African therapist, influenced by Steinhardt and by Solomon (2003), uses body maps to help children create "internal self-portraits," traced from their body outlines, into which they map felt experiences as they are forming (Mendel & Goldberg, 2012; Mendel & Khumalo, 2006). As Mendel (personal communication, December 5, 2013) explained:

> Resonating between the bodily sensation and its expression in the corresponding area of the artwork brings the felt sense into focus, visually and experientially. This allows children to get to know parts of themselves and their internal worlds, which are witnessed and worked with in this externalized form. This usually leads to bodily felt shifts that continue to be mapped in unfolding layers.

These drawings vary from literal presentations of physical appearance to visualizations that resemble experiential body maps (see Figures 6.1 and 6.2).

In Israel, focusing-oriented therapists (Perlstein & Frohlinger, 2013) developed a similar technique, called *Kol-Be* (Hebrew for "Everything that is in me" or "The voice within me"), a combination of Steinhardt's (2013) body outline drawing technique and the way she uses the bounded area in sandboxes. These therapists offer children a standardized picture of a human figure without gender or facial characteristics. The children can draw, write, and add different objects on that figure as symbols to stimulate and facilitate felt process.

Shirar (1996) introduced a cognitive-behavioral approach to body mapping in the diagramming of "part selves" in psychotherapy with dissociated children (see also Baita, 2011). She asked these children to

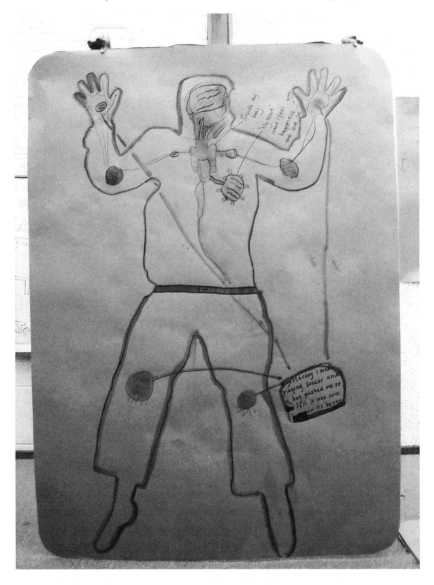

FIGURE 6.1. Body map by Rory, 9 years old (Mendel & Khumalo, 2006).

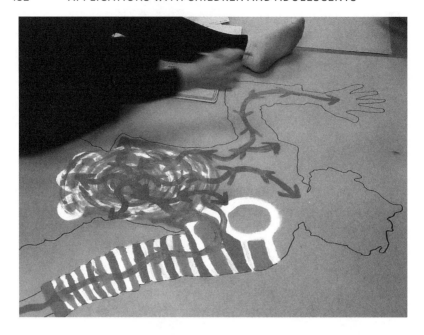

FIGURE 6.2. Body map by Elize, 19 years old (Mendel & Goldberg, 2012).

draw a picture of their inside world (e.g., as a house, divided in apartments) where their alters live, to get "a visual layout of the 'inner family' of personalities." "It helps both me and the child to get a better idea of how the child conceptualizes the personalities and their separateness or connectedness," Shirar explained (p. 159). "Once the inner world is made metaphorically concrete by a drawing, the drawing becomes the framework for the inner 'construction work' of building communication and cooperation" (p. 159). Baita (2007, 2011) also developed a drawing technique, called the "Inside–Outside Technique," to disclose the presence of dissociative parts. She offered children "a piece of white paper with a circle drawn on each side of it," and invited them to draw their "outside head" and their "inside head." Her goal is similar to that of Shirar: to help the child develop "a map of the internal dissociative system, by showing not only the parts but the kind of communication, or lack of communication, existing between them" (Baita, 2011, p. 61). Potgieter Marks (2011) and Silberg (2011, 2013) have children draw their brains and/or heads for similar reasons. These drawing techniques aim primarily at the cognitive-behavioral goal of exploring and explaining trauma and dissociation to the child.

EXPERIENTIAL BODY MAPPING

When I saw the drawings in Shirar's (1996) book, it came to me that a body outlined on paper might as well be used as a container for an *experiential* process that could manifest focusing-oriented work. Stone and Winkelman (1985) provided the link that made me aware of the handle (in focusing-oriented work, a *handle* is a word, phrase, or image that captures the quality of the concern felt in the body) I needed to materialize. They stated that "each sub-personality brings its own energy in our body. We can feel them inside" (p. 31). The plausibility of this assertion encouraged me to develop the technique described below.

General Guidelines

• *Clearing a space.* Clearing a space is the first step in focusing-oriented work and is a method of finding and putting aside each distress-producing feeling that is being carried by the body (Gendlin, 1996). Experiential body mapping has been derived from that step. It gives dissociated children, who find it very difficult to connect with any "feeling place," a framework that is strong enough to counteract their foggy state and secure resonation with the body. It provides an inevitable *out-there* (emerging body map) that can reflect and clarify the dynamics of the child's experienced reality inside.

• *Basic attitude.* In focusing-oriented psychotherapy, "welcoming" is a way of letting feelings, thoughts, and sensations arise; they are accepted as they are and invited to be recognized (Rappaport, 2009). What comes from underneath is protected against smothering inner attacks. The material is welcomed and received patiently by the person and the therapist; the felt bodily sense is emphasized over cognitive responses.

• *Materials.* Sheets of white paper (20 × 27.5 inches [50 × 70 cm]), and (optional) large sheets of paper longer than a human body; adhesive tape; pen and pencil; colored markers (red, blue, green, yellow).

• *Preparation.* The therapist adheres three sheets of white paper (20 × 27.5 inches [50 × 70 cm]) or uses one large sheet longer than a human figure and places the paper on the floor. The therapist then draws the outline of a life-sized human (not a tracing of the child's body) and asks the child to kneel down next to that figure.

Basic Instructions

1. "Travel slowly with one or more fingers of one of your hands across this paper body. Touch it lightly. Meanwhile, turn your attention to the middle of your own body and ask your body to signify where 'voices,' 'fear places,' or 'restless places' may be found on this paper body. Wherever your fingers are on the paper body, check inside yourself and notice if your body responds. If it responds when your fingers have arrived at a specific place, draw on that place on the paper body. Start traveling with your fingers again, until your body signals that another place should be drawn. Continue in this way until it seems that all the places you could find have been drawn on the paper body."

2. "Choose two of the places on the paper body on which you drew. You can decide for yourself which ones to choose. Let your fingers travel between the two on the paper to find out if a response inside your own body signals a pathway between them: straight or winding, however it runs. If you find a pathway, draw it between the two places as you have found it. Also, visit the spaces between all the scanned places on the map in the same way. Draw any additional pathways as long as you find them with your fingers."

3. "Choose one of the pathways that you have found to travel on it with one of your fingers. While your finger travels there, a response inside your own body may signal that there is traffic on that road; it can be either one-way or two-way traffic. If one of these is the case, draw that direction/those directions with an arrow on the map. Let your finger visit each of the pathways in the same way. Draw an arrow wherever your finger finds a direction."

4. "Here are four marker pens; each one has its own color. Use them one by one, with their caps still on. Choose one of the scanned places on the map, brush across it with one of the marker pens, then do this with the second marker pen, the third, the fourth. When your body signals that one of these marker pens fits, color that place with that marker pen after you have tried all the colors. Visit each of the identified places in the same way, one by one. Give them a color. Do the same with the pathways: touch each pathway with each of the four closed marker pens, then color that specific path if your body feels that one of the marker pens fits. Do this with each of the pathways."

5. "Notice if there is a part of the paper body that remained blank. Travel with one or some fingers of either hand across that region one

more time. Meanwhile, ask your body to confirm that this blank area really is blank, or if it signifies that in this part of the paper body there are places or pathways that are more deeply hidden. If you detect new places or pathways, treat them the same way you did with the ones you found before."

6. "Choose one of the triangles that are formed by pathways on the map. Travel with one or some fingers across the surface of that triangle to find out if your body tells you there is 'something in there.' If you find one, treat it the same way you did for the places and pathways you found before. You may also try this on another triangle."

Depending on the therapist's sense of what might fit for the child, a combination of verbal and pictorial ways can be used to clarify what the individual has found in the body map:

7a. "Look at that 'something.' Put your attention inside your body, and check inside if there is a word or words that seem to describe what this is. If something comes that seems to fit, try it by saying it out loud for yourself several times to check inside if it still fits or if a new description comes."

7b. "Look at that 'something' ('black hole,' 'hidden silence,' 'core,' 'something that should be kept inside,' or other words the child has found). Paint it, enlarged, on a big sheet of blank paper, just the way it comes, to find out what is really *in* this, what is at the center of this."

7c. Cutouts (described in the next section) can be made and included in the body map.

Making and Exploring Cutouts

Making a cutout is a way of giving renewed attention to a particular piece of a body map or drawing, in order to take a further step toward reconnecting with the felt sense and the original trauma. It is a way of obtaining access—step by step—to the deeper layers of a selected area within the body map or drawing, by mentally transferring the selected area to a clear space on a larger scale in which freshly arising drawings can be made. This therapeutic intervention can be repeated for each newly emerging image as long as it contributes to further steps of exploration. A cutout is explicitly *not* meant to render merely a regular enlargement of a selected area of a body map or of a drawing.

In order to create "cutouts," prepare several sheets of blank paper (20 × 27.5 inches [50 × 70 cm]) by giving them a border (by putting dotted lines along the edges, not by actually cutting the paper). Put one of these prepared sheets next to the child's body map. Give the child a pencil, select a section on the body map, and "cut it out" with dotted lines. Instruct the child as follows:

> "I cut out this area on the body map. Look at that section. Touch it with a finger. Imagine that you can empty yourself and forget what you have drawn there. Now direct your attention to the bordered separate sheet of paper that you have put next to the body map. Imagine that you can use this blank sheet to enter the cut-out area that you attended to just before on the body map. Travel across that blank paper with your fingers. Notice where your body responds and draw what emerges on those places on the paper."

This way of entering a map/drawing can be repeated wherever it seems useful.

BEYOND THE MISLEADING WALL: THE CASE OF HOWARD

Ever since Howard, age 13 years, came home with a story about an accident with his bike, he has suffered from headaches, lower back pain, and pain around his navel. No medical explanation was found. Howard became depressed and began to self-mutilate. He was subject to mood swings and reported that he heard voices inside his head. When his anxiety level increased, he stopped attending school. He was sent to a mental hospital for clinical treatment because of what was called "the onset of a psychotic process." Verbal therapy did not change his state of self-alienation.

Scanning a Body Map and Detecting "Something That Should Be Kept Inside"

At age 16, Howard was sent to my office for focusing-oriented psychotherapy. During our first contact he told me about his confusion, his blackouts, and his memory loss. He manifested a wide range of dissociative symptoms that disrupted his daily functioning. I told him my impression that these symptoms reflected a dissociative state and that I wanted to try a nonverbal method that could help detect the bodily impact of that situation. I drew the life-sized contours of an empty human body on paper and told him that we would use this as a container for his future explorations. Howard followed my instructions and during parts of four sessions his fingers scanned his body map (see Figure 6.3).

When he seemed ready, I asked Howard to explore the empty surface of two connected triangles in the abdomen area of the map. His fingers detected a spot in the middle of the lower triangle. When he had added that on his map, his fingers also found pathways that connected this spot with the surrounding corners. When I asked Howard if he had a word that emerged from what he saw, he told me that it made him think of a "machine." He bent over this part of his map and commented: "This machine keeps something inside. All feelings come in there and he holds them, but he shouldn't. I need to express them. He is in motion, so my feelings repeat themselves over and over." When Howard focused his attention on the spot in the middle of the "machine," he drew a small black circle on it and repeated: "In this black pit there is something that should be kept inside. I don't know what it is."

Entry into "the Black Spot"

Over the next months, I gradually guided Howard into his "black spot" through a series of steps. During the seventh session, Howard used a sheet of paper for a microscopic visit into that place of the "something that should be kept inside." His fingers pictured the "something," surrounded by scattered pieces (see Figure 6.4).

Howard revealed that the explorations by his fingers activated a struggle inside himself. "This conflict," he told me, "takes so much energy. When we do this work, the powers that want to reveal something grow, and then the likelihood that I will get overwhelmed increases. I guard it, but I do that unconsciously. Gradually, I will have to start daring to loosen that control. We need to continue, but we will always have to keep a very close eye on what I can and cannot handle."

I asked Howard to visualize the struggle that he talked about. He drew arrows that pushed outward. They bumped on arrows that pushed inward. When he looked at what he had pictured, he remarked: "Until recently, I did not know that this was going on. It is scary to know, but it is also a relief."

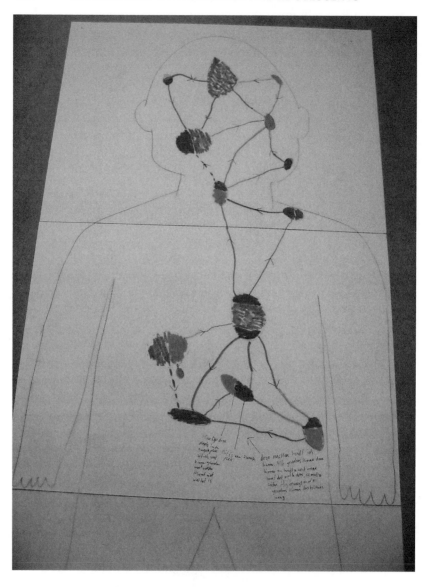

FIGURE 6.3. Howard's body map.

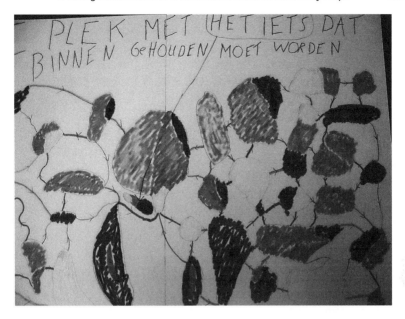

FIGURE 6.4. The place with the something that should be kept inside.

Revealing the Primary Split

Howard disclosed how his alter personality monitored his connection with the outside world; this alter accompanied him "like an older person who wants to be in charge":

> "I am present with my body, yet I am absent. He-in-me makes me believe that there is nothing around me and that I am not present either, that only he is there. When there are no other people, I feel helpless because then he—that black spot—takes over. Then I begin to think, and then he pulls the strings, takes power over my way of thinking. When I am scared, he grows bigger. When I am obliged to do things—like at school—that also makes him grow. What is happening here causes a bit of turmoil, and that makes everything even more difficult. He is the container of fear, that I open up when there are many incentives."

At this point, Howard temporarily stopped attending school. For a half year, the frequency of our sessions was increased to twice a week. During the 15th session Howard painted the feeling of the "something" (see Figure 6.5): imagery that conveyed restlessness, most of it encapsulated by a wall. He painted black dots at both sides of the wall, like monitoring eyes that were looking at him.

In the next session Howard transformed his painting in order to create a balance. He fortified the wall with a second wall and created more distance between himself and the black "eyes" by concealing them with blue paint. When he established more protection for himself through these images, he explained how the "black" influenced his emotional life: "The black figure is a troublemaker who spreads all over," he explained.

> "He feels like a disembodied spirit that takes over my body when I am alone. With the black figure I feel like a body that has a mind deep down inside. Me and he do not feel attached to each other but near each other. It seems that each of us wants a different thing. He is the leader who makes everyone restless. He scares me. He often floods me with emotions. The blue is calming. As long as the blue keeps the black inside, the emotions don't get worse."

This was a key moment for Howard. As he described later, it opened up his wall considerably, allowing emotions to touch him. After this,

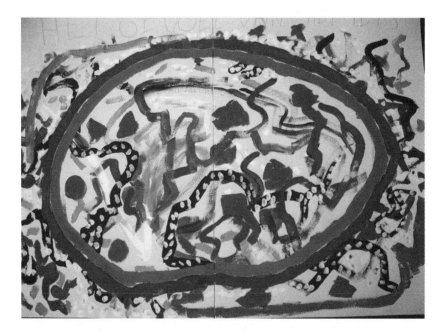

FIGURE 6.5. The feeling of the "something."

the black figure remained very present whenever the "something" was touched too strongly. Body mapping had exposed the existence and the feeling of what he called the "something"; now Howard might be ready to take small steps to expose his defensive layers. When I asked Howard if he would allow me to talk with "the black figure," he did not give me a direct reply. He warned me that "the black" wanted him to commit suicide. He felt that this would be better than disclosure because "when you are dead, there are no problems." "The black," Howard said, accused him of betrayal because of his engagement in the therapeutic process. "He distrusts everybody."

I asked Howard if there was a secret. He answered affirmatively. He said that "the black" wanted him to bury that secret with him in the grave. Somebody could not be betrayed "because that person is dangerous." Howard feared for his life if he would reveal the secret. "I think that that person also will want me to die." When Howard brought those words into the open, he was afraid that he might commit suicide right then. At this point, Howard and I took a short break in treatment. We consulted the psychiatrist and his mother, who both agreed that we should continue. That day Howard began to dismantle a number of layers of his defensive system; it was as if these layers emerged through a fog.

As a first step, I asked Howard to check inside himself to see if he felt ready to say anything concerning the secret or if he wanted to try to access it by drawing. He wanted to draw. During the hours that followed, he produced a sequence of pictures that linked him to his painful past. I asked Howard to make a drawing with the title "The secret and he" (see Figure 6.6). He drew a dozen rings around a core, and explained that the "black figure" was located near the outward boundary. The secret, Howard explained, was in the encapsulated core in the middle.

Entering the Cutouts: Retrieving Memory, Layer upon Layer

I delineated a rectangular area on the drawing "The secret and he" halfway "between" the walls as a first cutout to be entered. I gave Howard a big sheet of blank paper that he vcould use as a screen on which he could draw whatever his fingers found. Silently and without hesitation, his scanning fingers found a new picture (Figure 6.7). On his drawing, the blank secret was surrounded by a "misleading wall" that was in turn surrounded by a "protective wall." All this was walled off from the outside by "he."

Without comment on what had been created, I made another cutout, this time beyond the protective wall. Howard's fingers explored the

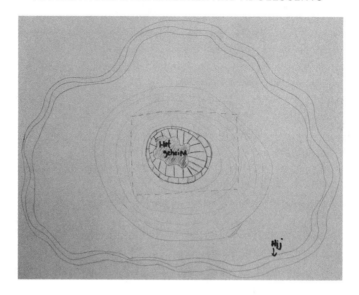

FIGURE 6.6. The secret and he.

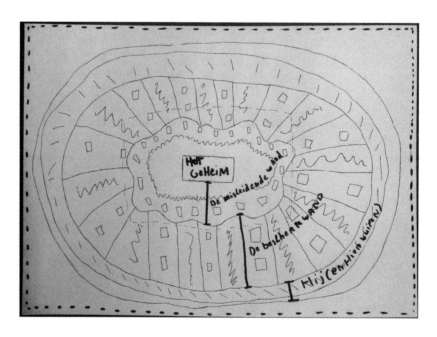

FIGURE 6.7. The secret, the misleading wall, the protective wall, and he.

next blank sheet of paper, imagining that it was an entry by which the area of the cutout could reemerge freshly. A new picture emerged. Behind a "misleading wall" filled with empty rectangles, the area of the secret was no longer empty. It appeared to contain circular shapes. Half of these shapes were gathered together by a line that surrounded them. Howard made a cutout again, this one of the area beyond the misleading wall, and used his fingers to let it reemerge on a next blank sheet of paper. Beyond the misleading wall a new wall ("the wall of the secret") appeared.

Howard made a new cutout that trespassed "the wall of the secret." His fingers explored the next blank sheet of paper. A new picture emerged, with 10 particles. He called these particles the "secret-inside-pieces." "There are five secret-inside-pieces," Howard explained. "Each of them holds a part of the secret, and they all have a duplication." I asked him to gather the "secret-inside-pieces" by drawing a line around them and to treat the five duplications in the same way. As a next step, his fingers detected which duplication mirrored which holder. With dotted lines he connected each of the holders with its duplication.

I asked Howard to explore each of the holders with his fingers to sense if it held something specific. In this way he recognized that each of the holders had a special function. He drew them enlarged on a blank sheet of paper (Figure 6.8): a holder of "the pain," one of "the emotions,"

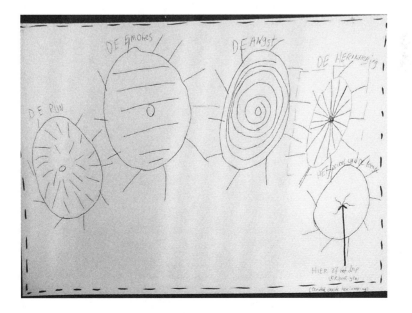

FIGURE 6.8. The holders.

"the fear," and "the memory" (left to right); the fifth one held what he called "the feeling of emptiness, where it is deeply hidden." He said that "part of the memory" was to be found there.

Howard continued in the same way. I guided him in making several additional cutouts. He made a cutout of "the holder called 'The memory.'" He also made a cutout in that holder of the encapsulating "chain" that appeared around what he called "the memory," and he made a cutout beyond that chain. His fingers found "the memory" (Figure 6.9). He observed his last drawing for a moment, then he reported, "There is a line between the images. The images have content, There is a mixture of colors. The images constitute a whole. They seem to be images of one event."

Howard made a cutout of one of the images. In the same way he had done with his cutouts before, his fingers explored its area on a separate piece of paper and found what he called "the lost picture" (Figure 6.10). I cut out the part of "the lost picture where the content had spread." He explored it with his fingers and called the curved lines that appeared "the dispersed content." Howard now felt physical pain; that was new to him. He said that on some places he could clearly sense the

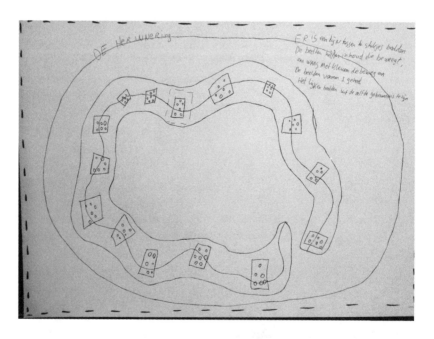

FIGURE 6.9. The memory.

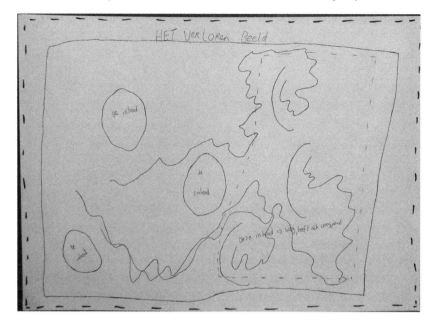

FIGURE 6.10. The lost picture.

presence of the contents of his memory. The other content was gone. When he touched this drawing with his fingers, new words came up: "I have been touched by a person. Someone I know. A boy from school. He said something."

Howard took a break. He felt exhausted, but safe. That same afternoon he continued where he had stopped. His fingers explored a cutout of part of "the dispersed content." When he entered that cutout in this way, a new figure emerged (Figure 6.11), which he called "the persecution." When Howard touched this figure with his fingers, he began to say words that seemed to refer to a situation he had been part of several years ago. He said that "the black shape" knew what had happened and that he was willing to tell me, but that he had to get used to the idea of doing that.

The week after he had made the drawing in Figure 6.11, Howard allowed me to have my first talk with "the black shape." During a sequence of talks this black shape revealed to me how Howard had been severely violated by a small group on several occasions. Howard heard those conversations on tape. Step by step, he unraveled the specifics of these assaults and gradually learned to accept the reality of what had

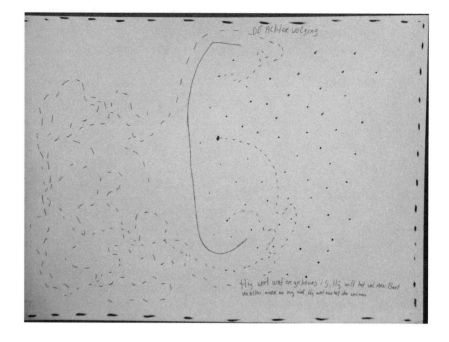

FIGURE 6.11. The persecution.

happened. His defensive system became obsolete and silent. A ritual burning of dolls that symbolized the offenders helped him "to allow and contain the extreme survival emotions of rage and terror without being overwhelmed" (Levine, 2010, p. 56). Howard's rage calmed down and his emotional condition improved considerably. The frequency of his sessions was reduced until therapy ended, 2 years after it had begun. The years that followed confirmed that his improvement was lasting.

CONCLUSION

In this chapter I have tried to show that body mapping, along with the element of touch that I described, can be a useful therapeutic intervention technique with dissociated children. If I were to ask the children I see in therapy to let their fingers explore dissociative phenomena on their bodies, those bodies would have kept them silent. In most of my sessions with dissociated children, body mapping has provided the connection to what these children's bodies already know. Their cases confirm that "knowing" exists at different levels. What could not yet become conscious or spoken out loud was recognized when their bodies were enabled to express the narrative aspects and emotional impact of their past experiences.

Eight months after body mapping had broken the silence, Howard reviewed what he had visualized. I was surprised by his comments. When his fingers pointed at "the machine" on his map, he remarked, "I think that these are the four offenders, and this is what they keep inside." When he saw his other visualizations, he knew in retrospect which cutouts had caused the walls to open up and allow the holders and their duplications to come closer to each other; the memory of what had happened had become clear. When he aligned with his body in the correct pace and from the correct distance, it was ready to tell him something, and he was able to receive what it told him.

Some children are skeptical about feeling a piece of paper with their fingers. It is hard for them to connect with a "feeling place." Not coincidentally, the word *feeling* stands for both experiences: "I *feel* hurt and I *feel* with my fingers" (Rothschild, 2000, p. 56). In most of the cases, however, feeling on paper stimulates the felt experience. In brief, body mapping helps dissociative children in two ways: (1) It reconnects them with their feelings and emotions and (2) it helps them to reconnect with and revisit their traumatic experiences, even when they are not yet ready to acknowledge them. As Emily would say (Santen, 2014, p. 89):

> "At first there is one big bubble of fear. Then you began to feel, slightly forced by the ostensibly innocent feeling on the body map and by beginning to identify. You can visualize the machine. That creates clarity. It outlines a structure. You can see that a system is operating that generates fear. Then you can discern that there is a core, a secret, that is protected."

REFERENCES

Baita, S. (2007, November). *What's inside my head?: How to explore and explain trauma and dissociation to children.* Paper presented at the annual meeting of the International Society for the Study of Trauma and Dissociation, Philadelphia.

Baita, S. (2011). Dalma (4 to 7 years old): "I've got all my sisters with me": Treatment of dissociative identity disorder in a sexually abused child. In

S. Wieland (Ed.), *Dissociation in traumatized children and adolescents: Theory and clinical interventions* (pp. 29–73). New York: Routledge.

Gendlin, E. T. (1996). *Focusing-oriented psychotherapy: A manual of the experiential method.* New York: Guilford Press.

Gendlin, E. T. (2003). *Focusing: How to gain direct access to your body's knowledge* (25th anniversary ed.). London: Rider.

Hornstein, N. (1998). Complexities of psychiatric differential diagnosis in children with dissociative symptoms and disorders. In J. Silberg (Ed.), *The dissociative child: Diagnosis, treatment and management* (2nd ed., pp. 27–45). Lutherville, MD: Sidran Press.

Janouch, G. (1965). *Gesprekken met Kafka.* Amsterdam: Querido. (Dutch translation of *Gespräche mit Kafka*)

Levine, P. A. (2010). *In an unspoken voice: How the body releases trauma and restores goodness.* Berkeley, CA: North Atlantic Books.

Malchiodi, C. A. (2008). Creative interventions and childhood trauma. In C. A. Malchiodi (Ed.), *Creative interventions with traumatized children* (pp. 3–21). New York: Guilford Press.

Mendel, A., & Goldberg, R. (2012, May–June). *Workshop "Mapping bodies: From inside out."* Surface Design Department of the Cape Peninsula University of Technology, Cape Town, South Africa.

Mendel, A., & Khumalo, N. (2006, April–October). *"Learning support group" therapy process.* Presentation given at the Child Guidance Clinic, University of Cape Town, Cape Town, South Africa.

Ogden, P., Minton, K., & Pain, C. (2006). *Trauma and the body: A sensorimotor approach to psychotherapy.* New York: Norton.

Perlstein, A., & Frohlinger, B. (2013, March). *Kol-be: Transforming the implicit into explicit integration of art and focusing.* Lecture presented at the conference "Arch of Arts in Health," Haifa, Israel.

Potgieter Marks, R. (2011). Jason (7 years old): Expressing past neglect and abuse. In S. Wieland (Ed.), *Dissociation in traumatized children and adolescents: Theory and clinical interventions* (pp. 97–140). New York: Routledge.

Putnam, F. (1997). *Dissociation in children and adolescents: A developmental perspective.* New York: Guilford Press.

Rappaport, L. (2009). *Focusing-oriented art therapy: Accessing the body's wisdom and creative intelligence.* London: Jessica Kingsley.

Rappaport, L. (2010). Focusing-oriented art therapy: Working with trauma. *Person-Centered and Experiential Psychotherapies, 9*(2), 128–142.

Rohde-Dachser, C. (1979). *Das borderline-syndrom.* Bern: Huber.

Rothschild, B. (2000). *The body remembers: The psychophysiology of trauma and trauma treatment.* New York: Norton.

Santen, B. (1993). Focusing with a dissociated adolescent: Tracing and treating multiple personality disorder experienced by a 13-year-old girl. *Folio: Journal for Focusing and Experiential Therapy, 12*(1), 45–58.

Santen, B. (1999). Focusing with children and young adolescents. In C. E. Schaefer (Ed.), *Innovative psychotherapy techniques in child and adolescent therapy* (pp. 384–414). New York: Wiley.

Santen, B. (2007). Into the fear-factory: Treating children of trauma with body maps. *Folio: Journal for Focusing and Experiential Therapy, 20*(1), 60–78.

Santen, B. (2014). Into the fear-factory: Connecting with the traumatic core. *Person-Centered and Experiential Psychotherapies, 13*(2), 75–93.

Shirar, L. (1996). *Dissociative children: Bridging the inner and outer worlds.* New York: Norton.

Silberg, J. L. (2011). Angela (14–16 years old)—finding words for pain: Treatment of a dissociative teen presenting with medical trauma. In S. Wieland (Ed.), *Dissociation in traumatized children and adolescents: Theory and clinical interventions* (pp. 263–284). New York: Routledge.

Silberg, J. L. (2013). *The child survivor: Healing developmental trauma and dissociation.* New York: Routledge.

Solomon, J. (2003). *How to body map: Instructions of body mapping technique.* Unpublished paper, Cape Town, South Africa.

Steinhardt, L. (1985). Freedom within boundaries: Body outline drawings in art therapy with children. *Arts in Psychotherapy, 12*(1), 25–34.

Steinhardt, L. (2013). *On becoming a Jungian sandplay therapist: The healing spirit of sandplay in nature and in therapy.* London: Jessica Kingsley.

Stone, H., & Winkelman. S. (1985). *Thuiskomen in Jezelf.* Amsterdam: Mesa Verde. (Dutch translation of *Embracing Our Selves*)

van der Hart, O., Nijenhuis, E. R. S., & Steele, K. (2006). *The haunted self: Structural dissociation and the treatment of chronic traumatization.* New York: Norton.

Waters, F. S., & Silberg, J. L. (1998). Therapeutic phases in the treatment of dissociative children. In J. L. Silberg (Ed.), *The dissociative child: Diagnosis, treatment and management* (2nd ed., pp. 135–165). Lutherville, MD: Sidran Press.

Wieland, S. (2011). Dissociation in children and adolescents: What it is, how it presents, and how we can understand it. In S. Wieland (Ed.), *Dissociation in traumatized children and adolescents: Theory and clinical interventions* (pp. 1–27). New York: Routledge.

CHAPTER 7

Therapeutic Stories and Play in the Sandtray for Traumatized Children

The Moving Stories Method

Susanne Carroll Duffy

How many of us have asked a child "why" he or she has done something? Most often, the answer is "I don't know." The child often really doesn't know. For a child, words come last. So, if words are not the primary language of a child, what is? A child's very first language is sensory—the world is understood through the experience of the body and emotions. From this sensorial beginning, the child moves toward play and finally alongside play, words. These layers of "language" hold the story of children's experience and for traumatized children, the path to their healing, because it is in these places that they are stuck.

Perry (2006) explains that for traumatized children, normal brain development has been disrupted due to chaotic and neglectful environments and caregivers. This disruption causes problems with emotional regulation and interrupts the ability of children to communicate, think, and relate to others. Perry states that interventions should match the developmental status of a child and that treatment should be repetitive and pleasurable. According to Perry, when a child is more regulated, the therapy can target higher and more complex parts of the brain.

The pleasurable and sensorial aspects of story, play, and sandtray help the traumatized child experience self-regulation, self-expression, and learning. The Moving Stories method (Carroll Duffy, 2014e) is an intermodal creative therapy tool that integrates the use of therapeutic stories (bibliotherapy) with sandtray and play therapies. This method offers traumatized children and their therapists, schoolteachers, and caregivers an engaging way to communicate positive therapeutic messages and to reflect the deepest feelings of children—in *their* language, the language that begins before words. As a therapeutic tool, it can be integrated into a range of existing models of child trauma treatment.

This chapter demonstrates how therapeutic stories come alive as the characters move in the theater of a sandtray (e.g., see Figure 7.1). The props used to tell the stories are housed in decorated story kits that are accessible to the children in a special kind of playroom—the Wonder Room. This chapter also describes the eight steps to consider in selecting stories, responding to the child's play, and documenting the child's response to the stories. Finally, applications of this method with traumatized children in individual therapy are presented.

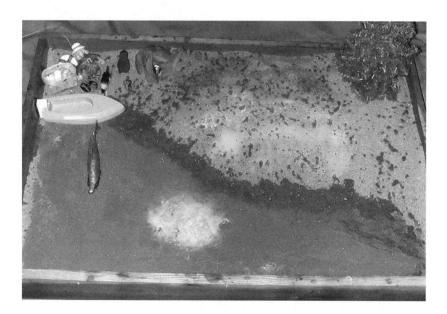

FIGURE 7.1. Moving Stories in the sandtray. Copyright 2014 by By The Sea Seminars/Susanne Carroll Duffy. Reprinted by permission.

THE USE OF STORIES IN THERAPY WITH CHILDREN

Storytelling as a way to teach and heal is ancient. In work with traumatized children, the story is both the one that they hear (well-selected therapeutic stories) as well as the one that they tell through their play or other creative medium. What is it about stories that are so powerful? Story provides a safe distance from a traumatized child's pain. Through story, children learn that they are not alone and that there are solutions for the challenges they face. Coping skills to better manage their feelings can be taught in engaging and fun ways through the use of story. In stories, children express more fully their emotions than is afforded by direct dialogue. Finally, therapeutic stories present hope—hope to feel better, hope to feel safe, and hope to function better in relationship to others.

The use of story/poetry/literature in therapy is its own discipline: bibliotherapy. Hynes and Hynes Berry (2012) describe bibliotherapy as the use of literature to promote mental health. They specify that the use of literature is an interactive process in which growth happens in the relationship between the participant, the facilitator, and the selected literature. There are two common phases in bibliotherapy: the receptive phase, when the story is shared, and the expressive phase, when individuals respond to the story (Kaufman, Chalmers, & Rosenbery, 2014). Or, as in the mutual storytelling technique (Gardner, 1993), there is an expressive phase (the child tells a story) followed by the therapist's response in the form of a therapeutic story.

SANDTRAY AND STORYTELLING

Integrating storytelling with sandtray therapy has many benefits for the traumatized child. Badenoch (2008) states, "Grounded in the body, sandplay unfolds through the limbic regions and cortex and spans both hemispheres as the symbolic world unfolds into words" (p. 220). The multisensory experience of hearing, seeing, and touching a story that occurs in a sandtray not only helps children to understand the story that they have heard, but also to respond to the story through the use of objects in the sand and to find words.

The sandtray is a naturally engaging, unintimidating medium for children. No skills are needed. A child can push the sand together to make a mountain or a cave, clear space to make a body of water, or add water and work with wet sand. In sandtray therapy, shelves of objects for the sandtray, representing every aspect of life, aid in communication (Figure 7.2). For example, a child could find animals, plants, houses, religious figures, cultural figures, cars, and people to add to the story in the sandtray. In essence, the sandtray provides the child with a multi-sensory symbolic language in which to understand the healing message in the story and in which to express his or her own feelings in response.

There are many approaches to the use of sandtray and story. Some practitioners use sandtray and story in school settings with academic and behavioral goals (Smith, 2012); others use sandtray and story from a Jungian ("sandplay") perspective (Turner & Unnsteindsdottir, 2011). The Moving Stories method is most closely aligned with more interactive uses of sandtray and story, such as those described by integrative arts psychotherapist Margot Sunderland (2008) and by Adlerian play therapist Terry Kottman (2001).

PLAY THERAPY AND STORYTELLING

The use of play, particularly after a child has heard a therapeutic story (expressive phase), enhances the child's ability to communicate and

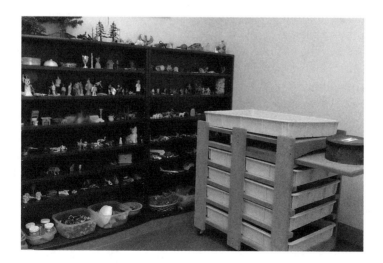

FIGURE 7.2. Sandtray shelves, multi-sandtray cart, and Moving Stories kit. Copyright 2014 by By The Sea Seminars/Susanne Carroll Duffy. Reprinted by permission.

process feelings in response to what he or she has heard. Landreth (2012) describes a child's play as the sensory–motor use of concrete objects that are symbols for something the child has experienced. The field of play therapy offers guidance in ways to be present with children in their play (particularly in the sandtray) from within the structure of a theoretical model (Drewes & Bratton, 2014). The therapist might take a nondirective stance (e.g., child-centered play therapy) or perhaps a more interactive stance (e.g., Adlerian play therapy). Joyce Mills, a play therapist and coauthor of the seminal book *Therapeutic Metaphors for Children and the Child Within*, developed an approach called Story Play™ in which she uses the power of metaphor in story and play within an Ericksonian orientation. In the Moving Stories method, if a child chooses to play after hearing a story, the play is understood as his or her story-response or play-story. The specific way in which a therapist interacts with the child likely depends on the therapist's theoretical orientation, the developmental needs of the child, the phase of therapy, and most importantly, attunement with the needs of the child in the moment.

THE MOVING STORIES METHOD

The Moving Stories method is a multisensory, developmentally attuned approach that integrates the disciplines of bibliotherapy, sandtray therapy, and play therapy. It meets the traumatized child within the safety of healing stories, gently approaching painful feelings and offering a new perspective. Therapeutic stories are housed in kits, making up a three-dimensional library. The stories are told with props in the sandtray. After experiencing the therapeutic story in the sandtray, the child is invited to play. Children can use props from the story in the sandtray or another expressive medium such as clay, painting, or imaginative play. As a child responds through play to the healing story told in the sandtray, he or she learns to express him- or herself in story as well: a play-story. All of this happens within the context of a safe and supportive relationship and an engaging and fun process.

The idea of creating story kits with thoughtful placement in a playroom came from the work of Jerome Berryman, an Episcopal priest who created "Godly Play" (2005). Trained in the Montessori method, Berryman brings Bible stories to life with props. The story props are kept in wooden boxes, trays, or baskets that are placed on low, well-organized shelves. The storyteller learns both the content of the story and the actions for telling the story—much like a play.

In the Moving Stories method the child's response to the story most often involves play in the sandtray. It is designed as a flexible model with choices ranging from directive to nondirective at each step. For traumatized children, Gil (2006) espouses a combination of both directive and nondirective play therapy approaches. As an illustration of one way to use the Moving Stories method, this chapter describes a directive approach to the selection of the stories and a nondirective play therapy approach during the time that the child responds to the stories.

USING THE MOVING STORIES METHOD WITH TRAUMATIZED CHILDREN

The eight steps in the Moving Stories method (Figure 7.3) provide the therapist with a flexible structure in which to tell, process, and document the use of therapeutic stories in the sandtray with children. The

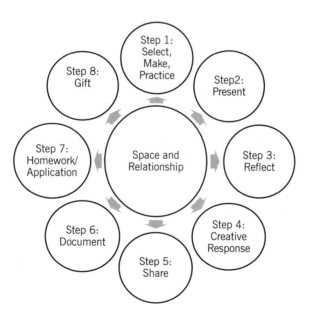

FIGURE 7.3. Steps in the Moving Stories method. Copyright 2014 by By The Sea Seminars/Susanne Carroll Duffy. Reprinted by permission.

way a therapist uses the steps for a group, or a classroom, differs from the way that they are used for an individual child or in a family session. The child, the context, and the relationship to the child inform each step; a therapist can use a directive or nondirective approach, depending on the child's needs and the therapist's orientation. Sensitive engagement may mean eliminating steps or moving flexibly along a directive to nondirective continuum. Following is a description of how the method could be used with a traumatized child seen in an individual therapy session.

CREATING THE SPACE AND THE RELATIONSHIP

The relationship to the child and the setting are central to the success of this method. In the Moving Stories method, the playroom is called the "Wonder Room," as mentioned. This name for the playroom captures (1) the feeling of awe that children experience when they walk into a room filled with creative storytelling possibilities, and (2) the "wondering" phase of the Moving Stories method when children begin to reflect on the meaning of the story for themselves. The defining features of a Wonder Room are the shelves of therapeutic story kits that together make a three-dimensional library (Figure 7.4). Each kit is labeled, and the pieces contained in the kit are listed on the lid so that it is easy to keep the story pieces together.

A Wonder Room also contains a cart holding multiple trays of different-colored sandtrays (Figure 7.2). The sandtrays are approximately 24 × 30 inches with a 3- to 4-inch depth. The bottom of the tray is blue to represent water. Some stories are enhanced by using a particular color of sand. For example, the story "Black Black Bear" (Carroll Duffy, 2014a) addresses feelings of sadness and is told in the black sandtray. There is also an "everything tray" where kids can mix sand colors. Saltshakers filled with different-colored sands and with water provide "special effects." For example, a child might use the saltshaker with water for a rainstorm, or the saltshaker with white sand for a snowstorm. "Special effects" might also involve music. Simple rhythm instruments such as a rain stick, rattles, bells, and drums can also be found in the Wonder Room.

Shelves of objects, such as you would find in sandtray therapy (Figure 7.2), are another key element of the Wonder Room. The objects represent all aspects of life, as mentioned, such as nature, transportation,

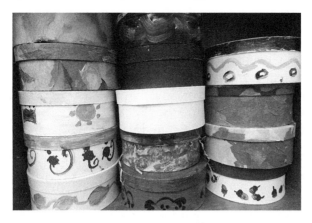

FIGURE 7.4. Therapeutic Moving Stories library. Copyright 2014 by By The Sea Seminars/Susanne Carroll Duffy. Reprinted by permission.

housing, animals, people, cultural pieces, mystical items, and religious artifacts. Art materials such as clay, markers, and paint are available. Finally, a Wonder Room offers play materials such as puppets, balls, a basketball hoop, costumes, and games.

In addition to creating the setting, the specific emotional and developmental needs of a child within a particular historical, family, and community context must be considered. This is a perspective supported by the ecosystemic play therapy model (O'Conner & Ammen, 2012). In this model, the therapist considers the developmental level, stage of therapy, and therapeutic goals when considering play interventions. In the Moving Stories method, the therapist is attuned to the child's response throughout the steps and remains flexible. For example, if the child wants a particular piece in the sandtray, it is included.

Step 1: Select, Make, Practice

The first step in the Moving Stories method involves thoughtful planning. The therapist selects a therapeutic story, makes a Moving Stories kit, and plans how to tell the story in the sandtray.

Select or Write the Story

When selecting stories, it is important to understand the cultural context of the child and the values of the family. For example, what meaning does an owl have? Many people would associate wisdom with an owl; however, for some Native Americans the owl is a harbinger of death. Stories should be consistent with cultural and family beliefs and values. According to Sunderland (2008), therapeutic stories offer hope and more creative ways of coping. Main characters should experience emotional challenges similar to the child's.

The therapist should also consider the goals of a particular stage of therapy. For example, in the beginning stages of therapy, if there is a suspicion of abuse, the therapist might select "Taffy and the Invisible Magic Bandage" (Davis, 1996). This story describes Taffy, a dog who goes into the woods and returns sad. She thinks she has an invisible bandage over her mouth and believes that if she speaks, she will disappear. Taffy learns that she feels better when she talks to trusted adults.

"Sammy Squirrel and the Nuts" (Greene, 2014) teaches coping skills and addresses feelings of safety, a common goal in trauma treatment. Sammy survives a storm, but is separated from her mother. Afterward she begins hoarding nuts. She learns through Bear how to feel safe again, and that she can talk with her family when she is frightened at night.

To teach the traumatized child affect regulation and relaxation, the story "Claude Flies an Airplane" (Simpson, 2014) might be selected. In this story, Claude (who is a rabbit) becomes angry, jumps in a plane, and takes off. He gets scared when he realizes that he is out of control and doesn't know how to land. Some geese hear his cries and teach him how to land the plane by breathing slowly in through his nose and blowing out through his mouth. With their guidance and support, Claude lands safely.

Many traumatized children need to see the trauma in perspective. A story that helps with this goal is "The Woman Who Saw the Good Side of Everything" (Tapio, 1975). A woman and her cat experience a series of apparent catastrophes due to the rain—a ruined picnic, the flowers drowning, the house floating away, and finally floating across the sea to China (where it starts raining). Through it all, the woman sees the positive side of what has happened.

At the end of therapy, the story "Emerging" (Carroll Duffy, 2014b) illustrates the therapeutic journey. Based on the popular story "The Struggle" (author unknown), a butterfly learns that the difficulty emerging from the cocoon provides the strength to fly.

The stories told in the sandtray should be brief and reflect the child's capacity to attend. A wonderful resource for stories that can be adapted to the Moving Stories method for traumatized children is *Therapeutic*

Stories That Teach and Heal (Davis, 1996) The stories use metaphors to address common issues faced by traumatized children, such as night-mares, fear of disclosing, fear of testifying, damaged sense of self, and problems with affect regulation. Another source of stories can be found in the Moving Stories online library located at *http://bytheseaseminars. com*. Therapists might also write their own therapeutic stories. Copies of stories should be kept in a binder in the Wonder Room for easy refer-ence to the Moving Stories library contents.

Make the Moving Stories Kit

Once the therapist has selected a story for a particular child, the next task is to create the Moving Stories kit. This can be a meditative process in which the therapist internalizes and owns the story. A box holds the story and is decorated with clear symbols of the story on the outside. Therapists can use oven-baked clay to make characters, or even sticks and stones and marbles to represent aspects of the story. For those who already do sandtray therapy, many of the objects needed for a story may be found on the sandtray shelves.

Each Moving Stories kit includes a symbol/gift. The gift is an inex-pensive representation of some important aspect of the story. Each time the story is told, there is a ready-made gift for each child. Gifts could be as simple as a piece of clipart representing a character in a story.

Practice in the Sandtray

Once the kit is complete, the therapist plans the layout and sequence of the story in the sandtray. There is no need to memorize stories, but it is important to have the sequence of events in mind and ideas about how to portray these events in the sandtray. The therapist is the director in a play—thinking about how to set the scene in the sandtray, where to place and move pieces, and how to create engaging special effects that include the participation of the child. After all of this planning, the therapist has to let go of expectations and place the child's response at the forefront.

Step 2: Presentation of a Story in the Sandtray

The next step is to present the story in the sandtray. Illustrating a directive approach, the therapist would say, "Today I have a story for you. Would you like to help me get the sandtray ready?" The child participates in preparing the sandtray. For example, if the story includes water as one of its elements, the therapist asks, "Where shall we put the water?" and allows the child to clear an area in the tray. Often a child will place an object from the sandtray shelves in the story. It is very important to include these items in the story. The therapist takes dramatic license to adapt the sex of the main character or emotional themes of any given story to the child. The attuned therapist will tell the story a different way to each child.

Once the sandtray scene is complete, the therapist invites the child to wonder about the story. The therapist might take a peek in the box and talk to one of the characters, or make the box jump to build anticipation. The therapist might also have a ritual before the story begins that prepares the child for the beginning of a story. For example, the therapist says, "Watch and listen to the rain stick. When it is done, the story will begin."

During the storytelling, the therapist pays attention to the child's response and looks for ways to involve him or her. For example, if rain is part of the story, the child might shake a saltshaker of water over the tray; or perhaps chant a particular line that is repeated throughout the story, or provide other sound effects. Movement and actions are another way to include a child in the telling of the story. When the story is over, the therapist thoughtfully and slowly waves his or her hand over the space above the sandtray and says, "That is the end of my story."

Step 3: Reflection upon the Story

After the story, the therapist asks reflective "wondering" questions. These questions deepen the meaning of the story for the child. In individual sessions, particularly with developmentally younger clients, the therapist may drop the reflection step. A child sitting next to the sandtray is eager to play.

"Wondering questions" can be tailored to the therapist's goals for the story. For example, the therapist might explore what was important to the child in the story, with special focus on the parts of the story the child liked or, just as important, the parts that he or she did not like. It is always interesting to ask children where they see themselves in a story or how they might change or continue the story. As the child responds, the therapist gives full attention to the part of the sandtray to which the child is referring and reflects back his or her response. There are no right or wrong answers. It is important that the therapist permit the child to take from the story whatever he or she needs . . . not what the therapist hoped the child would learn.

Step 4: Creative Response to the Story

The fourth step is to elicit or simply receive the creative response to the story. This is the expressive phase of the story dialogue between the therapist and child. In this phase, the therapist becomes the story-listener.

Again, there are a number of ways that a therapist might handle this phase, moving along a directive to nondirective continuum. Here is an example of a nondirective approach that provides the possibility of giving the child a choice about how to respond. After telling the story, the therapist might simply say to the child, "Now it is your turn to play." This is when the therapist becomes the story-listener, and whatever the child chooses to do in the playroom is considered their story-response.

Sometimes a child will start a completely different story in the sandtray; other times the child will expand upon the story and add characters from the sandtray shelf. As the story-listener, the therapist is present in whatever way the child seems to need. For instance, if the child is attempting to get a man to stay on a horse, the therapist helps this play by offering a bit of clay to make the man stick. Some children want the therapist to write their story down as they tell it. Others want the therapist to play with them in the sandtray or Wonder Room. Generally, the therapist does not ask questions, such as in child-centered play therapy (Landreth, 2012). Story listening means joining the process of children's play; it is *their* story no matter what creative expression they happen to choose. The therapist is an astute observer of every detail of the child's play-story.

Step 5: Sharing

In the fifth step, the child shares his or her creative response. In an individual session, this step occurs if the creative response resulted in a product—for example, a sandtray picture, a painting, a poem, or a written story. Verbal processing, or sharing, does not occur if the child's response to the story was active play that involved the therapist's playful participation or presence.

This step may look different depending on a therapist's orientation. For example, consider the approach common to Sandtray-Worldplay™ (DeDomenico, 2000). After listening to the child, the therapist might choose to reflect back to the child the creative process he or she just witnessed. The therapist can deepen the process further by giving different objects a voice and having them interact with each other, or by inviting the child to experience different symbols. Within this model, sharing involves the child in co-discovering, with the therapist, the meaning of his or her creation.

Step 6: Documenting the Story for the Therapist and the Child

After the therapist listens to the child's creative response/sharing, the therapist summarizes the experience as a story and writes it down to go with a picture of the child's creative response. Then the therapist asks, "What is the title of this story?" Over the course of therapy, the child's stories/pictures are kept in a binder. This document includes the name of the Moving Stories that the child heard, a picture of his or her creative response to the story, a summary of the child's story, a title, and the symbol/gift the child was given. The child may review the stories whenever desired, but most especially at the end of therapy. This collection of stories builds self-esteem for the child and is a journal of his or therapy experience. Over time, the process tends to move in the direction of the child taking the lead in storytelling, even making his or her own Moving Stories kits. When a child has difficulty leaving a session because his or her story does not seem to be finished, say, "Perhaps this is a chapter book that you can continue next session." Sometimes children do make a whole "book."

For the therapist, documentation also includes a description of the goal/theme addressed in the story, as well as the emotional themes of the child's play, the nature of the play and engagement, and any homework or symbols/gifts that were given. The therapist might also note ideas for future stories based on the child's play-response. In this way, the therapeutic story-dialogue continues.

Step 7: Homework/Application

The homework/application step encourages the therapist to think about ways that the story might be generalized beyond the therapy session.

The therapist might pose a thoughtful question for the child to ponder or give the questions as a specific assignment. Some stories easily lend themselves to homework. For instance, in the story "I'm Sorry" (Carroll Duffy, 2014d), the child learns the Montessori approach to solving conflict using the "The Peace Rose" (Jewell, 2006). As a way to generalize this skill, the child might be given homework to practice resolving a conflict like Maggie and Mucky moose do in the story. Caregivers might also have homework. For example, after hearing a story designed to encourage positive self-regard, the therapist might ask the parent to notice the positive qualities of his or her child.

Step 8: The Gift/Symbol

For the traumatized child, receiving a gift encourages relationship, conveys nurturing, and serves as a record of the therapy experience and a transitional object between sessions. After hearing a Moving Story, a symbol from the story becomes a gift, representing some aspect of importance to the child or perhaps symbolizing the experience itself. For example, in the story "Sammy Squirrel and the Nuts" (Greene, 2014) the gift might be an acorn.

Gifts need not cost money. Sets of ready-made symbols can be easily produced by using clipart or stickers. A "gift" might also be as simple as a picture of the sandtray story. If Moving Stories are a routine part of therapy, create a way to organize the gifts. For example, sandtray pictures can be printed on business-card-size stock and kept together in a business card contact sheet. A child can make a clay bowl or medicine bag to hold the gifts, or make a charm bracelet with a symbol from each story.

CASE EXAMPLE

This case example is based on a number of experiences with traumatized children using the story "The Giant" (Carroll Duffy, 2014c). In the story, Squirrel's forest friends leave when a fire approaches, and she is left hiding in the top of a giant sequoia. Squirrel experiences loneliness, sadness, and deep fear as she watches the forest burn. The world seems like it will never be the same, even after the fire is over. However, the fire brings something unexpected—baby sequoias and the beginning of a new forest. This story encourages resilience and hope in the

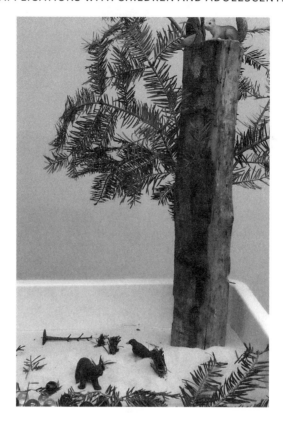

FIGURE 7.5. Sandtray scene from the story "The Giant" (Carroll Duffy, 2009b). Copyright 2014 by By The Sea Seminars/Susanne Carroll Duffy. Reprinted by permission.

face of loss and trauma. Figure 7.5 depicts a sandtray scene from the story.

Sarah's Moving Story Session

Sarah was a 10-year-old foster child whose mother had died. Exposed to domestic violence and substance abuse growing up, she presented with anxiety, nightmares, and depression. Sarah was in the middle stage of therapy. She had established coping skills, was showing less anxiety and depression, and she had made a friend. In the therapy room she found natural expression through stories in the sandtray. The therapist led the first part of the session, followed by a child-directed time where Sarah chose her response. Often her response was to fill the sandtray with many objects, sometimes expanding to a second tray.

Step 1: Story Selection, Kit Making, and Practice

"The Giant" was selected because it captured the emotional feelings of Sarah's trauma and loss as well as offered hope. The kit was made with a decorated box and filled with several forest animals from the sandtray shelves. The giant sequoia was made from a piece of firewood. A scarf was placed over "The Giant" so that Sarah would be surprised by the enormity of the tree when it was placed in the sandtray. The plan for the story was drawn on a piece of paper and rehearsed.

Step 2: Presentation

Sarah was told at the beginning of the session that there was a new story for her. She was excited and helped to set up the sandtray, creating the stream with a paintbrush to clear away the sand. As the story began, the therapist asked if she wanted to meet "The Giant." When she said, "Yes," with just a small bit of anxiety, the tree was presented and the scarf removed. Sarah was enthralled as the story unfolded. She helped by using red sand in a saltshaker to show the approaching fire. She used water from a saltshaker to show the cooling rains that put out the fire, and finally black sand to show the destruction left from the fire.

Step 3: Reflection

The therapist sensed Sarah's eagerness to play with the story and chose not to interrupt her engagement with "wondering" questions.

Step 4: Creative Response

After finishing the story, the therapist said, "Now it is your turn to play." Sarah chose to continue playing with the story in the sandtray in silence. She added water to the sand and made a cave for the forest animals. She made a bridge to cross the river. She found plants from the sandtray shelves and brought the forest back to life, filling the tray in her typical fashion. She found a fireman from the sandtray shelves and placed him by the animals. Sarah worked intently and quietly. The therapist mirrored her affect, also remaining quiet. Sarah had trouble getting some of the flowers to stand, so the therapist offered to help and she gladly accepted. Finally, Sarah looked up and said, "Done."

Step 5: Sharing

The therapist invited Sarah to tell her sandtray story. She described the animals coming back to the forest and needing new homes where they would be safe from all dangers. She liked the bear most because he was the strongest. She felt very sorry for the squirrel because she was left alone when the fire came. Then she thought about the giant tree, and decided the squirrel wasn't completely alone. As she talked, she decided to give them each food and went to the sandtray shelves to find nuts. The therapist listened intently and when she appeared to be done talking, said, "I wonder where you are in this story?" Sarah thought that she was "The Giant," having survived many storms.

Step 6: Documenting

After it was clear that she was done talking, the therapist invited her to take a picture of her story. The therapist summarized, "After the fire, each forest animal came back and made its own safe cave and ate nuts. The forest grew back." Sarah looked pleased with the summary and added, "Don't forget the fireman. He protects the animals and the forest so it does not happen again." The therapist added this important detail to her story and asked what to title it. Sarah replied, "Back Home." After Sarah left, the therapist put the picture, along with the story and title, in a binder together with Sarah's other stories.

Step 7: Homework/Application

Sarah was seen briefly with her foster mother at the end of the session. Given the theme of nurturing and home that arose from her story, they were encouraged to spend "special time" together during the next week. Sarah wanted to paint her bedroom with her foster mother.

Step 8: Gift/Symbol

Sarah was given a pinecone as a symbolic representation of the story experience and of "new beginnings." In future stories, the theme of safety continued as she made homes for other animals in the sandtray.

CONCLUSION

The Moving Stories method is an intermodal creative arts therapy process that provides an engaging approach for traumatized children to hear therapeutic messages and to respond in their own language—the language of play, symbols, and story. The eight steps in the method guide the therapist's interventions as both the storyteller and story-listener. It is a flexible tool that can be applied differently within a range of therapeutic models. While this chapter focused on the use of the method with individuals, traumatized children also benefit from it in the context of family sessions, groups, and the classroom. The first step in applying the method is opening oneself to the language of play, story, and sandtray. With a meaningful personal experience as a foundation, therapists can appreciate the profound and sacred language of our most vulnerable and resilient children.

REFERENCES

Badenoch, B. (2008). *Being a brain-wise therapist: A practical guide to interpersonal neurobiology.* New York: Norton.

Berryman, J. (2005). *The complete guide to godly play* (Vol. 1). New York: Church.

Carroll Duffy, S. (2014a). Black black bear. Perry, ME: By the Sea Seminars. Retrieved from: *http://bytheseaseminars.com/moving-stories-e-library.*

Carroll Duffy, S. (2014b). Emerging. Perry, ME: By the Sea Seminars. Retrieved from *http://bytheseaseminars.com/moving-stories-e-library.*

Carroll Duffy, S. (2014c). The giant. Perry, ME: By the Sea Seminars. Retrieved from: *http://bytheseaseminars.com/moving-stories-e-library.*

Carroll Duffy, S. (2014d). I'm sorry. Perry, ME: By the Sea Seminars. Retrieved from *http://bytheseaseminars.com/moving-stories-e-library.*

Carroll Duffy, S. (2014e). *Moving Stories method: A playful therapeutic storytelling method for the sandtray.* Perry, ME: By the Sea Seminars. Retrieved from *http://bytheseaseminars.com/moving-stories-e-library.*

Davis, N. (1996). Therapeutic stories that teach and heal. Available at *http://drnancydavis.org.*

De Domenico, G. (2000). *Sandtray-Worldplay^{TM}: A comprehensive guide to the use of sandtray in psychotherapy and transformational settings.* Oakland, CA: Vision Quest Images.

Drew, A., & Bratton, S. (2014). Play therapy. In E. Green & A. Drewes (Eds.), *Integrating expressive arts and play therapy with children and adolescents* (pp. 17–40). Hoboken, NJ: Wiley.

Gardner, R. (1993). *Storytelling in psychotherapy with children.* Northvale, NJ: Jason Aronson.

Gil, E. (2006). *Helping abused and traumatized children: Integrating directive and nondirective approaches.* New York: Guilford Press.

Greene, R. (2014). *Sammy squirrel and the nuts.* Perry, ME: By the Sea Seminars. Retrieved from *http://bytheseaseminars.com/moving-stories-e-library.*

Hynes, A., & Hynes-Berry, M. (2012). *Biblio/poetry therapy: The interactive process—a handbook.* St. Cloud, MN: North Star Press of St. Cloud.

Jewell, A. (2006). *The peace rose.* Santa Rosa, CA: Parent Child Press.

Kaufman, D., Chalmers, R., & Rosenberg, W. (2014). Poetry therapy. In E. Green & A. Drewes (Eds.), *Integrating expressive arts and play therapy with children and adolescents* (pp. 205–230). Hoboken, NJ: Wiley.

Kottman, T. (2001). *Partners in play.* Alexandria, VA: American Counseling Association.

Landreth, G. (2012). *Play therapy: The art of the relationship* (3rd ed.). New York: Routledge.

Mills, J., & Crowley, R. (1986). *Therapeutic metaphors for children and the child within.* New York: Brunner/Mazel.

O'Conner, K., & Ammen, S. (2012). *Play therapy treatment planning and interventions: The ecosystemic model and workbook.* Waltham, MA: Academic Press.

Perry, B. (2006). Applying principles of neurodevelopment to clinical work with maltreated and traumatized children. In N. B. Webb (Ed.), *Working with traumatized youth in child welfare* (pp. 27–52). New York: Guilford Press.

Simpson, L. (2014). *Claude flies a plane.* Perry, ME: By the Sea Seminars. Retrieved from *http://bytheseaseminars.com/moving-stories-e-library.*

Smith, S. (2012). *Sandtray play and storymaking.* Philadelphia: Jessica Kingsley.

Sunderland, M. (2008). *Using story telling as a therapeutic tool with children.* Milton Keyes, UK: Speechmark.

Tapio, P. (1975). *The woman who saw the good side of everything.* New York: Harper Collins Children's Books.

Turner, B., & Unnsteindsdottir, K. (2011). *Sandplay and storytelling: The impact of imaginative thinking on children's learning and development.* Cloverdale, CA: Temenos Press.

CHAPTER 8

Dance/Movement Therapy with Refugee and Survivor Children

A Healing Pathway Is a Creative Process

Amber Elizabeth Gray

Refugees, by definition, are displaced people. Whether they remain within the boundary of their own country as internally displaced people or have fled the borders of their country as refugees or asylum seekers, they have been exposed to some form of persecution, causing them to flee. These individuals have spent time in flight, are still in flight, or are being resettled in a completely new and strange world. For children, in particular, this is a harrowing, uncertain experience. Children's sense of safety, trust, and human relationship is undermined by this experience, and when family members, or the children themselves, experience torture, the foundations of safety, trust, and relationship can be devastated. This means that the experience of childhood—with its potential for healthy development and a strong foundation of what it is to be human—is marred by violence, fear, and even threat to life. Many of these children come from impoverished homes or they are literally abandoned by their own parents and experience the stigma associated with living on the streets. They also encounter ongoing rejection by the social body, compounding a long exposure to traumatic events and circumstances. All the magical, grounding, securing, and nurturing aspects of childhood that many of us take for granted are completely unknown to many refugee children and others who have survived adverse events.

It is often assumed that everyone who has been through a war, a hurricane, a flood, a shooting, or domestic violence is traumatized. Not all children exposed to traumatic events will be traumatized, however. But exposure to the experiences described in this chapter, especially during the developmentally critical period of life known as childhood, increases risks that children will meet diagnostic criteria for posttraumatic stress disorder (PTSD) or display trauma reactions; these children's lives are often altered in the short or long term.

Movement, as described by Perry (2014), may be a direct pathway to promote brain plasticity (or, literally "grow" our brains) and therefore promote learning capacities, healing, and a sense of well-being. This chapter addresses the application of dance/movement therapy (DMT) to work with children and adolescents, ages 6–18 years, who have experienced trauma. Most of the case examples described here occurred in two cross-cultural treatment settings: a former program for survivors of torture and war in Denver, Colorado, and in Haiti during the embargo years. After a brief theoretical introduction to DMT, case examples and references to theory and research, drawing from the fields of trauma-informed care, neuroplasticity, and the polyvagal theory (Porges, 2011), are offered as endorsement of this powerful somatic and creative arts therapy for children affected by exposure to traumatic events.

DANCE/MOVEMENT THERAPY

DMT is a holistic framework for a restorative process and a powerful therapy in the context of trauma-informed care. Describing the relationship between movement and the brain, Perry (2014) says that "the most powerful input into the lower part of the brain is from your body; the biggest feedback comes from somato-motoric information . . . [the] rhythmic loop of input and output between the body and the brain is soothing, regulating, and organizing. In a very real way, touch and movement grow the brain."

DMT is both a creative arts and a somatic psychotherapy. It is distinctly poised at the crossroads of these two classifications of therapies that are increasingly endorsed by neuropsychiatric research because it encompasses integration of bodily sensations, movement as a primary language, and the creative and expressive nature of dance. The arts, including dance, have been the voice of life experience far longer than medicine or psychology and have served people and communities as a means to process suffering, pain, celebration, and healing for eons.

DMT is defined as the psychotherapeutic use of movement to support integration of the mind, body, and spirit in the healing process (Levy, 2005). A core premise of DMT is that body movement reflects the inner emotional landscape (Kornblum & Halsten, 2006). Change on a physical level, such as change in movement behavior, posture, and muscular tension, have an effect on emotional functioning. Unlike practitioners of traditional forms of psychotherapy, dance/movement therapists believe that there is an intricate and undeniable connection between people's history, thoughts, feelings, and behaviors and their bodies (Levy, 2005).

DMT is a particularly powerful therapy for working with children affected by trauma who are actively engaged in achieving developmental milestones. Achieving these milestones can be seen as a creative process because a "successful" childhood is a rite of passage supported by structure, spontaneity, and exploration. One need only observe the soothing and regulating interaction between a loving caregiver and a distressed infant to witness the neurologically and affectively regulating structure provided by caregivers and a hopefully safe environment. This structure is enhanced by the periods of curiosity that guide a child's earliest movements, including lying on the floor; head orienting toward sounds or movements; and rocking, scooting, crawling, and eventually standing and walking. This sequential developmental movement process is actually a "spiral dance" between structure, as informed by our physiological development interacting with the environment, and a safe-enough environment where explorations and creative encounters with the space and people occur. These are the earliest underpinnings of our interoceptive and exteroceptive capacities. In fact, if we describe the developmental trajectory of childhood as a creative process, then the disruption to this process, instigated by wounding, trauma, or disease, can be restored only by engaging the child creatively. DMT allows people to "move through" the traumatic memories and experience the more benevolent memories as an aspect of embodied creative experience. In the words of Fran Ostroburski (2009), "Children tell their stories by using their bodies. Movement appears to be their preference. When an adult joins them in this preferred mode a child feels not only seen but heard" (p. 156).

DMT is a holistic approach to psychotherapy that integrates all aspects of the developing self: physical, emotional, cognitive, spiritual, and behavioral. It is also communal, social, and familial. To be alive is to be embodied and to move is to explore the most basic language of humanity: the language with which we all begin life. If movement is a primary language, than dance is the creative expression of our first language.

TRAUMA, MEMORY, AND DMT

Trauma memories in both adults and children are most often sensorimotoric and image-based memories (Herman, 1992; Rothschild, 2000; Terr, 1986; van der Kolk, 1994; van der Kolk, Hopper, & Osterman, 2001) or non-language-based "packages" (Siegel, 2012). Porges (2011) illuminates the root of these non-language-based memories as biological and physiological responses to danger and life threat during traumatic exposure that involves a reversion to more primitive behavioral and survival strategies. Siegel (2012) describes the instant of exposure as a moment when "the victim may focus his [or her] attention on a nontraumatic aspect of the environment or on his imaginations as a means of at least partial escape. Divided-attention studies suggest that this situation will lead to the encoding of parts of the traumatic experience implicitly but not explicitly."

As a body-based therapy, DMT can unlock the implicit memory of traumatic experience and access the imaginations that support a restoration of well-being. If the continuum of human language is described as beginning with sensation, sound, and movement (*in utero* and infancy) as a first means of communication and later moving to the world of symbols, imagination, and finally to spoken words, then movement and the imaginary, symbolic realms are valuable portals into a child's experience. Language development is the outcome of the sequential, somatically woven development trajectory from conception to personhood.

PORGES'S POLYVAGAL THEORY AND DMT

Polyvagal theory, proposed by Dr. Porges (2011), illuminates the evolution of the mammalian nervous system as an influence on human behavior. Polyvagal theory, from a clinical perspective, highlights the importance of safety and human relationship in the developmental process. Porges's work has restored and reinforced the notion that perhaps the most essential aspect of truly helpful, meaningful therapy is human connection in a safe environment. From a somatic perspective, our faces are the "go-to" place to detect features, or evidence, of safety in the interpersonal space. Porges describes the "rules of engagement" as dependent on prosody, gaze, facial expressivity, mood and affect, posture during social engagement, and state regulation (S. Porges, personal communication, May 25, 2010; Porges, 2011, pp. 191–192). Deficits in any of these components of social engagement may lead to disorders that are classified as mental illnesses.

Polyvagal theory describes social engagement as an emergent, adaptive behavior arising from the development of a branched (dorsal and ventral) nerve, the vagus nerve, also known as the 10th cranial nerve (formerly the pneumo-gastric nerve). This social engagement system describes the physiological, biological, and neurological processes that underpin and guide our interactions with the environment—all via the vagus nerve. (The term *social nervous system* refers to the five special efferents to striated muscles [somatomotor], cranial nerves [5, 7, 9, 10, 11] that innervate somatic muscles arising from the bronchial arches [which are descendants of primitive gill arches]). These more highly evolved structures are a result of the increased need for oxygen produced by evolution toward a more complex physiological system and the concomitant increase in metabolic demands. This social nervous system comprises the neural circuits involved in sucking, chewing, smiling, eye movements, vocalizations, and facial expressions, along with head turning and orientation and the heart–brain connection.

According to Porges's model, the vagus nerve (specifically, the *ventral* vagal neural circuitry associated with social engagement) has an inhibitory effect on the sympathetic adrenal neural circuit that guides our ability to mobilize when faced with danger. The ventral vagus nerve might be considered a "guiding star" in our ability to choose how we interact with an environment and those in it. This nerve pathway provides the neurological circuitry and cues that facilitate our social and relational capacity. Children, depending on their ages and developmental levels, rely on relationship and safety, as experienced through the facial expressions, eye contact, and smiles of others, as the way primary caregivers help them move in and out of the environment (space), their own bodies (weight), and their relationships with others (time) (see Table 8.1). Facial expressivity, gaze, prosody, and posture are primary nonverbal ways we communicate safety. In other words, it's not language but our *biology* that communicates safety. Somewhat more

TABLE 8.1. Practical Skills for Using Space, Weight, and Time Dimensions with Children

Considering how children use space, weight, and time is essential for assessment and intervention tools in DMT. These dimensions are the neurological, biological, and physiological basis of development and the abilities to socially engage, relate to others, and move and be in relationship with the world. The following activities combine these three dimensions and can be adapted for individual, family, or group work.

Space Bubble. For children and adolescents ages 4–18 years, the following activity can be tailored with age-appropriate language and enhanced with age- and culture-appropriate music.

1. What's your relationship to the space we are in, right now? Find the place in this room where you wish to begin. Establish your space bubble by standing on one foot and seeing how far your other leg and arms can extend into space. Imagine that your farthest reach is the edge of your personal space bubble.

2. Now, stand still inside your space bubble. If you want, imagine the color and shape of your space bubble. Make any adjustments to size you need to— perhaps you don't want it to extend as far as you can reach, for example. [With latency-age children, imagining their space bubble as the colors or shape or characteristics of an action character or hero can be helpful; with adolescents, heroes or favorite people or symbols can decorate or tattoo the space bubble.]

3. Remaining inside your space bubble, begin to look around you at the space outside your space bubble. How do you feel in this space? [If children need verbal cues, you can cue them using words such as *safe, comfortable, familiar, happy,* or *scared* in a questioning tone of voice.] Look at all the other people in our space bubbles. How do you feel knowing that all these other people are in the same space as you?

4. When you are ready, leave your space bubble and begin to walk through the space. As you walk, pay attention to your weight by noticing how hard or soft your feet land on the floor. Do you feel your whole foot on the floor? Does your whole foot land at the same time, or does the front or back of your foot touch first? How would you describe the way your foot lands on the floor? [Note: The contact between foot and floor is an expression of weight.] Does each foot land on the floor the same, or are they different?

5. Keep moving and feel yourself becoming very, very heavy. With every step (or every exhale) you get heavier and heavier. Now notice how your feet land on the floor. Has this changed?

6. Keep moving and getting heavier. Is walking getting easier? Harder? More or less comfortable? When you get heavier, how do you feel in [or relate to] this space? Remember how you felt inside your space bubble? Do you feel the same or differently now that you are heavy? Is it comfortable to move while you are heavy? Is it easy or hard to move when you are heavy?

7. Stand still. What's it like to be still and heavy? How long can you hold yourself up?

(continued)

TABLE 8.1. *(continued)*

8. Let that feeling of heavy go. Popcorn style, feel free to share any words or phrases that describe how heavy feels to you. [Note: The facilitator can jot down these words or phrases to refer to later in terms of the client's inner states, emotions, images, and beliefs.]

9. Begin to walk again and notice if your walking and the way your feet land has changed. If it has, this is a change in your sense of weight.

10. Now imagine that you are growing lighter and lighter with every footstep [or breath]. As you get lighter and lighter, notice what happens to your weight. Do your feet meet the floor the same way? Do your feet spend as much time on the floor? Pretend you can fly and notice the relationship between your feet and the floor. How does this experience feel? [Again, offer age-appropriate verbal cues, if necessary, such as posing possibilities like *free, scary, grounded,* or *ungrounded.*] For the next few moments, become as light as you can possibly be and feel what it's like to move through the space.

11. Does it feel like the space we are moving in is changing? If so, how?

12. Take a break from walking and be still. How do you feel, standing in this space? Can you remember what you felt like when you first stood in your space bubble? How do you feel now? How did being light affect you?

13. Now let's play with time. We are going to vary our speed as we move through space. Let's begin by going fast—as fast as you can go! Keep moving, faster and faster and faster! What's it like to move through this space, fast? Is it comfortable to be moving this fast, with all the other people in the same space? How do you feel moving this fast in a room full of other fast-moving people: Confident? Frightened? Joyful? Silly? Stressed?

14. Take a break from "fast" and be still for a moment. What do you notice in your body? How does moving fast affect your heart and breathing? If you want, share words or phrases that describe how you are feeling now. You can describe body feelings [sensations], body actions [i.e., physiology], emotions or feelings, or any thoughts you might be having. [Again, if verbal cues are needed, say possibilities such as *prickly* (sensation), *heart racing* (physiology); *excited* (feelings), and *crazy* (thoughts).]

15. Okay, now let's try "slow." Begin to move really, r-e-a-l-l-y, r—e—a—l—l—y slowly. How does your sense of weight change? Do you feel more or less of your feet on the floor? Does it feel different to move through this space safely, when you can only go slowly? Does the room full of people also moving feel different now, from when we moved fast? If so, how?

16. Now go as slowly as you can go—slower, slower, slower, until you stop moving. Stand where you are. Again, notice your body, your feelings, and your thoughts.

17. Look around. How does the space seem to you now? How do you feel in this space?

18. Go back to your original space bubble and get inside it. Notice if it seems the same or different as you look around this space from inside your own space bubble now. If it feels different, in what way? Is it in your weight? Your sense of time [i.e., do you feel faster or slower now]? Your body, feelings, or thoughts? Share anything aloud you want to about how you feel right now.

(continued)

TABLE 8.1. *(continued)*

19. Look around at the room of other people in their bubbles. What do you think or feel about all these people now?
20. Is your space bubble still the same size and color? With the same decorations?
21. Share anything you would like to about this experience.

For younger children (4–8 years) the activity can be simplified and more playful. For example, using imaginative language and music helps to stimulate movement. Choose a song the children like and that gets them moving. Then invite children to play, using cues:

- "Float like clouds . . . float like a buoy on the waves . . . float like an angel."
- "Pop! Like popcorn in an air popper!"
- "Walk like your feet are stuck in the mud. Or like you are barefoot on snow!"
- "Ride the waves of a storm."
- "Drift like an autumn leaf falling from a tree. Let the wind toss you around!"
- "Move like an elephant . . . a snake . . . a leopard . . . a kangaroo."

theoretically, I would add that because "vocalizations are a reflection of the vagal regulation of the heart" (Porges, 2013, p. 10), facial expression, prosody, and gaze might literally be considered as reflections of the heart. The neural connections that mediate social engagement are the same as those involved in states of health, well-being, and restoration. DMT directly accesses the neurological underpinnings of human behavior described by Porges because it incorporates facial expressivity, vocalization, listening, changes in the dynamics of movement (i.e., "movement prosody"), and muscle tonus and actions.

DEVELOPMENT, CHILDHOOD TRAUMA, AND DMT

Like developmental psychology, DMT posits that human development is a sequential process involving both inner and outer worlds. What DMT integrates, perhaps more dynamically and explicitly than other practices, is engagement with the body as the site of all human experience. An individual can communicate memory, even when it is not explicitly recalled, through posture, muscle tone, breathing, and movement patterns. Children exposed to and affected by trauma may carry these patterns well into adult life if they are not addressed and processed by literally moving "stuck" energy. Although there is tremendous power in all psychotherapies that are evidence-based or considered best or promising practices, only those with a strong creative and somatic basis truly engage the whole child.

Lewis's (1986) seminal writing about DMT describes this point in language similar to Perry's (2013) description of state-dependent development. Describing a holistic framework for development, Lewis writes that an individual develops in relationship to the self as "an integrated unity; mind and body reflect and affect each other" (p. 280)—an aspect of human development that dance/movement therapists observe in the links between muscle tonus and psychic expression. Furthermore, an individual's "mind, body, organic functioning, and behavior are interwoven with the environment" (p. 280). From a DMT perspective, development is described as organized and sequential: "Each phase of development has its somatic and physiological elements as well as its psycho-social aspects, all of which interrelate and are necessary for healthy development" (p. 280). Perry's description of the basis of development, learning, and memory reflects a neuroplasticity perspective; that is, "the more a neural system is 'activated,' the more that system changes to reflect that pattern of activation." In the language of DMT, learning and memory are:

> developmentally related, intermeshed somatic experiences, unconscious material and conscious behavior . . . stored in the body and . . . reflected in the breathing, posturing, and movement of an individual. Present experience may be influenced by and trigger past stored experience bringing past behavior to present. Movement, because of its neurologic historically primitive origins, can more easily tap into this developmentally based schema than other more sophisticated forms of communication such as verbalization. (Lewis, 1986, p. 279)

The previously described image of soothing and regulating interaction between an infant and caregiver is what Lewis describes as "development viewed within an interactional system" (1986, p. 280). Lewis's somewhat dated explanation of this interaction is strongly endorsed by the current theories and discoveries in the field of interpersonal neurobiology, which describe the science behind human behavior (Perry, 2013; Porges, 2011; Siegel, 1999, 2012, 2013). The language of human development is sensorimotoric and movement-based, and is facilitated through a relationship between the infant and the significant other (Lewis, 1986). Stern (1985) describes *affect attunement* using this very movement-based example:

> A nine month old girl becomes very excited about a toy and reaches for it. As she grabs it, she lets out an exuberant "aaaah!" and looks at her mother. Her mother looks back, scrunches up her shoulders and performs a terrific shimmy with her upper body, like a go-go dancer. The shimmy lasts only about as long as her daughter's "aaaah!" but is equally excited, joyful and intense. (p. 140)

Thus our earliest foundational relationship is carried out primarily through sensorimotor engagement. Because body movement is viewed as the most primary mode of communication, many dance/movement therapists contend that it can be applied to work with all individuals, no matter what the age, dysfunction, or cultural heritage (Lewis, 1986, p. 281). However, culture is a powerful mediating variable that will inform what movement looks like. Biology is the universal factor; culture is what varies our nonverbal communication styles and meanings.

Developmental Case Example: Amanda

This case example illustrates the major concepts presented in the previous section. A 16-year-old girl, Amanda, joined extended family in the United States after fleeing her home country's long-term civil conflict in which people were brutally slaughtered and their bodies regularly left in the open. She fled on foot to a neighboring country and, then with the help of family, came to the United States as an asylum seeker. Born and raised in East Africa, she grew up, and loved, dancing.

When I first met with Amanda, her body posture and movement were literally frozen from a series of immobilized moments during her terrifying flight, including multiple assaults and rapes. Her family brought her to me for treatment because she was not sleeping, dissociated frequently (or as they said, "just went away"), and was no longer the social, friendly girl they knew before they had moved to the United States. Her range of motion was limited, she had flat affect, and she often disappeared to her room when at home. She was disengaged from life.

Because she would not engage in movement or dance, we began with the symbolic or imaginary realm, and worked with a sandtray. The war began when she was 8 years old, during the period of childhood when the primary language of movement expands to include culturally relevant images and symbols. Because she seemed so afraid all the time, I decided that the sandtray might offer a relatively safe portal into the experiences that had captured her attentional, cognitive, and affective worlds. I have often found this imaginative portal to be as powerful as the body in both recalling and healing trauma, but it can literally feel like a minefield of painful and overwhelming sensory- and image-based shards if approached too quickly in the therapeutic process. As part of a trauma-informed and neurosequential approach, moving at the client's pace can mean approaching the integrative power of the body quite slowly. The first (and ongoing) phase of treatment, as endorsed by early research on complex trauma (Herman, 1997; van der Kolk, 2002), is to promote safety and stability. The relatively safe language of images can support this phasic process. Also, by beginning with a link to the "upstairs" (Siegel, 2012) or higher brain, it is safer to work toward the integration of the lower ("downstairs") brain, and more sensorimotoric aspects of the trauma memory.

Amanda's first two sandtrays contained large bugs and snakes, and she did not have much to say about them. She simply sat there, hunched over with flat affect and a distracted, faraway gaze, limply placing the objects in the sand. I observed quietly, asked a few questions, and did not push.

The third sandtray was much more complex. Amanda arrived with a little more energy in her step that day; movement of energy, as it flows through the body, is a key informant for assessment in DMT. She created a clear diagonal divide through the middle of the tray and created a river. On one side of the river there were images of war: soldiers and tanks, people fallen over, the color red spilled everywhere, and her usual large bugs and snakes. On the other side of the river was a bucolic village scene of a happy family, seated around a table inside a home that was surrounded by trees and gardens. When she finished, we looked at her creation together in silence and then I asked her how she felt looking at this tray. She immediately burst into tears, and continued to cry for the remainder of the session. When her brother arrived, she asked if he could come in and the three of us sat together; he also was moved to tears. She had never spoken of what had happened. In this moment she simply said: "The rest of them are gone; they came one day and killed my family."

When Amanda returned a week later, I asked if she was ready to move; she agreed. From a somatic and movement perspective she already appeared changed: The vertical dimension, as described in Laban movement analysis (Tortura, 2006), was more evident. This posture can be evidence of a more deeply inhabited sense of self and a willingness or ability to take a stand. Verticality reveals one's relationship to weight, which in my DMT-based trauma and resiliency framework (Gray, in press) is a measure of our presence. Amanda's movement already demonstrated more dimensionality. (The three most basic dimensions of movement are horizontal, vertical, and sagittal; these are common modes of assessment, diagnosis, and treatment in DMT; Tortura, 2006.) The "kinesphere" (essentially a "personal space bubble") is also an effective measure of an individual's comfort and ability to interact with the surrounding space (including the environment and those who inhabit it). A thorough explanation of the bodies of work that elucidate these dimensions (Laban movement analysis [Newlove & Dalby, 2004], body–mind centering [Bainbridge Cohen, 2012], and Bartenieff fundamentals [Bartenieff, 2002]) are beyond the scope of this chapter.

In order to document change, I asked Amanda to explore her kinesphere or personal space bubble with me. The easiest way to do this is to stand in one place, supported by one leg, if possible, and see how far you can extend your other leg, arms, and even head and tail into the space around you. This establishes your kinesphere, which can be indicative of social and relational capacity and a willingness or ability to explore the environment and relate to others. Once we had established Amanda's kinesphere, we agreed it was time to dance.

Amanda chose a favorite song, a cultural resource of hers from the group she also participated in: Congolese musician Papa Wemba's "Sala Keba." We began standing together and stepped our feet in unison. This matching of external tempos is a typical DMT "intervention": We are kinesthetically empathizing with the individual and promoting cohesion or relational connection through shared rhythm, intensity, effort (a Laban movement analysis concept), and movement. According to Schmais (1985), "rhythm helps to stimulate and to organize the individual's behavior as well as to put him [or her] in time and in step with others" (p. 30); in other words, moving in rhythm promotes shared experience and therefore relationship. Berrol (1992) summarizes several studies that demonstrate how rhythm affects physiological responses: "Emotional perception of music has a significant effect on autonomic responses—e.g., changes in pulse rate, galvanic skin response, and blood pressure. . . . Bodily rhythms and activities appear to regulate to external rhythmic stimuli, matching tempi" (p. 25), which can help regulate emotions. Soon Amanda began to swing, an early developmental movement that, like rocking, can soothe and regulate. Eventually she included her arms in the swinging movement, which began to bring her whole body into movement in place.

Although this movement did not flow sequentially through all of Amanda's body (i.e., there were "stiff," "stuck," and unmoving body parts), she *was* moving. She identified feelings of freedom and comfort, like being "a baby rocked by its mother." We worked with the imagined: rocking our babies together. We varied rocking from slow and small to large and fast; we varied the shape of the rocking (arced and curved vs. more "pointy" or staccato rhythms). This variance in rhythmicity helps clients negotiate the physiological underpinnings of the emotions that can get too intense to bear. The more variability in rhythm a person can tolerate, the more variability in expression and emotion. A primary tenet of DMT is that movement repertoire is directly related to our expressivity. As I encouraged, through mirroring her movements and altering them slightly (kinesthetic attunement), she moved a little more, included more of her body, made more eye contact, and even smiled a little.

I asked what Amanda wished to name her baby, and she gave it the name "Freedom." I named mine "Freedom 2" to underscore her metaphor of birthing freedom that we talked about as part of our discussion following the movement. She stated a desire to be free of the haunting feelings of grief and loneliness that often overwhelmed her. We finished this session by tucking our babies in until the next time. This process of imagining that began with the sandtray and moved into the rocking of imaginary babies related our dance to the memories she had of a happy family where there was a baby (her youngest sister, killed in the massacre). Rocking may stimulate vagal tone if it is based on a pelvic tilt (Cottingham, Porges, & Lyons, 1988) because it is a movement that engages the natural tilting, rocking, and "wheel-like" movement of the sacrum (DMT pioneer Liljan Espanak used this rocking motion extensively for movement diagnostic tests; Levy, 2005).

In our next session, we resumed by "untucking" the babies and continuing the rocking, which soon turned into a dance of flying—and we became birds. We playfully moved in place, and eventually, several sessions later, around the room together, playing with being birds flying through different types of wind and weather. The dimensionality of her movement had shifted visibly; all three dimensions and the movement planes described in Laban movement analysis were evident. We closed by rocking ourselves instead of our imagined babies. A final exploration of Amanda's kinesphere was very different; she now inhabited a larger space bubble and moved more freely and fluidly within it. She soon began to invite friends over after school, joined the soccer team, and enthusiastically went on to college after she graduated high school. She also provided her own testimony at her asylum hearing, and bravely recounted what had happened to her family multiple times for the judge.

This example of movement and dance exploration demonstrates that giving symbolic and movement "language" to the experience helps dampen the unbearable affect (Siegel, 2012) and support a process of meaning making, the third phase in Siegel's (2012) somatic and movement-based framework for children. Children make meaning through sensory- and image-based cues and memories to which they connect (both traumatic and benevolent cues/memories). Amanda and I spent several sessions talking about birds from her area of the world and how their ability to fly offers them a means to escape; she was the only one in the family who escaped the massacre.

We spent many sessions working through the grief and loss, verbally and through sandtrays full of images of birds flying toward freedom and away from the war images she still created in the tray, albeit with engaged affect and a willingness and ability to talk about what had happened. She actually described the massacre that had befallen her family, and we realized that the river was the divide that she had created between her happy childhood and the horrors of that day and the ongoing war. The sandtray images served as the portal into the sensorimotoric memories and their physical expression through movement, which reconnected fragments of memory with a coherent narrative about her life, allowing her to place the trauma in the context of a broader history and to make meaning of that past and the present—and even begin to think about a future.

CULTURE, TRAUMA, AND DMT

Cross-cultural psychotherapy is an increasingly relevant endeavor for anyone working with trauma. An important aspect (it may even be the most important) of trauma-informed care is cultural sensitivity. An open, inquiring mind that allows the therapist to engage with a child through learning as much as possible about that child's culture may "make or break" the therapy.

Children's cultures, especially those children displaced from homes, families, countries, and all the contexts that provide regulating familiarity, human relationship, and comfort, are essential ingredients to the fundamental experience of human connection that supports a positive attachment in the therapeutic encounter. In a cross-cultural context, the Western perspective on resistance or "stuckness" in therapy can often be reframed as a clash of cultures. What is relevant in our worldview may not be as relevant to another person, especially a child. Although children may not have the complex understanding of, or ability to describe, culture, what they carry in their nonverbal, somatically enmeshed physiological memory is an interoceptive aspect of that very culture.

Figure 8.1, from the "*Poto Mitan*" (Haitian Kreyol for "The Center Post" or "Center Space") Trauma and Resiliency Framework for refugees and survivors of war and torture, illustrates a revision of the cognitive-behavioral triangle. This figure represents the basis of many of the effective evidence-based and trauma-specific practices for child trauma: the basic premise that our thoughts and feelings influence our behavior. The focus on cognitive interventions places thoughts at the apex of the triangle. Figure 8.2 is a more conceptual framework that acknowledges some of the principles of trauma-informed care. Central to this framework is *culture* as an important mitigating influence in both a person's resiliency or available resources and his or her understanding of the meaning of traumatic experience. The memories, our coping skills, and our healing resources restore our place in the world; a sense of "belonging" after traumatic experience is significantly linked to culture. "Belonging and meaning making" (Phase 3 in treatment) might be considered the ultimate treatment goals for those who seek therapy due to displacement. A sense of displacement may not be limited

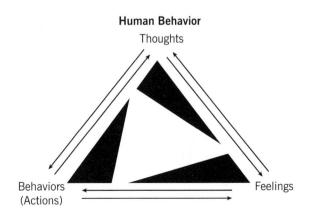

FIGURE 8.1. A traditional cognitive-behavioral triangle.

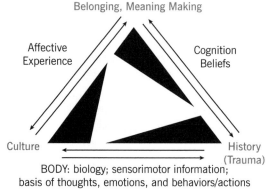

Human Behavior:
Adjusting the Framework
for Culture, Context, and the Body

FIGURE 8.2. The restorative process triangle.

to those with life experience as refugees; many people who come to therapy, especially children, can be conceptually understood as feeling "alone," "unsupported," "not sure where or why I am in the world." The question of meaning underscores most therapeutic inquiries. In a sense, all young clients can be perceived as seeking a way to belong, whether its learning to be comfortable in their own skin, or to participate in a family, social, or communal system that feels uncertain, strange, or unsafe to them now.

Cloitre, Cohen, and Koenen (2006) speak about the necessity of placing the trauma in the context of the broader history of a child's life. In doing so, we encourage a person not to be identified as his or her trauma. When using DMT, we are literally delving into cultural history through body and movement; the human body is literally how we know where we are.

Cross-Cultural Case Example: Emmanuel

Emmanuel is a 12-year-old Haitian male who was found on the streets during the embargo years (1990–1994), which were particularly violent in Haiti. Many street children like Emmanuel were imprisoned and brutally beaten, tortured, and abused, both in prison and on the streets. The culture of street children, sadly, is a mainstay of Haiti's collective culture due to the immense conditions of impoverishment and lack of educational opportunities there.

When I met Emmanuel, he was living in a group home for boys who were either developmentally challenged or traumatized by their experiences, or both. Group homes of this sort are also part of Haiti's unique culture; the term *lakou* refers, simplistically, to a gathering space that can be neighborly or spiritual. (After the earthquake of January 12, 2010, many demolished neighborhoods gathered in their *lakous* to collectively strategize food gathering and cooking, watching children unable to go to school, and conducting night watches. Households are large and exist in small spaces in Haiti. Group living is a common cultural response to displacement.) Even at the age of 12, Emmanuel was nonverbal; he communicated with sounds (grunts, snorts, laughs, etc.) only. He had an eternal smile on his face that literally looked as if it were pasted on. His gaze was distracted; he would only make eye contact for a moment and then look around, sometimes wildly. His affect was monotonous and his movement very stiff and disconnected. He moved robotically.

It bears noting that fluid movement is an aspect of culture in Haiti. Although it is never possible to generalize a movement style to an entire population, Haitian dance, which is core to the history and context of Haiti as the first black republic in the world, has as its central movement style a fluid and ongoing undulation of the spine. It is truly uncommon to see stiff body movement in Haiti, even among those who spend long days physically laboring.

When I entered the space in which Emmanuel lived, which was run by a home for former street boys who had "adopted" this residential program when a French nongovernment organization (NGO) was about to abandon it, he would follow me, even if I were working with other children. My role was to train local staff in simple movement-based therapeutic interventions for this household of abandoned children.

When I turned my attention fully to Emmanuel, he would smile a little more; this smile seemed more embodied. He followed closely, often entering my kinesphere, and would attempt to imitate almost any movement I made. So I began to do a kinesphere exploration, which along with his stiff smile and movement, defined his baseline response. His first kinesphere exploration was unstable, fragmented, and tight.

Over several weeks, we spent time each day in movement explorations that I intentionally invited, nonverbally, so that Emmanuel could expand his movement repertoire, increase the fluidity of his movement and negotiation of space, and increase his facial expressivity. Facing one another, we began with shaping our smiles. I would intentionally change my smile to be bigger, smaller, open-mouthed, close-mouthed, or round-mouthed and invite him to mirror me. Eventually I shifted from leading to following him, and attuning, rather than mirroring, my facial expressions to his explorations of different shapes and sizes of smiles.

Over a series of several visits, we began to expand these movement explorations to include more of the body. Using stretch bands, I faced Emmanuel and with the band under my feet, stretched it side to side (horizontal) "as wide as I possibly can!" and then let it come back in. We varied the direction of shaping our bodies in space from the horizontal (side–side; space), vertical (up–down; weight), and sagittal (front–back; time) dimensions of movement, which follows a natural developmental progression.

Eventually I began mixing up the sequencing of these dimensional movement explorations, increasing the complexity of our movement from dimensions to planes (planes consist of two dimensions) and then into more multidimensional movement sequences that resembled free-form dancing. We then took this movement into locomotion, alternating who led and who followed and alternating rhythms between slow and fast, heavy and light, tight and free. Oscillations of rhythms, especially when they are reinforced by externally changing tempos (as can be facilitated with the use of culturally congruent music) can provide a feedback loop to internal or endogenous rhythms of the human body. The three most influential endogenous rhythms of well-being are heart rate, respiration, and vascular feedback (related to blood pressure) (Porges & Gray, 2002). These rhythms all change in states of social engagement, mobilization (i.e., fear due to danger; energizing or pleasure in non-fear-related states of play), and immobilization (i.e., due to life threat or blissful surrender to deep safety and relaxation) (Porges, 2011; Porges & Gray, 2002).

Occasionally we paused and faced one another, intended to foster a sense of relational capacity and reciprocity. I added sounds to mirror and attune with the movements, and sometimes we stopped and vocalized sizes and shapes instead of moving. We always ended sessions with a kinesphere exploration; Emmanuel's kinesphere expanded and his movement exploration was more fluid and coherent. He no longer followed me closely and stiffly; he eased in and out of differing spatial relationships to me and began to show some initiative and innovation in his leadership of facial expressions and movements. Over time (multiple visits over a period of 2 years, working with myself and others), Emmanuel's smile softened and the range of his facial expressivity increased. Eye gaze, prosody of his vocalizations, and his overall movement expanded. He was able to lead other children in the home in similar movement explorations after a year of these sessions.

Summary of Case Example and Interventions

Initially, Emmanuel's smile appeared almost as if he were being forced to smile; there was no affect connected to it. My first intervention was literally to expand the repertoire of his smile, both to promote attachment and to stimulate or invigorate the social nervous system (Porges, 2011, p. 37) and promote social engagement. Emmanuel's robotic movement style was imbalanced, according to the Laban system (Tortura, 2006); he moved indirectly and seemed incapable of direct movement approaches; he had no levity in his movement, so was always moving in chunky, strong efforts rather than fluidly, which lighter movement effort might afford him; and whether standing, sitting, or in motion, his movement was bound and unflowing. His movement repertoire was limited to a very stiff, heavy lifting of the arms and stomping; the energetic sequencing did not go beyond his knees. His upper legs and pelvic floor appeared to be uninvolved with his locomotion. Even though he tried to interact, he would continue to smile in his disengaged way while playing ball, mirroring my movements, or interacting with the other children.

My work with Emmanuel typifies DMT goals of facilitating an expansion of and connection to his expressive capacity through a movement repertoire. I used mirroring as a classic intervention in DMT; it offers an opportunity to see, and be seen, which is the basis of reciprocity and relationship. In order to provide the structure that was likely missing from his development, I used props to create a safe transitional space in therapy. Using stretch bands, I performed simple horizontal and vertical shaping exercises, and using my voice (prosody) and face (expressivity), I invited Emmanuel to imitate exactly what I was doing. Initially, he did so with minimal expression and engagement. By using my voice as a cue and by expanding my movement repertoire with simple verbal cues and fluctuating my intonation ("Let's make it R—E—A—L—L—Y B—I—G"; "Let's make it R—E—A—L—L—Y S—M—A—L—L"), Emmanuel began to smile and maintain eye contact more regularly. He also began to move the muscles of his face more, and as he did, his movement repertoire expanded (i.e., he made bigger movements) while maintaining his core support. Instead of falling or teetering to the side, he was able to stay centered and continue to make a variety of movements that ranged in size and shape. These changes evidenced an increased ability to move with his natural fluidity, to play with and relate to other children in his environment, be in relationship, and to socially engage.

CONCLUSION

DMT is a deeply embodied therapeutic modality that engages mind, body, and heart in a restorative process. The interventions presented in this chapter vary from (1) inviting and mirroring developmental movements, to (2) making expressive faces and smiles, to (3) engaging children in the symbolic realm at the earliest phases of treatment, and to (4) using vocalizations and sound as an extension of movement. DMT promotes social engagement and a restoration to well-being for children, regardless of age or culture. The stimulation of the social nervous system that occurs through the promotion of reciprocal exchange between child client and therapist engages the underpinnings of our capacities to relate and be in the world (i.e., relational and social capacity). Movement is the most fundamental and primary mode of communication that is the root of all other modes of human connection and communication, and dance is its most potent expression. DMT has the potential to assist young clients in making meaning of both terrible and wonderful childhood experiences, integrating these experiences into the long or short trajectory of their lives, and restoring their deepest sense of belonging in the world.

REFERENCES

Bainbridge Cohen, B. (2012). *Sensing, feeling and action: The experiential anatomy of body–mind centering.* Toronto: Contact Editions.

Bartenieff, I. (2002). *Body movement: Coping with the environment.* New York: Routledge.

Berrol, C. (1992). The neurophysiologic basis of the mind/body connection in dance/movement therapy. *American Journal of Dance Therapy, 14*(1), 19–29.

Cloitre, M., Cohen, L. R., & Koenen, K. C. (2006). *Treating survivors of childhood abuse: Psychotherapy for the interrupted life.* New York: Guilford Press.

Cottingham, J., Porges, S., & Lyons, T. (1988). Effects of soft tissue mobilization (Rolfing pelvic life) on parasympathetic tone in two age groups. *Journal of American Physical Therapy,* 68(3), 352–356.

Gray, A. E. (in press). The broken body: Somatic perspectives on surviving torture. In S. L. Brooke & C. E. Myers (Eds.), *Therapists creating a cultural tapestry: Using the creative therapies across cultures.* Springfield, IL: Charles C. Thomas.

Herman, J. (1997). *Trauma and recovery.* New York: Basic Books.

Kornblum, R., & Halsten, R. L. (2006). In school dance movement therapy for traumatized children. In S. Brooke (Ed.), *Creative arts therapies manual: A guide to the history, theoretical approaches, assessment, and work with special populations of art, play, dance, music, drama, and poetry therapies* (pp. 144–155) Springfield, IL: Charles C. Thomas.

Levy, F. (2005). *Dance/movement therapy: A healing art.* Reston, VA: National Dance Association, American Alliance for Health, Physical Education, Recreation, and Dance.

Lewis, P. (1986). *Theoretical approaches in dance-movement therapy* (Vol. I). Dubuque, IA: Kendall/Hunt.

Newlove, J., & Dalby, J. (2004). *Laban for all.* New York: Routledge.

Ostroburski, F. (2009). Dance movement therapy as primary treatment. *Dance Therapy Collections,* 3, 151–157.

Perry, B. D. (2013). *Integrating principles of neurodevelopment into clinical practice: Introduction to the neurosequential model of therapeutics (NMT).* National Council for Behavioral Health webinar.

Perry, B. D. (2014). *The moving child: Supporting early development through movement* [Film]. Vancouver, Canada. Available at *www.themovingchild.com.*

Porges, S. (2011). *The polyvagal theory: Neurophysiological foundations of emotions, attachment, communication, self-regulation.* New York: Norton.

Porges, S. (2013, February). *Body, brain, behavior: How polyvagal theory expands our healing paradigm.* NICABM Webinar Session, New Brain Science 2013 Webinar Series.

Porges, S., & Gray, A. E. (2002, October). *DMT and the polyvagal theory.* PowerPoint presentation at the annual conference of the American Dance Therapy Association, Burlington, VT.

Rothschild, B. (2000). *The body remembers: The psychophysiology of trauma and trauma treatment.* New York: Norton.

Schmais, C. (1985). Healing processes in group dance therapy. *American Journal of Dance Therapy,* 8, 17–36.

Siegel, D. J. (1999). *The developing mind: How relationships and the brain interact to shape who we are.* New York: Guilford Press.

Siegel, D. (2012, March 28). *Bringing out the best in kids: Strategies for working with the developing mind*. Webinar session of the National Institute for the Clinical Application of Behavioral Medicine (*www.nicabm.com*).

Siegel, D. (2013, January 16). *The mind lives in two places: Inside your body, embedded in the world*. Webinar session of the National Institute for the Clinical Application of Behavioral Medicine (*www.nicabm.com*).

Stern, D. (1985). *The interpersonal world of the infant: A view from psychoanalysis and developmental psychology*. New York: Basic Books

Terr, L. (1990). *Too scared to cry*. New York: Basic Books.

Tortura, S. (2006). *The dancing dialogue: Using the communicative power of movement with young children*. Baltimore: Brookes.

van der Kolk, B. (1994). The body keeps the score?: Memory and the evolving psychobiology of post traumatic stress. *Harvard Review of Psychiatry, 1*(5), 253–265.

van der Kolk, B. (2002). The assessment and treatment of complex PTSD. In R. Yehuda (Ed.), *Treating trauma survivors with PTSD* (pp. 127–156). Arlington, VA: American Psychiatric Press.

van der Kolk, B., Hopper, J. W., & Osterman, J. E. (2001). Exploring the nature of traumatic memory: Combining clinical knowledge with laboratory science. In J. J. Freyd & A. P. DePrince (Eds.), *Trauma and cognitive science: A meeting of minds, science and human experience* (pp. 9–31). Binghamton, NY: Haworth Press.

CHAPTER 9

The Clay Field and Developmental Trauma in Children

Cornelia Elbrecht

Touch is the most fundamental of human experiences. Infants rely on touch to feel safe and loved; to be rocked and held soothes them and regulates their nervous system. We comfort each other through a hug; friends are "in touch" with each other; we relax with the touch of a massage. Our body rhythms synchronize through touch (Orbach, 2009). Love and sexuality, as well as violence, are primarily communicated through touch. Our skin boundary is invaded through inappropriate touching such as abuse, and accidents and medical procedures may also be experienced as invasive. The vast majority of traumatic memories involve some form of touch.

Work at the Clay Field® as a therapeutic modality was developed by Heinz Deuser (2004, 2006, 2007, 2009) over the past 40 years in Germany for children from 2 years of age through adulthood. The Clay Field is a rectangular flat wooden box that can hold up to 33 pounds (15 kg) of smooth, nongritty clay. A bowl of warm water is supplied along with a sponge. Some cups of different sizes and tools such as an ice cream scoop are also provided. The clay offers children a world to explore: It is pliable, yet has weight; presents resistance; and is a mass much larger than the hands. The box as a safe container is a crucial element in this setting, providing permanence and boundaries.

For many children trauma is a preverbal experience. Failures of infant–caregiver attunement, early medical procedures, and abuse experiences are imprinted in implicit memory and are nonconceptual and nonlinguistic. Stored in implicit memory are the memories of shapes and forms; of motor skills, habits, and routines; and of our emotional and relational responses (Heller & LaPierre, 2012, p. 112). Implicit memory makes us "feel" who we are; it defines our identity and it does not feel like a memory. When young children's *bodies* have been mistreated, they *feel* bad and therefore *think* they are bad, but do not know why. A top-down cognitive approach is rarely effective with implicit memories. Through establishing a bottom-up, sensorimotor way of working at the Clay Field, no story needs to be remembered. However, lost or neglected aspects of the self can gradually be repaired and reclaimed through the felt sense (Gendlin, 1981).

Work at the Clay Field is grounded in theories of human development, object relations, sensorimotor perception, and haptic perception. Although the Clay Field is a specific therapeutic approach that requires years of training, it is important for therapists who use creative arts in treatment to become more aware of the impact and importance of using clay work with children, as well as the necessity for body-focused approaches. This chapter explains the basic premises that form the foundation of Clay Field therapy, emphasizing the unique role it can play to help children who have experienced developmental trauma.

DEVELOPMENTAL TRAUMA

From infancy throughout early childhood, children need consistently attuned caregivers to help them regulate their nervous systems (Gerhardt, 2004; Orbach, 2009). Neglect, separation, loud noises, and quarreling are traumatizing for an infant that has no option to fight or flee (Levine & Kline, 2007). Global high-intensity activation (GHIA) describes the experience of an all-surrounding, prolonged, inescapable threat, such as is caused by fetal distress, birth trauma, early surgeries, suffocation, drowning, high fevers, and anesthesia (Heller & LaPierre, 2012, p. 134), which leaves children in states of high stress that have otherwise only been experienced by soldiers after years in combat. The result is hyper- or hypoarousal and dysregulation of the central nervous system. Such children respond globally to each new stimulus with a mixture of extreme fear and strong psychosomatic symptoms, causing a domino effect of multiple adverse and overwhelming life experiences and interpersonal violence (van der Kolk, 2003).

Developmental trauma is a term used to describe multiple experiences of traumatic events, such as insecure attachment, neglect, and/ or emotional, sexual, or physical abuse, especially during early to midchildhood. Developmental trauma is linked to scores of psychosomatic symptoms, such as environmental hypersensitivities, asthma, digestive problems, allergies, and chronic pain. Relational misattunement reinforces implicit body memories and is the cause for emotional dysregulation disorders such as substance and alcohol abuse, eating disorders, bipolar mood swings and depression, attention-deficit/hyperactivity disorder (ADHD), anxiety, and panic attacks. All share emotional and nervous system dysregulation, which has not been sufficiently supported early in life (Gerhardt, 2004; Heller & LaPierre, 2012; Levine & Kline, 2007; Schore, 2001).

CLAY WORK AND DEVELOPMENTAL TRAUMA

The sensorimotor system connects our limbs and organs to the brain and the spinal cord in the central nervous system (Heller & LaPierre, 2012, p. 96). The sensory division detects information in our external environment and internal organs and relays this information to the brain so that it can then organize an appropriate motor action. At the Clay Field children are encouraged to use the physical, emotional, and social building blocks of infants' hand movements to connect to these neurological pathways in order to explore and rewrite implicit memories. When children gain sufficient resources in the form of consistent experiences of order and safety at the Clay Field, they eventually find an active response to a formerly overwhelming event. Trauma expert Peter Levine (2010) researched how such sensorimotor actions can turn fear-based patterning into empowerment, and thereby help individuals begin to regulate their hypo- or hyperaroused brainstem. Interventions enhance sensory discrimination to support a reevaluation of past identifications. Of course, during the process, children need the witnessing presence of a supportive professional. Heller and LaPierre (2012) explain:

> Sensory–motor functions develop simultaneously with emotional, relational, and social capacities, and all build on each other. From

this perspective I believe it is important to view the body as *having its own reality* and its own struggle to come into being. When children miss their developmental markers *at the sensory–motor level,* the physiological foundation is not in place to support the emergence of their emotional and relational capacities, and they have no alternative but to compensate and work around the compromised capacities. (p. 242, original emphasis)

Children who have experienced developmental trauma often do not know how to adequately protect themselves, lack social skills, and become easy scapegoats for abuse.

Research on what Heller and LaPierre (2012) term *neuroaffective touch* is still in its infancy, but it suggests that it can repair synapses in the brain that either could not develop in the first place or suffered setbacks due to developmental trauma. As a medium for self-expression, clay has the unique ability to mirror every imprint made into the material. It provides tactile feedback; in other words, as I touch it, it touches me, and as I affect it, it affects me. Hands touching clay simultaneously experience their positions as subjects doing the touching and objects being touched (Paterson, 2007). Sholt and Gavron (2006) also observe that clay work enables children to encounter the constructive and destructive aspects of the self as processes of psychic change and identity formation.

The Clay Field empowers children to explore a manageable world in a safe setting. The therapist witnesses the child's expressions of crisis and success and serves as an "auxiliary cortex" helping to regulate and modulate arousal (Ogden & Minton, 2000). In such a supportive environment children's hands become capable of creating new implicit memories through sensorimotor experiences that are incorporated in the same way as learning to swim or ride a bike; such implicit memory will not be forgotten.

The material in the Clay Field is both limited in its amount and unlimited in its possibilities. The smooth surface becomes available for creation only through an act of destruction; it requires the courage to take an existing order apart. By building blocks up, tearing them down, over and over again, toddlers learn to survive change and acquire trust and object constancy (Winnicott, 1971). Children who have been overwhelmed by destructive experiences, however, lose their ability to create; they no longer believe in the possibility of repair. They do not dare to *grasp and handle* life; instead, their hands retreat and freeze in terror, or blindly act out. Their ability to relate is impaired. Work at the Clay Field builds sensorimotor resources that will eventually allow an active response in the clay that deals with the physical and emotional injuries incurred. Such an active response is capable of undoing the patterns of dissociation in the nervous system without the need to concentrate on "what happened" (Heller & LaPierre, 2012; Levine, 2010; Levine & Kline, 2007).

In recent years neurological research has discovered that psychology, with its medical emphasis on malfunction and disease, has created therapies that focus overly on the pathology of the psyche. This therapeutic emphasis often creates even more instability and dysfunction in individuals (Heller & LaPierre, 2012, p. 2). The brain is endowed with neuroplasticity, which means that experience can change the physical structure of the brain (Siegel & Bryson, 2012, p. 7). It is possible to strengthen the nervous system; it is possible to build resources and learn emotional regulation through sensorimotor activities; it is possible to reach children in their need to heal early infant trauma through touch. Work at the Clay Field is one effective way to do so.

The following sections describe the two main concepts of sensory perception and haptic perception.

SENSORY PERCEPTION

Body awareness is determined by *exteroceptors* (touch, taste, smell, sound, sight) and *interoceptors* (connective tissue, muscles, viscera) (Rothschild, 2000, p. 40). Body memories are stored in the interoceptors whereas exteroceptors are focused on the environment outside of the body. The proximal senses of touch and taste are designed to assess events close by, whereas smell, sound, and sight deal with stimuli that are more distal. Interoceptors perceive stimuli emanating from inside the body; they include the vestibular sense of balance, proprioception (ability to locate ourselves in space), the kinesthetic sense of movement, and the internal sense that gives feedback on body states such as heart rate, respiration, internal temperature, muscular tension, and visceral discomfort (Rothschild, 2000).

In traumatized individuals it is the internal sense that often becomes overactive, communicating anxiety through increased heart rate, cold sweat or hot flashes, as well as muscular and visceral tension. Intense anxiety can diminish the functional effectiveness of the exteroceptors to the extent that the here-and-now reality of the outside world becomes seriously distorted and the inner sensations begin to define an individual's reality. External danger can no longer be assessed adequately; the day-to-day environment becomes easily overwhelming and retraumatizing. Individuals in the grip of fear need to strengthen their exteroceptors in order to check the external reality around them.

Both exteroceptors and interoceptors find their particular expression in the hands and significantly contribute to what is called *haptic perception*. Unlike any other body part, our hands are extraordinarily complex sense organs. Every square inch of skin on fingertips has about 16,000 touch sensors that communicate with the brain (Murphy, 2010). Touch can strengthen the feedback loops between the nervous system, viscera, and cortical functions (Heller & LaPierre, 2012).

HAPTIC PERCEPTION AND HAPTIC OBJECT RELATIONS

Haptic perception refers to the perception through touch. The proximal sense of touch is instrumental in cortical development (Wilson, 1999). Through decades of research, Deuser discovered that the hands act as neurophysiological sensory organs (Deuser, 2009; Elbrecht, 2013; Grunwald, 2008; Paterson, 2007). He structured haptic perception into three core domains:

1. The *skin sense*, which develops in infancy.
2. *Balance*, which is acquired in the second year of life.
3. *Depth sensibility*, which healthy children discover between the ages of 3 and 4 years.

Understanding haptic object relations allows therapists to identify developmental needs and assist children in a unique sensorimotor healing process.

Haptic perception was briefly researched in the 1800s and produced, for example, Braille for the blind. In the visually overloaded 21st-century lifestyle, however, touch is a neglected sense. There is a paucity of research in the art therapy literature describing the potential of haptic perception to heal, particularly with developmental trauma. In addition, many therapists fear the regressive qualities of clay, its connection to our earliest experiences of touch, of smearing and squishing that has neither structure nor words. However, it is exactly these qualities, given insight through haptic perception, that allow therapists to address relational trauma through the bottom-up, "brainwise" approach (Badenoch, 2008). Neuroaffective touch enables children to "form meaning from bodily experience" (Heller & LaPierre, 2012, p. 269).

Observing the movement of children's hands in the Clay Field allows diagnostic conclusions about clients' degree of embodiment or patterns of dissociation. The term *haptic object relations* refers to how infants and children learn about their world and how they discover the environment around them. At every stage developmental needs demand satiation; these are developmental building blocks that can be clearly observed at the Clay Field. Their sensorimotor fulfillment has neurophysiological repercussions. Brockmann and Geiss (2011) state: "If the sensory and motor basis remains fragmented due to biography or social circumstances, hand actions remain instable and fragile. The lack of a haptic and bodily basis will then be substituted through the activation of fantasies and imaginations, which lack the vital intensity of the physical, in order to gain stability" (quoted in Elbrecht, 2012, p. 43).

At the Clay Field children regress whenever a developmental need has remained unfulfilled or has been compromised by traumatic experiences. The hands unerringly reflect exactly that developmental stage that requires attention. In such cases even the hands of adult men may look like the hands of small infants as they explore the clay.

The next three sections explain Deuser's core concepts of skin sense, balance, and depth sensibility as they relate to the Clay Field therapeutic approach.

Skin Sense

Imagine an infant from birth to 12 months of age. Safety, love, and emotional regulation, as well as violation and neglect, are primarily communicated through touch and how one is held. Skin contains and surrounds the entire human body; it divides our inside from the outside. To awaken a rudimentary sense of self, something needs to come to the skin from the outside. Only then can the perception of a felt boundary emerge as a layer of contact between the self and the other. At the Clay Field children's hands search for contact, for tangible support; children may lean up to their elbows on the clay, cuddle into it, even rest their head on it as if on a pillow. It is clearly visible, when the clay is "not there" for children's hands, when they cannot connect with the field.

These children may be incapable of grasping any of the material; their hands desperately or aimlessly scratch along the surface of the clay, but cannot take anything from it. Or they hit and throw it rather than relate to it.

The addition of water can significantly enhance contact, especially when the clay is turned into a soft smooth bog into which the hands can sink or that can be creamed onto the hands, arms, and face (Figures 9.1 and 9.2). Children need to feel surrounded, warmed, and caressed by their caregivers. The active delight of such self-touch leads to deep bodily reassurance that self-fulfillment is possible.

Children who have experienced insecure attachment can benefit from having their hands encased in clay and being held in it. In this case the therapist assists in fulfilling a developmental need. Clay is gently packed around the child's hands; warm water can be poured into

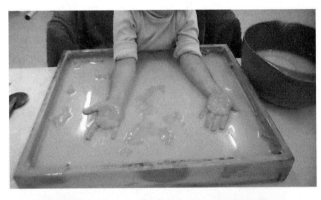

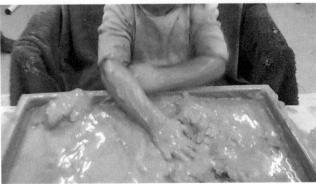

FIGURES 9.1 and 9.2. Skin sense: A 3-year-old girl relishes the support of the field, which she filled with lots of water and then used the diluted clay to cream her underarms with delight.

the cavity to create a "womb" that is similar to a prenatal environment. Inner tensions may be released as the hands experience a nurturing, all-encompassing environment. As a result, restless, unfocused children often settle into this holding space, become calm, and enjoy spending extended periods "playing" inside such a container (Figure 9.3).

Once a basic sense of trust has been gained, children often begin to explore the clay, similar to an infant left alone with a bowl of mashed potatoes. They will pat and smear, squish and squirt, relishing how the clay can ooze through the fingers. All of these experiences are sensual delights. Trust is gained through experimentation with fast and slow patting, tapping rhythms, and through repetition while being witnessed by the therapist. Images such as nest, skin, dough, or breast are stimulated through wiping and circling movements. An infant's primary interest at this stage is the skin of the parent or caregiver; baby hands search for something soft, graspable, movable, stable, and lasting. The clay survives it all; it does not disappear. The temperature of the material and water should be warm to the touch to encourage engagement with the clay.

The hands of older babies have more intense motor impulses—they want to *have* the clay, grab it, move it, and push it around. These actions resonate in the entire body and awaken tonus and awareness. If a piece of clay is lifted out and shown to the therapist, the child is demonstrating, "Look! I have got something." In the context of the skin sense, it is purely about sensory experience, not about creating an object. All these actions have no permanence. Object constancy is acquired through

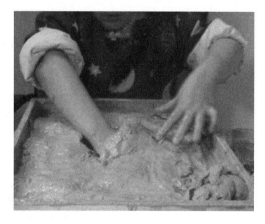

FIGURE 9.3. Skin sense: This 9-year-old boy's mother was dying. His right hand is looking for containment. From Elbrecht (2013). Reprinted with permission from Jessica Kingsley Publishers.

building *up* and tearing *down*, digging *out* and filling *in*. Emphasis on any sensory or tactile discovery happens through rhythmic repetition, through tapping with fingertips, banging with the fists, patting with the open hand, and poking with the index finger. Repetition helps the interoceptors to remember achievements. This process should not be interrupted through introducing "meaning" because this skin-sense level of meaning is sensory in nature.

Children may need several sessions to complete developmental milestones that were not fulfilled as infants. In particular, children with learning and behavioral difficulties often suffer from a relational deficit in their early infancy. Because of the calming qualities of clay, many otherwise erratic children spend surprising amounts of time caressing smooth mounds of clay, humming happily and contentedly, and enjoying their relationship with the clay.

Eventually it is necessary to help children retrieve something permanent from the primal, slushy bog of the Clay Field. If children cannot find something more structured and solid by their own explorations, the therapist may introduce marbles or crystals into the clay to provoke the haptic experience of something firm. In response, children create solid "islands" that are permanent and tangible; these creations may require safekeeping by the therapist in order to survive intact until the following session.

At this stage the clay frequently evokes memories of a sensual and sexual nature. Since trauma almost always affects an individual's skin boundary, traumatic body memories are easily provoked through the skin sense. In such cases individuals have difficulties touching the clay and connecting with it with the entire hand; dissociation manifests as partial use of the hands, such as contact with just one fingertip. Traumatized hands look frozen, rigid, like a "dead spider"; they cannot move. It can be helpful to encourage children in such a case to work with their elbows and underarms, which usually hold less sensitive memories, and the posture is a reminder of the first impulse to be upright and empowered, when they learned as babies to crawl.

Balance

From an object relations perspective, between 1 and 2 years of age healthy children begin to leave the relational "oneness" of the skin sense and discover the world of duality. The ability to walk now, along with a powerful curiosity about what is predominantly an unfamiliar environment, changes children's worldview. They realize that there is a world out there that is somehow "other-than-me," and that realization provokes differentiation between self-perception and object perception.

In the Clay Field this encounter between the self and other is acted out through touching and letting go and through connecting the hands with, and disconnecting them from, the clay. Trust is gained through distancing and connecting (caregiver leaving and returning); the Clay Field becomes an entity that gives the moving hands and the moving body a reliable hold. For children, rhythmic repetition with clay helps with integration just as drumming a beat can give stability as well as resonate throughout the body down into the legs (Figure 9.4). If children explore such rhythmic discoveries, they become aware that there are two sides and a center in the field and thus two sides of their body and the central axis of the spine. The sensorimotor discovery of the spine as a felt sense is crucial at this stage. It correlates with a rudimentary sense of identity; from now on children begin to refer to themselves by name and say "I." To integrate the perception of spinal awareness and that of duality, children experiment with seesawing movements, weighing bits of clay in each hand, or their hands "walk" across the field holding balls of clay.

In their attempt to negotiate the changed dynamics of attachment, children between ages 1 and 2 years explore duality and balance by picking bits out of a big lump of clay. The picked-out bit becomes separated from the whole. Such separation from oneness is as existential as the separation of the hands from the ground. In order to survive this, children play the age-old game of "peek-a-boo": picking a bit out and then reuniting it with the whole. Separation and contact has now been

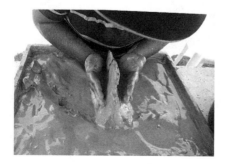

FIGURE 9.4. This boy is in balance. His hands are coordinated, and he is aligned with the field. His elbows are extended simultaneously to both sides.

transferred onto a substance, a thing, or an object (Elbrecht, 2012). In this context high and low, empty and full become spatial orders of a mass in space.

Parental unison manifests as balance in a child, whereas power struggles between parents (e.g., divorce, absence through death or abandonment) causes *im*balance. The child's experience of internal balance becomes apparent in the Clay Field as coordination between the hands (or lack thereof) (see Figure 9.4).

In older children, parental disharmony shows up as incoordination of the hands and misalignment of the body with the Clay Field and the extent to which the entire field is landscaped and handled. For example, if only sections of the field are moved and explored, while others are being ignored, aspects in the psyche are also being ignored. If the body is twisted sideways or one hand only is used, part of the child's psyche is "twisted" or has learned not to get involved. Imbalance shows as one hand dominating the other such as one hand remaining inactive (e.g., underneath the table). In my experience, children whose parents undergo divorce often build trenches, ditches, rivers, walls, or fences that divide the field. When one parent is physically or emotionally absent, parts of the field tend to be filled with life and movement, whereas the other lays dormant (Figure 9.5).

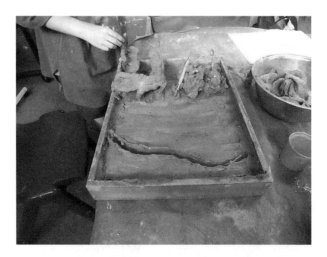

FIGURE 9.5. This is the imbalanced scenario of an 11-year-old boy whose parents were separated. He continued to build dramatic battle scenes of two armies fighting along the banks of a river.

Traumatic events cause serious imbalances in individuals and their interpersonal relationships. Brain functions are impaired and the connection between the brain hemispheres can be seriously affected (Gerhardt, 2004; Levine & Kline, 2007; Schore, 2001; Siegel & Bryson, 2012). Emotional and cognitive regulation is often disrupted; in the case of traumatized infants, important connections may have never actually developed. Even if these connections were not encouraged at home, children can find balance within themselves. At the Clay Field their hands will build bridges or tunnels that connect the two hemispheres of the field. The involvement of both hands in the creative process at the Clay Field, cooperation between both hands, and eventually a use of the entire field assists children in resetting their balance.

Depth Sensibility

Depth sensibility develops between the ages of 3 and 4. It is connected to the child's sense of power, competence, and the ability to do things. In an object relations perspective, it grows with the emergence of ego when a child realizes that he or she has a separate identity from his or her surrounding. In brief, the child begins to internalize, "I am me."

Depth sensibility, according to Deuser, requires the "experience of a relationship with something that is experienced as other than me" (Elbrecht, 2013, p. 51). As children's hands experiment with pressure, they get to know their strength and ability (Figure 9.6 on the next page). In other words, children learn "here are my hands" and recognize their strength to apply them to action outside of the self. Developmentally, joints, muscles, ligaments, and the skeleton become one integrated organism with growing flexibility.

Depth sensibility develops in the following ways:

1. *Pressure.* Pressure is directed toward another and affects that other. When the hands apply pressure, the spine becomes erect, and the feet dig into the ground and gain a firm standpoint. Fearful children or those who lack self-confidence benefit surprisingly from simple experimentations with pressure, including digging with the base of their hands, their fists, or their elbows into the clay, or leaning on them in order to gain trust in their bodies and their abilities.

2. *Impressions.* Impressions are the intentional execution of pressure. This expansion of tonus and the body communicates solid

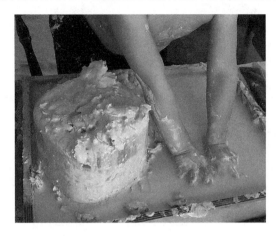

FIGURE 9.6. Depth sensibility: This 4-year-old boy is discovering his strength and competence. All clay has been collected into a container, then emptied out again and refilled. His arms show strength, tonus, and bodily organization. He can move it ALL! From Elbrecht (2013). Reprinted with permission from Jessica Kingsley Publishers.

positioning within the physical self. Children may need to test their endurance at times through impressions in the clay ("Look how long I can push down!") and thus experience their "impressive" power and simultaneous grounding in their bodies.

3. *Imprints.* Imprints expand the haptic gestures into visible, traceable marks. Similar to handprints in prehistoric caves, the intention here is to leave a mark, a concrete effect in the clay; such marks invite a story. The hands and fists create dints, furrows, ruts, and grooves with the intention of creating a record of "me."

4. *Pushing.* Pushing is directed from the center of the hand and center of the body toward something on the outside; it also creates distance. Pushing is far more dynamic than exerting simple downward pressure because it also includes mass and resistance. Children's hands create new space in the clay and cause separation through pushing. In brief, they cause the encounter with an opposite. In terms of developmental trauma, children who have been physically violated often relish the opportunity to push the "other-than-me away," often out of the box, even until the clay drops onto the floor. It is not important to name whom they are pushing away or to engage in the story, but to experience and witness the physical strength that they can do it. Some children

may need the assurance from the therapist at this point that such assertiveness is safe and will not attract punishment.

5. *Pulling.* Pulling brings in material, retrieves it, and brings it close to the body. For example, the clay sometimes is pressed against the chest and given a hug. Once push and pull have become integrated patterns, children can experience the entire mass of clay and the hands become more potent.

6. *Drilling.* Drilling is a movement that investigates the inside of the clay, usually through poking into it with the index finger, or through tunneling. The bottom of the box becomes tangible as depth of space.

7. *Differentiating.* Differentiating includes dividing the mass of clay into high and low or small and large bits; separating amounts from the whole allows the experimentation with separate identities. Bits are bull-dozed out, shoveled out, cut out, raked, or drilled out. Initially such bits are squashed back into the whole and then retrieved and pushed and pulled. Eventually, the bits survive as something special and are gathered in a ball and placed into a central space in the field. The child's hands know now that they can create something and that their creation has lasting stability. This is reflected in how the child holds his or her body, which has now gained stability within, direction, and a place in space.

OLDER CHILDREN'S WORK AT THE CLAY FIELD

During the first 3 years of life children are right-hemisphere dominant. In subsequent years, the left hemisphere and cortical areas develop. "When the toddler begins asking 'Why?' all the time, you know that the left brain is beginning to really kick in" (Siegel & Bryson, 2012, p. 16). At this point, children develop images and stories in relation to their action cycles at the Clay Field. Skin sense, balance, and depth sensibility, however, remain the core haptic tools. All further age-specific stages characterized by creating objects and attaching meaning and stories to them rest on these developmental foundations. If early childhood and developmental trauma have thwarted healthy development, it will manifest in older children; they will display less resilience, little emotional tolerance, and are unable to take what they need with confidence. The clay, as a symbolic world, is not "there" for them. In my observation this trauma is the basis for many symptoms later diagnosed on the spectrum of attention-deficit/hyperactivity disorder (ADHD) (Hölz, 2013).

However, with encouragement these children will unerringly regress to the age that remains incomplete and needs attention (Figures 9.7 and 9.8). It is really important that older children are allowed to engage with incomplete developmental cycles, without judgment and pressure to act more grown up. Once the need for skin sense attachment or self-perception through balance has been satiated, these children will move on in their own time, having gained trust and reliable self-awareness. For example, Mustafa, age 7, has witnessed his father beating his mother severely on many occasions. He hits and bashes the clay relentlessly, announcing that his father is the strongest man on the planet. Eventually the therapist suggests that his hands might feel tired and offers him the warm water bowl in which to rest them. He follows her suggestion with relief; while gently creaming his hands with liquid clay, he can finally begin to feel himself. It is okay to be "weak."

Fearful children, whether they behave in a hypo- or hyperaroused manner, need support to find a way to feel safe. Trusting support may take time, especially if safety was not part of their upbringing. Once they have gained trust in the setting, however, their hands will unerringly discover whatever is developmentally required to master the offered world in the Clay Field. Over time children will acquire age-specific social integration, self-esteem, and competence through sensorimotor actions. Emotionally they will build identity, certainty, and consistency and claim their own ground as opposed to a diffuse identity and feelings of inferiority.

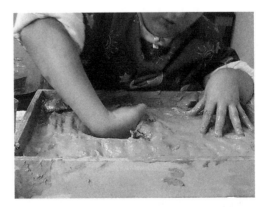

FIGURE 9.7. Depth sensibility: This 9-year-old boy diagnosed with ADHD is still struggling to find sufficient strength in his hand. The wrist is bent, his shoulder is twisted, and his body is not aligned. Later in the session he stood up and could then experience better alignment, which gave him a growing sense of strength and allowed him to fulfill his intention and dig out the material.

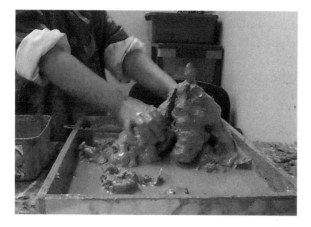

FIGURE 9.8. Depth sensibility: The same boy in the same session, now toward the end. He has stood up, and the alignment of his arms and hands with his body is obvious. Now he radiates confidence and intention, rather than collapse and weakness. Less frustrated, this confidence translated into a more focused behavior at school and improved his social and learning ability significantly. From Elbrecht (2013). Reprinted with permission from Jessica Kingsley Publishers.

This brief vignette illustrates an older child who has experienced developmental trauma and how the Clay Field helped her in her recovery from sexual abuse. Lindy is 10 years old; she has been removed from her family due to sexual abuse. The perpetrator was the mother's boyfriend. Initially she can barely touch the clay, except for tiny indentations. Eventually she begins to pour water into these indentations and to caress them with one finger, and then moving on to landscape the surface of the field. Seven Clay Field sessions are dedicated to gaining trust through strengthening her skin sense, balance, and depth sensibility. In the following encounter, right at the start, she places a disproportionally large phallic shape into the left bottom corner of the field. The therapist does not address it and just waits. The girl then avoids it for most of the session while she concentrates on bulldozing material into various places, building it up and smashing it down, placing bits outside of the box, thus gaining increasing confidence and competence. All of a sudden she jumps up, rips out the phallic object, holds it up to her mouth, and begins belting out her favorite pop song. It is a microphone! She skips out of the session, elated.

This is the transformation from feeling overwhelmed to self-empowerment; in brief, the work in the Clay Field "settles the nervous system" after a traumatic event. It was not important to address again the sexual abuse that had happened, but Lindy had to gain the sensorimotor competence and confidence that she could turn a situation around and that she had the power to do so. The effect of trauma does not depend on the severity of the incident, but on the experienced level of helplessness (Levine & Kline, 2007). What Lindy needed was a strengthening of her inner resources and to gain the trust that she had the power to actively respond to what had happened (Biebrach & Larsch, 2014).

HAPTIC RECOMMENDATIONS

The Clay Field is a therapeutic process that requires formal training. This chapter points out the importance of the haptic and sensorimotor building blocks that shape our sense of self. Therapists do not necessarily need to work with clay if they want to rebuild developmental resources in children, even though the sensory quality of the material is wonderfully suited to do so.

The acquisition of trust is learned through safe touch. Thus skin sense can also be strengthened through playing with water and sand, through finger paints, or through caressing a blanket and leaning into cushions. Many children can integrate this sense of safe touch by holding teddy bears, as long as therapists focus on how much contact the children's hands have with the chosen objects and if the objects are emotionally available for them. Balance can be encouraged through various ways, such as drumming, knitting, and dancing, or through drawing with both hands simultaneously, as long as the hands learn to coordinate their movements and work together. Whatever supports the physical perception of the spinal axis as a source of identity will be beneficial. To gain confidence and competence, depth sensibility can be encouraged through sculpting or participating in sports, martial arts, or resistance training—anything that involves pressure to strengthen and align the joints and ligaments in the body. This is, after all, how life teaches us these skills.

CONCLUSION

Children tend to be resistant to, and can often be incapable of, recalling traumatic memories. Focus on distressing events also adds to their experience of destabilization. In addition, all learning in the first 3 years of life is predominantly sensorimotor, rather than cognitive, in nature. Early developmental trauma creates implicit memory that becomes part of our physiological identity and is not perceived as explicit memory of specific events. However, this implicit memory impacts on children's sensorimotor responses, which compromises their emotional, relational, and social capacities. Work at the Clay Field supports the body's own reality in coming into being by creating new synaptic connections in the brain through sensorimotor actions in the clay and within a secure relationship with the therapist.

Children who embody sensorimotor developmental milestones, as described in this chapter, gain age-specific resiliency through being able to "handle" their world. Such a sense of competence supports nervous system regulation. Thus equipped, these children will be capable of responding adequately and creatively to adverse situations occurring in their lives.

REFERENCES

Badenoch, B. (2008). *Being a brain-wise therapist.* New York: Norton

Biebrach, M., & Larsch, P. (2014). Work at the Clay Field: Recognising potential, awakening resources, furthering development. Available on YouTube at *www.clay-field.com.*

Brockman, A. D., & Geiss, M. L. (2011). *Sprechende hände: Haptik und haptischer sinn als entwicklungspotential [Speaking hands: Haptic and haptic sense as developmental potential].* Berlin: Pro Business.

Deuser, H. (Ed.). (2004). *Bewegung wird gestalt [Movement becomes gestalt].* Bremen, Germany: W. und W. Döring Verlagsgesellschaft.

Deuser, H. (2006). Die arbeit am tonfeld [Work at the clay field]. In G. Tschachler-Nagy & A. Fleck (Eds.), *Die arbeit am tonfeld nach Heinz Deuser: Eine entwicklungsfördernde methode für kinder [Work at the clay field based on Heinz Deuser: A method for children, adolescents and adults to support development]* (pp. 19–33). Keutschach, Germany: Tschachler-Nagy.

Deuser, H. (2007). Ich berühre und werde berührt [I touch and am touched]. In G. Tschachler-Nagy (Ed.), *Im greifen sich begreifen: Die arbeit am tonfeld nach Heinz Deuser [Grasping through grasp: The work at the clay field by Heinz Deuser]* (pp. 19–29). Keutschach, Germany: Verlag Tonfeld-Anna Sutter.

Deuser, H. (2009). *Der haptische sinn [The haptic sense].* Keutschach, Germany: Verlag Tonfeld-Anna Sutter.

Elbrecht, C. (2013). *Trauma healing at the Clay Field*. London: Jessica Kingsley.

Gendlin, E. T. (1981). *Focussing* (4th ed.). Toronto: Bantam Books.

Gerhardt, S. (2004). *Why love matters: How affection shapes a baby's brain*. New York: Routledge.

Grunwald, M. (Ed.). (2008). *Human haptic perception: Basics and application*. Berlin: Birkhauser.

Heller, L., & LaPierre, A. (2012). *Healing developmental trauma*. Berkeley, CA: North Atlantic Books.

Hölz, B. (2013). *Untersuchung der psychotherapeutischen wirkung der haptisch orientierten therapiemethode arbeit am tonfeld bei kindern mit der diagnose AD(H)S* [Examination of the psychotherapeutic effect of a therapy method with an haptic orientation through work at the clay field with children with a diagnosis of AD(H)D]. Tübingen, Germany: University of Tübingen.

Levine, P. A. (2010). *In an unspoken voice: How the body releases trauma and restores goodness*. Bekerley, CA: North Atlantic Books.

Levine, P. A., & Kline, M. (2007). *Trauma through a child's eyes*. Berkeley, CA: North Atlantic Books.

Murphy, P. (2010). *The hand book*. Palo Alto, CA: Klutz.

Ogden, P., & Minton, K. (2000). Sensorimotor psychotherapy. *Traumatology*, 6(3), 149–173.

Orbach, S. (2009). *Bodies*. London: Profile Books.

Paterson, M. (2007). *The senses of touch: Haptics, affects and technologies*. Oxford, UK: Berg.

Rothschild, B. (2000). *The body remembers*. New York: Norton.

Schore, A. (2001). *Early relational trauma: Effects on the right brain development and the etiology of pathological dissociation*. Paper presented at the conference "Attachment, the Developing Brain and Psychotherapy: Minds in the Making," University College London.

Sholt, M., & Gavron, T. (2006). Therapeutic qualities of clay-work in art therapy and psychotherapy: A review. *Journal of American Art Therapy Association, 23*(6), 66–72.

Siegel, D., & Bryson, T. (2012). *The whole-brain child*. New York: Bantam Books.

van der Kolk, B. A. (2003). Posttraumatic stress disorder and the nature of trauma. In M. F. Solomon & D. J. Siegel (Eds.), *Healing trauma: Attachment, mind, body, and brain* (pp. 168–196). New York: Norton.

Wilson, F. R. (1999). *The hand: How its use shapes the brain, language, and human culture*. New York: Vintage Books

Winnicott, D. W. (1971). *Playing and reality*. New York: Basic Books.

PART III

Applications with Families and Groups

CHAPTER 10

Creative Crisis Intervention Techniques with Children and Families

Lennis G. Echterling
Anne L. Stewart

Not far from our community is a cornfield that has been transformed into a maze, filled with dead ends, blind spots, and disorienting twists and turns. The cornfield maze is a wonderful metaphor for how children and families find their way through life's challenges, whether the challenges are anticipated developmental tasks, unexpected family changes, or natural or human-made disasters. In the cornfield, some children cling to their parents as they enter the maze, but most run ahead, exuberant and enthusiastic about this new adventure, skipping along, laughing, and shouting. When they reach a turning point or stray too far ahead, children typically return to the security of their parents. They grab an adult's hand, accompany him or her for a few steps, share impressions about their surroundings, wonder about possible options, and then rush headlong down the path once again. The children rely on their own problem-solving capacities and their caregivers' reassurance and guidance to playfully create a pathway through the maze.

To gain an appreciation for the power of creativity and the resources you have to use in times of confusion and chaos, take a look at Figure 10.1. At first glance, it may appear to be a maze like the cornfield, except this one doesn't seem to have any particular beginning or end—just a

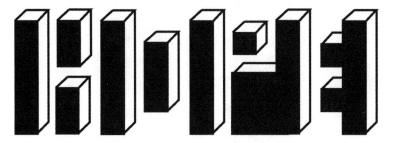

FIGURE 10.1. Create a vision of hope.

meaningless assortment of block-like shapes. Nevertheless, your challenge is to find something meaningful here. You may feel the same sense of doubt and apprehension that you have when you look at one of those Magic Eye pictures and cannot see any hidden figures, but as you explore the terrain of this puzzle, keep in mind that you can rely on your internalized base to find hope. As you may recall from your own experiences of creativity in times of chaos, you do not need to force the process. Instead, just relax and focus your eyes on one specific point in the figure. It doesn't matter where, as long as you stay focused. By keeping your attention tuned into one spot for 20 or 30 seconds, something meaningful seems to pop out of the chaos—you create a unified vision of hope. If you didn't have much luck with that strategy, you can also gain some perspective by moving 4 or 5 feet away from the figure. What word appears?

CHALLENGES OF CREATIVE CRISIS INTERVENTION

In other chapters in this volume, you have learned creative techniques that you can readily apply to your traditional therapeutic relationships with traumatized children. Typically, your counseling and therapy work takes place at appointed times, during regular working hours, for 50-minute sessions, in professional offices that provide a sense of safety and privacy, and with therapeutic tools that are not easily portable. You are surrounded by trappings such as diplomas, certificates, and books that speak to your legitimacy as a therapist. Moreover, you normally have the opportunity to complete a comprehensive assessment, develop a treatment plan, and establish therapeutic goals before you decide how you will apply these interventions.

In this chapter we focus on crisis intervention, in which the circumstances are often dramatically different from the typical therapy session. *Crisis intervention* is any rapid, brief collaboration to assist someone in surviving and resolving a crisis (Echterling, Presbury, & McKee, 2005). The creative techniques we describe can be used in the immediate wake of a crisis event and under adverse conditions. In the midst of the chaos and confusion of a personal or community crisis, encounters with survivors are likely to be unscheduled and take place any time, day or night. They often occur in a nontraditional setting, such as a disaster assistance center, emergency room, or temporary shelter. Without any diplomas on the walls, the therapist must rely solely on actions to demonstrate his or her ability to help, and the intervention may last a couple of minutes or go on for several hours.

Wherever and whenever crises confront children and families, you nevertheless can offer creative interventions with materials you are able to take with you. The purpose of this chapter is to help you engage children and families in creative experiences that promote reaching out, making meaning, taking heart, and moving on to resolve their crisis. The techniques we describe require minimal materials, can be done with little or no special preparation, and can be implemented in virtually any setting, however primitive the conditions. The activities can take any form of creative expression—playing, drawing, singing, sculpting, dancing, or making music. Whatever the form, the active, potent ingredient in every technique is you.

Outside a temple compound in Sri Lanka, one of us (A. S.) conducted play-based activities with child survivors of the 2004 tsunami. Neither the children and families nor the therapists had any of their/ our familiar surroundings or tools. As the therapists entered the gated temple area, we were introduced to the caregivers and children and listened to the children perform songs about daily life and their hopes for the future. We then participated in play-based activities to enhance the children's ability to identify adaptive coping behaviors, to focus, and to regulate their emotions. We taught and sang songs about healthy coping with engaging gestures, including the sign language gestures for "I love you." A few days later we returned to the temple, where the children came running to greet us, laughing, smiling, shouting our names, and signing "I love you." The intervention was unconventional, powerful, and genuine.

We believe that crisis intervention competencies are vital elements of effective mental health practice, but this does not mean that each practitioner should provide services in the midst of a disaster area. It is neither necessary nor advisable for all therapists to be on the scene of a crisis. Most therapists offer excellent services to traumatized children and families in more traditional settings and do not choose to work under primitive or unconventional conditions. As with all the services you provide, in times of crisis it is important to critically evaluate your knowledge, skills, and abilities as you determine your professional response. We recommend that you consult with colleagues and refer to your discipline's professional practice standards and code of ethics to inform your decision making. It is imperative that you do not compromise the well-being of your current clients, students, employer, or employees as you make your decision about how to respond. Of course, it is necessary to consider the impact of how you choose to respond on your family and other personal relationships. Last, carefully consider your tolerance for discomfort, ambiguity, distractions, and confusion. If you are willing to accommodate to these circumstances, then you may be a good match for providing interventions in the "ground zero" type of environment.

THE CONCEPT OF CRISIS

There is an important distinction between the concepts of trauma and crisis. *Trauma*, which comes from the Greek word for *wound*, refers to a serious psychological injury that results from a threatening, terrifying, or horrifying experience. Psychological traumas can have a profound impact on a person's cognitive abilities, emotional reactivity, behavior, and even neural functioning (Endo, Shioiri, & Someya, 2008; Gaskill & Perry, 2012). However, studies have found that resilience is much more commonly expressed than was once believed (Ryff & Singer, 2003). For example, Kessler, Davis, and Kendler (1997) documented that the majority of children who experienced severe traumas, such as sexual assault or death of a parent, did not develop psychiatric disorders such as posttraumatic stress disorder (PTSD). In fact, many people report posttraumatic growth (PTG) (Calhoun & Tedeschi, 2006). Concepts such as trauma can be useful by calling attention to particular phenomena, but they may limit our focus and reduce our attention to supporting healthy striving if we rely only on trauma to provide our entire conceptual framework.

The concept of crisis provides a useful complement to that of trauma. *Crisis* comes from the Greek word for *decision*, and its Chinese symbol combines the figures for danger and decisive moment. A crisis is a pivotal turning point that involves both peril and promise. Not everyone in crisis is dealing with trauma. For example, a refugee child facing the crisis of entering an American school is going through a major turning point in life that presents both dangers and opportunities; however, that child is not likely to be traumatized by this particular event. On the other hand, orphaned and homeless Sri Lankan children who managed to survive the tsunami were not only suffering trauma, but also facing a crisis (Catani, Jacob, Schauer, Kohila, & Meuner, 2008). At this brief but crucial point in their lives, how they and their communities dealt with this traumatic event had far-reaching consequences, either positive or negative.

The purpose of crisis intervention is not to achieve a cure. Instead, it is to promote resilience by supporting the potential for hope and resolve that survivors possess. Because you intervene at such a crucial point in a child's life and a family's history, a seemingly small intervention can make a profound difference for years to come.

SYSTEMIC CONSIDERATIONS

In crisis work with children, you will want to keep in mind several important points regarding families. First, you may be intervening with an individual child, but the family is always present psychologically (Baggerly & Exum, 2008). Children bring along their families in their hearts and minds; family beliefs, expectations, voices, images, and histories are fixtures of a child's inner world. As a crisis intervener, you need to respect and build on this family context, especially when you are working with the child alone.

A second significant point is to recognize and appreciate the exciting and dramatic changes that are taking place in family constellations across the United States and throughout the world. In your work with children, you will encounter families that do not conform to the stereotyped and traditional models of the past. Same-sex partners, stepfamilies, single parents, blended families, and other forms are becoming more common. In fact, the conventional family of a married man and woman living together with their biological children is now the minority.

Third, families form a dynamic system. If one member is in crisis, then the entire system is likely to be in turmoil. Like individuals, family systems in crisis face both dangers and opportunities. If they fail to resolve a crisis, family members may come away with a sense of alienation from one another, in a state of confusion and chaos, and on the verge of disintegration. If they cope successfully, family members can emerge from crises feeling closer, having a greater sense of commitment to one another, and working more effectively as a system. The stakes for both individuals and systems are high.

Another important consideration is that families also function within the context of other systems. Your most important intervention may be to connect a family in crisis to those systems with the particular resources that can address their needs, such as social services, formal counseling and therapy, and financial support. Related to this consideration is the fact that these broader systems may also be in crisis. Violence, catastrophic accidents, natural disasters, and acts of terrorism can throw entire schools, churches, neighborhoods, communities, and societies into a state of crisis. Nevertheless, these broader systems also demonstrate social resilience (Keck & Lakdapolrak, 2013). You will need to design your creative interventions and, likely, broaden your ideas about your role with the child and family to accommodate these different conditions.

Finally, just as you take into consideration the developmental level of the child when you intervene, you also need to recognize the stage of the family's development in the family life cycle. As families grow and change, they negotiate many developmental tasks and face turning points (Kanel, 2012) that produce a range of emotions—anxiety, joy, heartbreak, compassion, and hope. Families rarely seek crisis intervention for such developmental crises as marriage, birth, and empty nest, and are more likely to contact you regarding specific situational crises that confront them. You will find it helpful to keep these broader developmental crises in mind as you work with families. These issues form the backdrop to the precipitating event and provide the context for exploring possible resolutions that lead to both personal and family growth.

BASIC PRINCIPLES

Before focusing on specific techniques, we want to mention several basic principles of effective crisis intervention. First, always intervene with LUV. The acronym *LUV* stands for *listen*, *understand*, and *validate*, which form the foundation of any successful helping relationship

(Echterling et al., 2005). Recent research has documented that such a resonating therapeutic relationship can enhance brain functioning and promote the creation of new, adaptive neural pathways (Badenoch & Bogdan, 2012; Siegel, 2012). As you practice LUV and the other principles, we encourage you to reflect on your own theoretical orientation. Evaluate the degree to which these principles of crisis intervention are congruent with your understanding of the emotional life of children and families as well as your conceptualization of your role.

When you offer LUV, you are actively *listening* to the child's verbal and nonverbal messages, communicating your empathic *understanding* of the child's thoughts and feelings, and *validating* unconditionally the child's innate worth. When someone does not feel heard, understood, and accepted, then your creative interventions, however elegant, can appear to be only scheming manipulations or, at best, meaningless gimmicks. You are not the expert with all the answers, the sage who dispenses advice in troubled times. Instead, by offering your supportive presence, you offer a safe space, a psychological refuge in this threatening storm. Fundamentally, an intervention takes place whenever a person in crisis is able to make contact with someone who cares. Your LUVing encounter with a child in crisis is the most powerful intervention of all.

Another basic principle of crisis intervention is to recognize and value the resilience of children and families—to presume that they are survivors, not pathetic and passive victims (Echterling & Stewart, in press). When you encounter young people in crisis, you may feel tempted to be the knight in shining armor who rescues them from any emotional turmoil, but your job is more like the carpenter's assistant, helping children and their families to use the tools they may be overlooking as they begin to rebuild their lives. Of course, people in troubled times feel overwhelmed and distressed, but they also possess undiscovered strengths, overlooked talents, and unnoticed resources. As children and families begin to experience empowerment, recognize their untapped capabilities, and reconnect to sources of sustenance and nurturance, they build the scaffolding for a successful resolution to the crisis.

CREATIVE INTERVENTIONS

Children and families are more likely to be resilient when they reach out to others for support, make meaning of the crisis experience, take heart by regulating their emotions, and move on by creatively coping with these challenges (Echterling et al., 2005). Therefore, we have organized our recommended creative interventions according to these four essential processes that promote resilience and facilitate successful resolution.

Reaching Out

Especially in times of crisis, people are not islands. Research on social support has shown that relationships offer survivors many vitally important resources, such as affection, advice, affirmation, and practical assistance (Reis, Collins, & Berscheid, 2000). Although the experience of victimization can initially provoke a sense of isolation and alienation, survivors quickly turn to others (Berscheid, 2003). The purpose of these interventions is to help children and families connect with one another to find support, comfort, and nurturance as they embark on the journey toward resolution. An underlying, and often overlooked, assumption of these techniques is that children are also resources in times of crisis. Providing children with the opportunity to make a positive difference during troubled times can promote their own sense of resilience.

From My Heart to Your Heart

This group activity is a playful and quick way to connect children to others and promote a sense of community after a disaster. Begin by inviting the children to pair up. Demonstrate how you want them to encounter one another by acting out the words as you chant. You can begin this introductory activity by saying, "From my heart to your heart, I wish you well," while pointing to your own heart and then pointing to the heart of your partner. Then go on to other body parts, such as, "From my elbow to your elbow, I wish you well," while connecting to another person at the elbow. Respecting personal privacy, you can facilitate a playful encounter among participants by leading them through other connections—toe to toe, knee to knee, shoulder to shoulder, hand to hand, and ear to ear. In Sri Lanka after the tsunami, children found this welcoming activity an appealing way to connect with a team of international interveners. Because the activity relies on gestures to communicate, you can use it even if you do not speak the same language. (This activity is based on the song "I Wish You Well," on the CD by Bailey and Hartman, 2002, titled *It Starts in the Heart*.)

Helping Hands

You can easily adapt this intervention to use with individuals, families, or even large groups. Briefly talk about how all of us need and offer helping hands to one another. Give all present a pencil and a piece of paper and invite them to draw the outline of one of their hands. In each finger, they then can make a drawing or write the name of a person, thing, or organization that has helped them through the crisis so far. The survivors can also make another helping hand to describe five ways that they have been a resource to others. If no materials are available, survivors can just show their hands and describe the help they have received from, and given to, each other.

This activity invites children to explore how they have been making a positive difference during this difficult and painful time. It encourages them to become conscious that they are playing an active role in contributing to the resolution of the crisis.

Rituals and Routines

Families and broader systems have many traditions that bring people together, affirm their collective identity, and celebrate their roots. As a crisis intervener, you can explore with children and families the customs that offer structure, meaning, and connectivity in their lives. You can then help them to be creative in designing new rituals and routines that preserve, as much as possible, these traditions while accommodating to new circumstances. These experiences—whether they are special occasions, such as birthdays and holidays, or daily routines, such as greetings in the morning and bedtime rituals—offer children and adults a sense of connectedness and normalcy.

For example, after Hurricane Katrina, school counselors in Pascagoula, Mississippi, implemented a communitywide project to help children and families reach out to one another at Halloween. The disaster had destroyed many homes, left dangerous debris scattered throughout the city, and made it impossible for many families to purchase costumes and candy for their children. To promote a sense of community, the high school students and other volunteers organized "Trunk or Treat." They arranged for children to receive donated costumes and publicized that families could bring their little trick-or-treaters to the community's high school parking lot, where more than 70 decorated cars had trunks of candy to disperse. Children and families were able to celebrate a traditional holiday, experience a sense of normalcy, and reach out to one another in a safe space.

Making Meaning

When children and families are in crisis, they are also experiencing a crisis of meaning (Janoff-Bulman, 1992). Using creative activities to tell their crisis stories offers them an opportunity to begin to give form to raw experience, gain some sense of cognitive mastery over the crisis, and make important discoveries about possible resolutions (Federal Emergency Management Agency, 2012). Children tell their stories in a variety of ways—by talking, playing, drawing, sculpting, singing, and writing—but whatever form their stories take, the process helps children create meaning from the destructive event that has taken place.

The themes that emerge from these stories eventually shape the storytellers' sense of personal identity and family legacy. In other words, the narratives that children and families create do more than organize their life experiences; they affirm fundamental beliefs, guide important decisions, and offer consolation and solace in times of tragedy (Neimeyer, 2000). Using the following creative activities, you can help children transform their crisis narratives into survival stories. In the process, you not only facilitate a successful resolution to a particular crisis, but also give them the opportunity to go on to thrive in their lives.

Art of Surviving

Children often become absorbed in using art to give form to their life experiences. When those life experiences are painful, frightening, or tragic, many spontaneously draw pictures of the crises they face and the ordeals they suffer. You can also invite children to give expression to their own resilience during these troubled times. Drawing pictures about their perseverance, resourcefulness, and creativity gives children an opportunity to recognize their strengths and contributions to the resolution process. They can also use drawings to portray the help that others gave them, the lessons they have learned from this experience, and the ways that they are stronger now that they have survived.

Children's art may take many forms. It could be a scene showing how they escaped danger, a depiction of something new that they have learned, a portrait of themselves as survivors, an illustration of how they helped others, or an example of how they overcame an obstacle. For example, when asked to draw a picture of a lesson that he had learned from coping with a flood to offer advice for other children who might be faced with a similar experience, a boy drew a rainbow over a river and wrote the caption, "You will be surprised what you can live through." You may invite them to design a poster showing what children could do to be better prepared for a disaster or what children could tell themselves as they face a crisis.

When you have a conversation with children about their art, you want to empathize with their victimization and be curious about their survival. In other words, acknowledge the crisis and ask questions to create opportunities for them to talk about their endurance, courage, compassion, joy, and hope. You can say, for example, "I notice that this boy and his mama are smiling at each other in your picture. How are they able to smile even though their house was destroyed?" Or you might wonder, "What is this girl feeling as she helps with cleaning up after the fire?" Such questions invite children to become more aware of the depth and richness of their own resilience.

Family Crisis Crest

This activity can be done with one child, a group of children, or an entire family. With individuals or groups, you can invite them to work alone to create their own family crisis crests. If you are working with a family, you can invite all the family members to collaborate in designing a single crest to share. See Figure 10.2 for an example of a blank template that you can use. One segment of the crest could be an animal that symbolizes family traits that have helped the family members through challenges. Another section could display a flower, tree, or plant that represents the family's roots and potential for growth. A third part could show a symbol, such as a mountain or threatening scene, that portrays the crisis event. Finally, the fourth portion of the crest could be a sign or symbol that expresses the family's hope for the future. Below the crest is a space for the family's motto, which should summarize one of the family's basic values.

Survival Diary

Many older children keep diaries or journals, finding satisfaction in the process of transforming their life experiences into words. In troubled times, you can invite children to give voice not only to their crisis

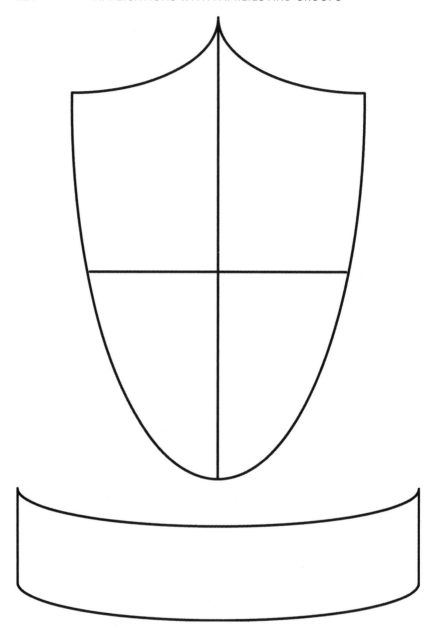

FIGURE 10.2. Template for family crisis crest.

narratives but also to their stories of survival. Instead of focusing on the details of the crisis event, you can encourage children to elaborate on how they have been facing these challenges, managing the many changes in their lives, and making sense of what is happening. The theme here is that children may have been victims of a crisis, but they are now survivors who have shown determination, courage, and compassion.

Through the child's disaster diary, you can hear the child's story, see the representations of the disaster, recognize its impact, and acknowledge the ways the child made it through this challenge. As with any encounter with someone in a crisis situation, you will want to leave the child on a positive note, feeling a greater sense of hope and resolve.

Playing to Strengths

Many children act out their crisis experiences and demonstrate their resilience through their play (Dugan, Snow, & Crowe, 2010). Moreover, adult survivors find play to be a wonderful opportunity to experience their own vitality and to savor the joys of life in spite of the sorrows and hardships of tragic events. Through play, children and families recreate themselves by expressing their feelings, enhancing their self-esteem, gaining self-control, acting out possible resolutions, and reinvigorating themselves. Play is one of your most powerful crisis intervention tools (Jordan, Perryman, & Anderson, 2013).

Play offers several significant benefits. By supporting children's independent play and creating specialized play-based interventions, you can normalize reactions, invite children to try out new coping strategies, modify cognitive distortions, increase self-soothing, enrich relationships, enhance social support, and leave children and families with a sense of hope (National Child Traumatic Stress Network—Terrorism and Disaster Branch, 2005). Although you typically will not have the luxury of a well-stocked play therapy room when you do crisis work, you can create a portable bag of toys and other materials for play-based intervention (Landreth, 2002). As you can see in Figure 10.3, you can assemble an impressive variety of materials to help people express themselves through different forms of art, engage in nurturing and family-life behaviors, play out fantasies, enact rescue operations, and vent feelings of aggression and destruction. Keep in mind that although these toys can be a helpful aid in your creative crisis interventions, the most

EXPRESSIVE ARTS
    Crayons, colored pencils, markers
    Drawing and construction paper, scissors, pipe cleaners
    Balloons, bubbles, queen-size sheet

NURTURANCE AND HOME LIFE
    Baby bottle, cups, dishes
    Cardboard box dollhouse, furniture
    Doll family, including baby doll

FANTASY
    Magic wand
    Royalty- or magical-themed puppets or figures

RESCUE
    Telephone
    Emergency vehicles and workers, airplane
    Construction blocks
    Bandages, medical kit

DESTRUCTION AND AGGRESSION
    Popsicle sticks, egg cartons, or sheets of bubble wrap
    Nonrealistic plastic dart gun, rubber knife
    Toy soldiers and aggressive puppets

YOU!

FIGURE 10.3. Basic materials in a tote bag for creative crisis intervention.

important tool is you. The fields of crisis intervention and play therapy are growing and changing rapidly, so you must make a commitment to obtain and maintain your skills through periodic education and training in order to effectively intervene with children and families.

Taking Heart

As a crisis intervener, your job is not to provoke emotional catharsis. Instead, you should help children regulate their emotions by reducing distress, soothing themselves when they are upset, enhancing feelings of resolve, and staying "in the zone" (Echterling et al., 2005). Successful athletes talk of being "in the zone" when they are performing at their best. At these times, they are energized yet focused, emotionally charged yet poised. Children and families are more likely to survive troubled times if they are in this ideal state of emotional arousal. The purpose of the following creative interventions is to help children and their families to take heart and manage their emotions productively.

A crisis is invariably a time of intense emotions, but a common assumption is that individuals in crisis have only negative feelings, such as fear, shock, and grief. Recent research has demonstrated that they actually experience not only painful crisis reactions, but also feelings of resolve (Larsen, Hemenover, Norris, & Cacioppo, 2003). These feelings of resolve include courage, compassion, hope, peace, and joy. Acknowledging and giving expression to the gamut of emotions, both negative and positive, can promote a positive crisis resolution (Stein, Folkman, Trabasso, & Richards, 1997). In other research, Emmons, Colby, and Kaiser (1998) explored how some survivors were eventually able to transform their losses into gains. They found that, even during the crisis experience itself, these future thrivers were able to take pleasure in savoring the few desirable events that took place, appreciating discoveries that they had made, and celebrating small victories. The following creative activities can help a child regulate emotions by reducing distress and enhancing feelings of resolve.

Sharing Your Worries

One way to help children regulate their emotions is to involve them in activities in which they use long, slow, deep breathing. For example, you can give balloons to children and other family members, ask them to imagine a worry or concern they would like to blow into the balloons, and have them allow the tension to flow into the expanding balloons as they slowly exhale. (You may need to inflate the balloon for young children.) This activity combines the relaxing process of deep breathing with the imagery of externalizing a concern. Once children and family members have inflated their balloons, they can play with them however they like, illustrating how they can share their worries and have fun along the way. They may want to toss them in the air, play catch with one another, or bounce the balloons.

If you are working with a group or family, you can add another creative activity that involves a sheet. Gather the participants around a sheet that you have spread on the floor. Invite them to place their balloons on the sheet, grasp the edge of the sheet, and lift it as a group in order to carry these worries together. The group may want to work together to guide all the balloons to the center or one of the corners of the sheet. They can collaborate to raise and lower the sheet while walking in a circle. They will enjoy shaking the sheet to toss their worry balloons into the air. At the end of the activity, some may decide to keep their balloons, exchange them with others, or even pop them.

Blowing Bubbles

Another breathing activity for emotional regulation can involve blowing bubbles, using commercial products, homemade materials, or even imaginary ones. You can begin by asking children what happens if they blow too hard when trying to blow bubbles. Then invite them to participate in the activity, either real or imagined, of softly, slowly, and gently blowing air to create bubbles. You may also want to encourage children to say one thing to themselves that helps them keep their hopes afloat as they prepare to blow bubbles.

Singing a Song of Resolve

Children love to sing, and one song you can offer them in times of crisis is a form of self-talk and reassurance that they can use later to regulate their emotions by themselves (Shelby & Bond, 2005). To the tune of "Twinkle, Twinkle, Little Star," you can lead children in the following song:

> I am safe and I am strong.
> Take a breath [take a deep breath and exhale] and sing this song.
> I am growing strong each day.
> Everything will be okay.
> I am safe and I am strong.
> Take a breath [take a deep breath and exhale] and sing this song.

When you sing the words "Take a breath," you can model slow, deep breathing for the children. You can also engage the children in acting out the other lines by making a muscle to show strength and giving a culturally appropriate sign for things being "okay."

Expressing Collective Resolve

Families and communities often spontaneously give expression to their collective resolve. These expressions may include tying yellow ribbons to trees, wearing bracelets, flying the flag, and building spontaneous shrines at the scene of a traumatic incident. Other examples include family activities, street performances, displaying survivors' drawings, painting murals, making posters, collecting survivors' stories, and participating in commemorations. Such public expressions can create a powerful synergy because their performance requires an audience. One of the classic symptoms of PTSD is a flashback, when some reminder triggers the traumatic experience. The power of these expressions of collective resolve is that they can become triggers for resolution to reconnect survivors to their experiences of success and triumph in coping with the crisis.

Moving On

Crises rob children and families of their dreams for the future, at least temporarily. As a crisis intervener, you can use these activities to help children and families envision new possibilities by inviting them to create positive goals. Once articulated, goals serve as beacons that light the way for the journey to resolution. In this section, we describe creative activities that can help children and families begin the process of rebuilding their lives. Once they begin to see a future, survivors gain a sense of direction and hope, become more motivated, and increase their momentum toward resolution. Studies have found that people who strive to attain positive goals have higher levels of well-being than those who merely try to avoid negative goals (Emmons, 1999).

Keep in mind that even though children and their families may not have resolved a crisis, somehow they have successfully survived it. You can invite children and families to explore the achievements that they have already accomplished. By drawing attention to these instances of taking flight, dealing with challenges, and finding refuge, you can assist survivors in discovering unknown strengths, appreciating unrecognized resources, and achieving a sense of hope. These strengths and resources form the foundation for a successful resolution.

Out of the Ashes

Begin this activity by giving everyone a small piece of paper and a pencil. Invite them to name or draw the crisis event that they experienced. Then, in a safe container, burn the paper and mix the ashes into a piece of modeling clay. Invite the participants to think of one of the hopes they have for the future. Using what they have learned and discovered in dealing with their crisis so far, the participants can mold a symbol of hope from the ashes and the clay.

Growing Garden

The growing garden activity is a story you create about flowers that grow up to live in a lovely garden. One version of the story follows, but feel free to improvise.

Tell the children to pretend to be tiny flower seeds under the soil [children curl up in a little ball with their legs tucked under them]. The sun warms the soil and the rain falls down on the seeds [tap your fingers on the children's heads and shoulders]. The seeds soak up the rainwater and begin to get bigger and bigger [children uncurl], and a stem begins to sprout [children raise one hand over their head and continue to uncurl]. The stem grows and grows and leaves appear on it [children slowly stand up and spread their arms for leaves]. Then a lovely blossom begins to bloom on the flower [children make big bright smiles]. A big storm comes, and the rain and wind come to the garden [children sway and bend]. The storm ends, the sun appears, and all the flowers admire the strong and beautiful flower friends in their neighborhood garden [children nod and smile at one another].

This activity highlights for children the resilience of living things withstanding adversity and the support friends and family provide.

Rebuild Your Village

This activity is particularly useful when there has been significant or widespread destruction in an area. First, acknowledge the disaster that has occurred and the loss of familiar homes, parks, schools, or neighborhoods. Share that you know many people are busy planning ways to rebuild and that you are interested in the children's ideas about how to rebuild. Children can create their village using objects from the immediate area (scan for safety) or by using blocks. A version of this activity can also be done with children and families who have lost their home, school, neighborhood, etc.

Hope Quilting Bee

This activity is like an old-fashioned quilting bee, in which different members contribute their personal material and the entire group then sews individual pieces into a collective patchwork. You can use different-colored construction paper, crayons, pencils, and tape to connect the pieces into a hope quilt. Begin the activity by inviting members to draw the things that give them hope in this troubled time. What are their hopes and dreams for the future? If they could look into a magic mirror that showed what they would look like, how they would feel, and what they would be doing 6 months from now, what would they see? What can emerge from this process is a complex and rich portrait of collective survival.

CONCLUSIONS

At the beginning of this chapter, we used the metaphor of a maze to discuss the dynamics of children and families in times of crisis. Exactly which turn survivors decide to take in troubled times is uncertain, but we can use play-based interventions to help them find comfort, make meaning, take heart, and move on to follow the path that courage, hope, and compassion lead them down.

RESOURCES

All Family Resources
www.familymanagement.com
All Family Resources is a comprehensive website that provides information and services to enrich families. The topics include aging, providing child care, communicating, parenting, and dealing with catastrophes.

Association for Play Therapy (APT)
www.a4pt.org
The mission of this interprofessional association is to promote the value of play, play therapy, and credentialed play therapists. The APT works to advance the psychosocial development and mental health of all people by providing and supporting those programs, services, and related activities that promote the therapeutic value of play across the lifespan.

Federal Emergency Management Agency (FEMA)
www.fema.gov
The FEMA website contains education and training materials and modules for emergency personnel, teachers, clergy, and parents. See also FEMA for Kids

at *www.fema.gov/kids*. This is a fun and interactive site for children to learn about disaster preparedness and response through stories, games, and activities.

National Child Traumatic Stress Network (NCTSN)
www.nctsnet.org/nccts
The mission of the NCTSN is to raise the standard of care and improve access to services for traumatized children and their families and communities throughout the United States. The website offers a wide variety of resources for caregivers, teachers, and mental health providers.

National Institute of Child Health and Human Development (NICHD)
www.nichd.nih.gov/publications/pubs.cfm?from=
This site provides an activity book for African American families to use to help their children cope with crises.

National Institute of Mental Health (NIMH)—Helping Children and Adolescents Cope with Violence and Disasters
www.nimh.nih.gov/health/publications/helping-children-and-adolescents-cope-with-violence-and-disasters-rescue-workers/index.shtml
This portion of the NIMH website describes the impact of violence and disasters on children and adolescents, with suggestions for minimizing long-term emotional harm.

Substance Abuse and Mental Health Services Administration (SAMHSA)
www.mentalhealth.samhsa.gov/dtac/default.asp
This site provides up-to-date information about disasters as well as a guide to "psychological first aid" in times of crisis.

REFERENCES

Badenoch, B., & Bogdan, N. (2012). Safety and connection: The neurobiology of play. In L. Gallo-Lopez & L. C. Rubin (Eds.), *Play-based interventions for children and adolescents with autism spectrum disorders* (pp. 3–18). New York: Routledge.

Baggerly, J., & Exum, H. A. (2008). Counseling children after natural disasters: Guidance for family therapists. *American Journal of Family Therapy, 36*, 79–93.

Bailey, B. A., & Hartman, J. (2002). I wish you well: Loving Guidance website. See *It starts in the heart* [CD recording]. Retrieved from *www.beckybailey.com*.

Berscheid, E. (2003). The human's greatest strength: Other humans. In L. G. Aspinwall & U. M. Staudinger (Eds.), *A psychology of human strengths: Fundamental questions and future directions for a positive psychology* (pp. 37–47). Washington, DC: American Psychological Association.

Calhoun, L. G., & Tedeschi, R. G. (Eds.). (2006). *Handbook for posttraumatic growth research and practice*. Mahwah, NJ: Erlbaum.

Catani, C., Jacob, N., Schauer, E., Kohila, M., & Meuner, F. (2008). Family violence, war, and natural disasters: A study of the effect of extreme stress on children's mental health in Sri Lanka. *BMC Psychiatry, 8*(33), 1–10.

Dugan, E., Snow, M., & Crowe, S. (2010). Working with children affected by Hurricane Katrina: Two case studies in play therapy. *Child and Adolescent Mental Health, 15*, 52–55.

Echterling, L. G., Presbury, J., & McKee, J. E. (2005). *Crisis intervention: Promoting resilience and resolution in troubled times*. Upper Saddle River, NJ: Merrill/Prentice Hall.

Echterling, L. G., & Stewart, A. (in press). Promotion of resiliency in early childhood. In T. Gullotta & M. Bloom (Eds.), *Encyclopedia of primary prevention and health promotion* (2nd ed.) New York: Springer.

Emmons, R. A. (1999). *The psychology of ultimate concerns: Motivation and spirituality in personality*. New York: Guilford Press.

Emmons, R. A., Colby, P. M., & Kaiser, H. A. (1998). When losses lead to gains: Personal goals and the recovery of meaning. In P. T. P. Wong & P. S. Fry (Eds.), *The human quest for meaning: A handbook of psychological research and clinical applications* (pp. 163–178). Mahwah, NJ: Erlbaum.

Endo, T., Shioiri, T., & Someya, T. (2008). Post-traumatic symptoms among the children and adolescents two years after the 2004 Niigata–Chuetsu earthquake in Japan. *Japanese Society of Psychiatry and Clinical Neurosciences, 63*, 253.

Federal Emergency Management Agency. (2012). Helping kids cope with disaster. Retrieved from *www.fema.gov/coping-disaster*.

Gaskill, R. L., & Perry, B. D. (2012). Child sexual abuse, traumatic experiences, and their impact on the developing brain. In P. Goodyear-Brown (Ed.), *Handbook of child sexual abuse: Identification, assessment, and treatment* (pp. 29–47). Hoboken, NJ: Wiley.

Janoff-Bulman, R. (1992). *Shattered assumptions: Towards a new psychology of trauma*. New York: Free Press.

Jordan, B., Perryman, K., & Anderson, L. (2013). A case for child-centered play therapy with natural disaster and catastrophic event survivors. *International Journal of Play Therapy, 22*(4), 219–230.

Kanel, K. (2012). *A guide to crisis intervention* (4th ed.). Pacific Grove, CA: Brooks/Cole.

Keck, M., & Lakdapolrak, P. (2013). What is social resilience?: Lessons learned and ways forward. *Erdkunde, 67*(1), 5–19.

Kessler, R. C., Davis, C. G., & Kendler, K. S. (1997). Childhood adversity and adult psychiatric disorder in the U.S. National Comorbidity Survey. *Psychological Medicine, 27*, 1101–1119.

Landreth, G. (2002). *Play therapy: The art of relationship* (2nd ed.). Muncie, IN: Accelerated Development.

Larsen, J. T., Hemenover, S. H., Norris, C. J., & Cacioppo, J. T. (2003). Turning adversity to advantage: On the virtues of the coactivation of positive and negative emotions. In L. G. Aspinwall & U. M. Staudinger (Eds.), *A psychology of human strengths: Fundamental questions and future directions for a positive psychology* (pp. 211–225). Washington, DC: American Psychological Association.

National Child Traumatic Stress Network—Terrorism and Disaster Branch. (2005). Tips for helping school-age children. Retrieved from *www.nctsnet. org/nctsn_assets/pdfs/pfa/TipsforHelpingSchool-AgeChildren.pdf.*

Neimeyer, R. A. (2000). Searching for the meaning of meaning: Grief therapy and the process of reconstruction. *Death Studies, 24*, 541–558.

Reis, H. T., Collins, W. A., & Berscheid, E. (2000). The relationship context of human behavior and development. *Psychological Bulletin, 126*, 844–872.

Ryff, C. D., & Singer, B. (2003). Flourishing under fire: Resilience as a prototype of challenged thriving. In C. L. M. Keyes & J. Haidt (Eds.), *Flourishing: Positive psychology and the life well-lived* (pp. 15–36). Washington, DC: American Psychological Association.

Shelby, J., & Bond, D. (2005, October). *Using play-based interventions in Sri Lanka.* Paper presented at the annual conference of the Association for Play Therapy, Nashville, TN.

Siegel, D. J. (2012). *The developing mind: How relationships and the brain interact to shape who we are* (2nd ed.). New York: Guilford Press.

Stein, N., Folkman, S., Trabasso, T., & Richards, T. A. (1997). Appraisal and goal processes as predictors of psychological well-being in bereaved caregivers. *Journal of Personality and Social Psychology, 72*, 872–884.

CHAPTER 11

Vanquishing Monsters
Group Drama Therapy for Treating Trauma

Craig Haen

> What drew me to the story and what I wanted to show people,
> is that even in the midst of trauma, children play.
> —MAURICE SENDAK (cited in Fosha, 2001)

My first internship as a drama therapist was spent working with adults in a hospital day treatment program. When I initially sat in on group therapy sessions, I found myself amazed at the frequency with which these patients spoke about their painful childhood experiences. The memories of traumatic events seemed to have a particularly tenacious grip on these adults: locking them into their past as they played out familiar relational patterns in an unsuccessful bid to rework the experiences. Indeed, research speaks to the tremendous power trauma wields over the human psyche; it is often resistant to intervention and connected to a range of long-term physical and mental health repercussions (Green et al., 2010; Irish, Kobayashi, & Delahanty, 2010). Research also suggests that the greatest hope for people who have been traumatized lies in the implementation of trauma-specific treatment during childhood (Perry, 2006; Schore, 2012). However, therapists who work with this population are continuously charged with the difficult tasks of engaging and building trust with young people whose abilities to connect with an adult and process what has happened to them are routinely compromised.

Drama therapy is a modality that integrates role play, stories, improvisation, and other techniques derived from theatrical performance with the theories and methodology of psychotherapy. The result is an embodied, experiential process that draws on the patient's capacity for play, utilizing it as a core route for accessing and expressing internal conflict, achieving insight, rehearsing alternative choices, and cognitively reworking habitual patterns of response to stressful situations. At its essence, drama therapy works with and through the imagination, making it an advantageous modality for therapists who treat traumatized children. In van der Kolk's (2005) words, trauma represents "a failure of the imagination" in which the past overtakes the present and patients become plagued by their own internal imagery, unable to foresee other possibilities for themselves. As Bloom (2005) wrote, "It is this ability to create possibility, to envision alternative universes, that must be unfrozen if an ill child is to re-enter the stream of life" (p. xvi). Contemporary neuroscience research is underscoring the potential, suggesting that imagination is central to meaning making, and that imagining an action can enhance one's ability to perform it (Marks-Tarlow, 2012).

In a previous article (Haen, 2005b) I described a game that spontaneously developed during my work with young children who lost parents in the terrorist attacks on the World Trade Center. In this game, one child would pretend to be a monster and chase the other group members around the room. Upon catching them, he would attack them in a grotesque fashion, gnawing at their limbs and eating their body parts. This game seemed a clear metaphorical representation of the traumatic deaths of their parents, whose bodies had been similarly torn to pieces. Eventually, the group was able to work with me to develop a safe space under a table where the monster was not welcome. In this space, they discussed what made them feel safe in real life. After connecting with one another and internalizing the safe space, they went out to face the monster. Together, they vanquished him, taking control of the game and experiencing a collective sense of accomplishment.

This clinical vignette provides an illustrative example of the drama therapy process with traumatized children. The first stage involves externalization, in which the traumata are projected out, separated from the patient, so they can be viewed from a safe distance. During this externalization process, some children feel the need to embody the perpetrator/traumatizing agent, as did some of the group members who chose to take on the role of the monster. In the second stage, a psychological safe space is built, either obliquely through the group process or more tangibly, as in this game, through the creation of an actual secure base in the room. In the third stage, there is connection as members begin to join together as a working group, finding strength, validation, and purpose. Finally, there is vanquishment of the monster—the stage in which members find ways to gain mastery over their traumatic material, to combat and contain it. In defining these stages, I am not articulating a progressive model, as stages may evolve at any point in the process and groups may return to them, as is often true of the cyclical nature of children's recovery. Indeed, in the aforementioned group, a great deal of work was done on creating safety before the members felt ready to invite a monster into their play.

This chapter illustrates how drama therapy processes can be used for externalization and containment of trauma material, as well as for the purposes of creating safety and building connection in groups. Group therapy has a long history in the treatment of children, particularly in trauma treatment where groups help to counter the isolation resulting from traumatic exposure (Ford, Fallot, & Harris, 2009). It is important to understand that the techniques presented here are not for application in a cookbook fashion. Rather, they are offered as additional tools that group leaders can access. The most resonant interventions tend to be those that reflect the therapist's attuned response to patients' readiness and needs, and that emerge naturally from the evolving treatment process (Blaustein & Kinniburgh, 2010; Gil, 2010).

ON THE EFFICACY OF DRAMA THERAPY INTERVENTION

Coalescing largely in the 1960s and 1970s, drama therapy is a young discipline relative to its counterparts in the mental health field. The vast majority of research in the field is qualitative (Jones, 2012), a state not unusual across the creative arts therapies (Goodman, Chapman, & Gantt, 2009). In the area of trauma, there have been a handful of outcome studies on drama therapy. These studies (Haste & McKenna, 2010; Johnson, Lubin, James, & Hale, 1997; McArdle et al., 2002, 2011) showed tentative evidence for greater effectiveness of trauma treatment when drama therapy was part of the treatment framework.

Research advances in the fields of traumatology, developmental psychopathology, neurobiology, and attachment studies, however, provide strong support for drama therapy as a treatment method for traumatized children. The integration of these related fields has led to a paradigm shift in psychotherapy from primarily cognitive models of clinical intervention to those that increasingly focus on embodied emotion and the regulation of psychobiological states (Bromberg, 2011; Perry, 2009; Schore, 2012). This shift has helped to define goals that drama therapy is uniquely suited to achieving, making it a promising practice in trauma treatment. Developmental researcher Trevarthen (2009) offered an example of such interdisciplinary support:

> Infant research supports the use of nonverbal intersubjective therapies, such as music therapy, movement or dance therapy, drama therapy, pictorial art therapy, and body psychotherapy because these approaches accept that we are all equipped with a sensitivity for movement and qualities in movement, not only in our own bodies but in the bodies of others we touch, see, and hear. Moreover, "arts therapies" have the benefit of accepting the assumption that we are story-making creatures, and that our own autobiography, and its main supportive characters, is the story that affects us most deeply. (p. 84)

GROUP TREATMENT OF TRAUMATIZED CHILDREN: A SERIES OF RETURNS

Galatzer-Levy (1991), in considering therapy with adolescents, advocated that the central goal of working with young people was not the amelioration of symptoms but the resumption of development. This perspective is readily applicable to trauma treatment with children. Trauma has the effect of freezing young people in the midst of psychological, neurological, social, and biological growth trajectories (D'Andrea, Ford, Stolbach, Spinazzola, & van der Kolk, 2012; Van Horn, 2011). Therapy, particularly in the initial stages, must aid in returning them to normal developmental pathways (Pearce & Pezzot-Pearce, 2007). As the effects of trauma are multifaceted, successful treatment usually involves a series of returns.

A Return to Safety

One of the paradoxes of trauma treatment is that patients are asked to access emotions and thoughts related to the very events from which their bodies and minds are now working to protect them (Muller, 2010;

Silberg, 2013). Children's exposure to trauma can rupture notions of safety at a time when they often lack the developmental capacity to verbalize cohesively what has happened to them or how they feel about it (Van Horn, 2011). Even when traumatized children are able to put experiences into words, concurrent hyperarousal and physiological dysregulation can render the treatment experience a failure (Fisher & Ogden, 2009; Levine, 2010). Although they may gain insight and develop a narrative that organizes the experience, many children's internal reactions continue to leave them feeling unsafe (Perry, 2006; Porges, 2011).

Research points to the need for patients to establish psychological distance from the affectively charged trauma material so that an internal sense of safety can be achieved (van der Kolk, 2003). Drama therapists regularly utilize distance as a central concept (Jones, 2007). By working through metaphor, patients are able to explore a problem from a depotentiated place safely removed from reality (Dix, 2012; Landy, 2010). From this position, the traumatized child can bring cognitive processing back online and view the situation more clearly (Pearce & Pezzot-Pearce, 2007; Wise & Nash, 2013). Ramachandran (2011) has suggested that metaphor also has the capacity to connect the differential processing modes of the left and right brain.

As the child internalizes the therapist's interventions, she learns to negotiate distance for herself, gradually responding to distress in a self-protective yet active way. Casson (2004) articulated this process:

> This play with distance creates the space between therapist and patient: space for the growth and expansion of the self. Such play enables us to discover that we can feel, think, move, achieve control, let go of control, choose, negotiate, change, lose and find self and other. (p. 125)

Providing distance opens the door for trust to develop. When children begin to trust the therapist and the group itself, they can step into a process that requires taking emotional and psychological risks that are in opposition to the stifling, self-protective barriers they have established (Hodermarska, Haen, & McLellan, 2014). In new groups of young children, I frequently bring a stuffed animal, usually a dog, to function as my veritable co-therapist. As a warm-up, the kids pass the dog around and tell him how they are feeling or what they would like to talk about that day. Through this small piece of projective work, the intensity of being in the group and talking to a therapist is lessened.

Distance is also achieved through the method used in creating characters. For example, I always have children who are engaging in dramatic play create characters with names other than their own or those of anyone in the group, so that these characters can function as both similar to the actor and different from him. Defining the boundaries of the dramatic space also helps to establish distance. The "stage" can be physically marked by the use of furniture, tape, the boundaries of the circle, and so on. The process of entering into a scene is similarly important in distancing the action from reality, with greater degrees of ritual or structure supporting a clearer boundary between the imagined and the actual. I often use the device of having the group collectively shout, "One, two, three, action!" to serve as a catalyst for a scene to begin.

Trauma practitioners regularly stress the importance of developing a safe space in treatment, an anchor patients can summon when they begin to experience distress in therapy or in life. The notion of a safe space harkens back to childhood attachment, in which safety is learned through the experience of attuned dyadic regulation with a trusted caregiver (Hart, 2011; Jennings, 2011). In the caregiver–child relationship, safety is communicated largely through the visual and sensory aspects of interaction: breath, touch, soothing sounds, facial expressions, singing, and prosody, leading to a "felt" sense of security that the child can summon when distressed (Caldwell, 2012; Holmes, 2010). Steele and Malchiodi (2012) asserted that the creative arts therapies, by engaging visual and sensory input, have the added advantage of enhancing attachment within the therapy relationship. For example, the building of a safe space in drama therapy can be actualized in the creation of that space in the room, allowing the patient to not only verbalize what it is like to be safe but to feel it *in vivo*.

During group sessions, particularly when it appears that the members are becoming dysregulated, I will often ask them to find a space in the room. Once there, I invite them to imagine themselves in a place that feels safe and to take on a pose of themselves in that place. One by one, I tap them and allow them to demonstrate what they are doing in that space, what it looks like there, and how it is similar to and different from the space of the group. We might also find a way to capture the essence of that space—by shrinking it and storing it within the body so it can be located through a somatic marker such as warmth in one's chest or strength in one's shoulders (Fisher & Ogden, 2009).

A lasting sense of safety is one that is sustained over time through experiences in which the child is able to summon trauma memories while simultaneously having newly generated experiences of grounded-ness, trust, pleasure, and affect modulation (Blaustein & Kinniburgh, 2010). This pairing results in the trauma memory gradually being asso-ciated neurologically with greater degrees of internal regulation and social engagement, and thereby creating the potential for reconsolida-tion (Ecker, Ticic, & Hulley, 2012; Porges, 2011). Van der Kolk (2005) asserted that theater is adept at providing this pairing for children because, by engaging in enactments in which they assume stances of power, freedom, and safety, they gain "the physical experience of how things can be different." In a recent outcome study, van der Kolk and colleagues (Kisiel et al., 2006) found that improvisational theater work had a significant impact on increasing prosocial behaviors and prevent-ing aggression, while decreasing hyperactivity and internalizing symp-toms, in inner-city fourth graders.

In groups with older children from traumatized families, I often invite someone to create a family portrait, casting other members in a bodily sculpture representing how the person creating the portrait per-ceives things to be in his family. I then ask the group member to stand in for himself in the picture, and to speak about how it feels to be in the picture. Next, the member is asked to step out of the picture and to make adjustments to show how he wishes it would look. He then steps back into it to talk about how it feels to be in this revised version of fam-ily. This activity can be adapted for younger children or group members who need greater distance by asking them to create a fictional fam-ily in which there are problems, or families of animals, wizards, or any other fantasy character. In addition to providing the impetus to voice changes, the family portrait allows the child to experience these differ-ences and highlights the internal sensations that develop as a result.

Finally, by working with children's imaginations, drama therapists can help them learn to regulate their fantasies. There are many rituals for containment in a group that can assist in teaching mastery over trauma material. Among those I've used most frequently are the magic box (Johnson, 1986) and fortunately/unfortunately stories. In the for-mer, an imaginary box is brought down from the ceiling, and the group members take turns putting something from their lives they would like to get rid of in the box where it can be safely kept. The box is then packed away through the closing and locking of the lid and other group efforts. In the latter, group members engage in collective storytelling, each contributing a line to the story in turn. Lines alternate between those that begin with "Fortunately . . ." and "Unfortunately. . . ".

The second exercise works with cognitive flexibility and particularly transformation, which usually resonates with traumatized children. The group can be accessed to transform overwhelming, violent images that arise into safe ones (Haen, 2005a; Haen & Brannon, 2002). The children might be asked to wave a magic wand to turn a monster into a mouse or to use an imaginary remote control to change the channel on a violent scene to another show "fit for family viewing." I have sometimes engaged groups in which members have been abused in pushing their imagined perpetrator out of the room or in building a jail to contain scary memories while they are in the session. These rehearsed pieces of mastery can be generalized outside the group into learning how to alter intrusive thoughts, nightmares, and other internally generated imagery. They also lend themselves to the practice of oscillation techniques in which children learn to move from triggering to manageable affective states (Ogden & Gomez, 2013).

A Return to the Body

More than just a psychological disorder, trauma is also a biological phenomenon with enduring effects on the body and brain (D'Andrea et al., 2012; Ehlert, 2013; Emerson & Hopper, 2011). Childhood trauma occurs at a time of rapid growth and development. This collision can result in the child's discomfort with being present in the body and aware of bodily sensations (Koch & Harvey, 2012), particularly those that convey what Tinnin and Gantt (2013) referred to as the "nonverbal truth" of the traumatic experience (p. 46). During my time working in a psychiatric unit, I encountered many traumatized children who went into hiding in their bodies or waged war against them: sexually abused girls who attempted to disguise their developing feminine features; recipients of physical abuse who disengaged from activities and resisted any form of touch or sensory stimulation; witnesses of traumatic deaths who stopped eating so they wouldn't grow up; abused and neglected children who engaged in self-harm or disordered eating. These responses can all be understood in the context of their trying to achieve a sense of control, regulate affect, or symbolically communicate what they have endured (Silberg, 2013).

Creative arts therapists have long appreciated the importance of engaging the body in the therapy process. Indeed, all the creative arts therapies involve some degree of kinesis, sensory input, or bodily rhythm (Armstrong, 2013; Steele & Malchiodi, 2012). Drama therapists work with degrees of embodiment: from the small, controlled movement of manipulating miniature toys or objects, to the partial embodiment of taking on a role utilizing a puppet, to the less distanced experiences of full-bodied role play, sculpting, and mask work (Haen, 2011).

Vigorous physical play has tremendous potential for reshaping traumatic experiences and allowing for reconsolidation of traumatic memories within a context of effective action and shared joy (Harvey, 2011; Panksepp & Biven, 2012). Trauma is constricting, rigidifying, and inflexible (Hodermarska et al., 2014), and therefore calls for interventions that promote somatic inhabitance and the expansion of windows of tolerance (Levine, 2010; Ogden, 2009; Siegel, 1999). In addition to increasing children's comfort with embodiment, drama therapy groups can gradually desensitize them to being looked at, a particular trigger for individuals who have endured abuse or bodily injury.

Often, simple drama games can begin this process. Because these games are fun, many children readily participate, despite their fears. One game in particular that I have used to get children and adolescents warmed up is Exploding Red Light, Green Light. This game is an enhancement of the children's game Red Light, Green Light, in which players must attempt to be the first to reach the leader who calls out "Green Light" to indicate when players can start moving and "Red Light" when they must stop. When the leader catches a child moving after she has called out "Red Light," she says that child's name and he must return to the start line. In this version of the game, while returning to the line the child is asked to "explode." Many types of explosions are celebrated, from uttering the words "Boom!" or "Kapow!" to letting out a noise of frustration, to yelling at or challenging the leader. This simple game playfully engages group members in practicing self-control, as well as expressing emotion through sound and movement. When the leader encourages explosions directed toward her, she gives permission and a context for the expression of anger and resistance in a contained structure. By engaging in this game, children are being brought safely into their bodies.

Sculptures have endless applications and are an easy initiation to role play, as well as to being in the body. I have asked group members to create brief, individual poses that reflect different feelings and situations. I have also asked groups to create sculptures together to reflect pertinent themes. One group of preadolescents would begin each session by casting members to create a picture from their day, from which full scenes were later built. In another group that took place in a school, the members played a game called Wax Museum in which they created a series of thematically similar sculptures for another member to walk through as though visiting a wax museum. Like Exploding Red Light, Green Light, some of the focus is on participants moving when the person walking around isn't looking. In this group, the game became a format for gradual exposure to material related to the violent death of a fellow student that had recently occurred at the school. With repeated sessions, the group members created Wax Museums related to the themes of death, reporters, suicide, mental hospitals, rage, protection, and heaven.

Drama games not only return children to their bodies but also integrate kinesthetic experience with verbal and iconic learning. In doing so, drama builds the children's sense of competency by internalizing the locus of control (Macy, Macy, Gross, & Brighton, 2003). Role-play activities also provide a natural lead-in to teaching body-based self-regulation skills such as diaphragmatic breathing, resourcing, mindfulness, body scanning, and deep pressure/release self-touch (Curran, 2013; Leahy, Tirch & Napolitano, 2011; Levine & Kline, 2007), which can easily be incorporated into *deroling* from dramatic scenes or the ritual closure of a group session. These techniques are designed to fine-tune traumatized children's faulty biological alarm systems and to encourage trust in their own capacity for self-repair (Ford, Albert, & Hawke, 2009).

A Return to Connection

Though the drama therapy field is a young one, it is rooted in the ancient tradition of the theater, dating back to early Greece. Since its beginnings, theater has been an art form based in community, in which people of all classes and backgrounds would gather to see life reflected on the stage. Integral to the narratives of many of the earliest recorded plays were traumatic events involving grief, loss, murder, violence, and war. Drama therapy is a natural extension of Ancient Greek theater, drawing upon the power of representation, identification, and communal experience in connecting people.

Social connectedness is vitally protective and reparative for traumatized children (Ludy-Dobson & Perry, 2010), and groups provide the opportunity for the formation of a literal support network (Ayalon, 2013). Drama therapy targets the most basic components of connection: mirroring, validation, empathy, and universality. Macy and colleagues (2003) articulated the process in this way: "When a child moves to music, he experiences connection; when that same child moves to music and experiences peers mirroring that movement, affiliation is experienced; when vocalization accompanies the shared movement, integration may begin" (pp. 65–66).

Recent research (Ramseyer & Tschacher, 2011) using video imaging software to analyze psychotherapy sessions found that bodily synchrony between patient and therapist positively correlated with patient ratings of the strength of the therapeutic relationship as well as with clinical outcomes. Mirror exercises, in which one member literally mirrors the movements and sounds of a partner, or in which the group serves as a collective mirror for the expression of an individual, are powerful ways to forge resonant interpersonal connections (Koch & Harvey, 2012). There are many variations of these exercises, including having two children work together, each trying out being leader and follower. In the warm-up, I will sometimes have members pass a movement around the circle. There are two components to this process. First, the member mirrors the movement that the child next to him has demonstrated, then she makes that movement her own and passes it to the next person. As the movement travels the circle, the group can witness the ways in which each person transforms it. As a facilitator, I often encourage the members toward effective mirroring, helping them notice subtleties of expression and accurately represent them, honoring the contributions of peers.

Objects can be used in the group to solidify connection. The passing of a ball or toy from person to person not only engages members, but also makes the process of sharing focus tangible. I will verbalize this process by saying, "Throw the ball to someone you'd like to check in with" or "Pass the bear to someone whom you think understands how you feel." In a group of very resistant teenagers, I once passed around a miniature, stuffed Sigmund Freud. When the members received the toy, they were asked to identify the worst thing a therapist or adult had ever said to them. In residential settings, I often ritualize the beginning of the group by having members send a greeting to someone in the circle, encouraging eye contact and authentic connection.

Finally, sociometric exercises that emphasize commonalities among members are helpful in underscoring that the group is an entity built on shared experience and emotions (Haen, 2005a). There are endless variations of these exercises, but they all involve marking similarities between members through action. For example, group members might be asked to cross from one end of the room to the other if they like pizza, to stand up from their seats if they have had nightmares, or to switch chairs if they sometimes cry when they think about their families. In each variation, the action is repeated: "Now cross the room if you hate getting up in the morning. . . . Now, everybody who thinks this group might be boring, cross the room." The expressions of connection are brief and nonverbal, allowing members to take risks quickly. For example, I have been in groups where a child might pose the statement, "Cross the room if you've been raped." Since the group learns that exposure is minimal, they often take the risk.

Fonagy and colleagues use the term *mentalization* to refer to the ability to see oneself from the outside and others from the inside (Allen, Fonagy, & Bateman, 2008). Mentalization is intimately tied to children's capacities to empathize, organize, self-regulate, self-protect, articulate feelings, develop a sense of agency, integrate self states, control impulses, and understand the impact of their actions on others (Hart, 2011). Not surprisingly, early exposure to trauma compromises mentalization processes, whereas a robust capacity to mentalize is thought to mitigate the impact of traumatic events (Allen, Lemma, & Fonagy, 2012).

Attachment theorists believe that mentalization is developed in part through the process of pretend play (Allen et al., 2008). During play, the child learns to link internal and external realities and to test out different possibilities (Irwin, 2005). Drama therapy can assist in reinvigorating this developmental milestone in traumatized children, particularly in a group (Barrat & Kerman, 2001). When children engage in dramatic play, they are externalizing aspects of the self to be examined, organized, and reintegrated (Armstrong, 2013; Holmes, 2010). Similarly, when they play roles, they are taking another's perspective and reflecting on thoughts, feelings, and intentions (Allen et al., 2008; Haen & Weber, 2009). Drama therapy may have unique advantages over other creative arts therapies in this domain. Preliminary research (Goldstein & Winner, 2012) suggests that ongoing exposure to acting, as opposed to visual art and music, correlated with increased empathy and theory of mind in children and adolescents.

When children are asked to give representation to the feelings of another, a connection is forged that is supported by mentalizing activity. I might ask children to create a sculpture representing something a group member has expressed, or to act out another member's story using puppets. I often use the psychodrama technique of doubling (Hoey, 2005) to encourage mentalization. In doubling, group members are asked to speak as if they are another member, giving voice to something that person might be thinking or feeling but unable to express. For example, an avoidant child might say, "I'm not talking today." When group members double, with the permission of the child, they stand behind him and say things like, "I'm bored" or "I'm afraid to talk" or "I'm not sure if I like this group." The child is then encouraged to share with the group which doubles came closest to articulating his true feelings.

Mentalization can be encouraged through taking on roles that are distant from who the child is in real life. For example, a passive group member can be encouraged to play an authority figure, or an angry member might be cast in a scene in which her task is to keep an angry character calm. Finally, the group can be engaged in reflecting back to a child her many facets of self as seen by peers. In an activity that I frequently used with hospitalized children (Haen, 2005a), the members would each sculpt different aspects of one child, choosing a part of her with which they related. When tapped by the leader, they might say, "I am the part of Stephanie that feels insecure" or "I am the part of Stephanie that wants to beat everyone up."

A Return to the Present

When a traumatized child's system shuts down in order to protect him, it often closes him off to the present moment. Trauma memories enter the mind without temporal anchoring, experienced as a reliving in the present rather than a remembering of the past (van der Kolk, 2003). Children who have been exposed to trauma thus show impairment in their abilities to be present, to take in new information, and to connect to what is happening around them from moment to moment (Emerson & Hopper, 2011). As Caldwell (2012) pointed out, trauma treatment, at its essence, is aimed at helping patients live in a present that is not continually intruded upon or dictated by past experience.

Stern (2004, 2010) devoted a great deal of attention to the clinical importance of the present moment. He cited the creative arts therapies, particularly those rooted in embodiment, as unique in their ability to focus the patient in the present. He also hypothesized that metaphor might serve to both connect and separate past and present, providing continuity and coherence for traumatized children. As an improvisational actor, I often felt a sense of heightened perception and connection when engaged fully in the experience. As Levine (2009) pointed out, improvisation is not without a level of risk as it hinges on uncertainty balanced by faith or trust in the process and others—a repeated experience of rupture and repair. In fact, a therapist's ability to stay focused and responsive to a patient in the midst of interpersonal turbulence has many parallels to the skills needed for theatrical improvisation (Kindler & Gray, 2010).

Drama therapists frequently ask patients to reflect on their *in vivo* experience and to represent it through metaphor or action. A much-used exercise involves asking members to express a sound and movement to reflect how they are feeling right then and there. I often begin groups with teenagers by asking them metaphorical questions, such as, "If how you are feeling inside right now was a type of weather, what would be the forecast?" or "If you were a kind of food today, what kind would you be?" Similarly, I might call a patient's attention to something his body is expressing but his words aren't. A member who is saying he's happy while his hands are making fists might be asked to talk as his fists. If I notice a patient who is rocking in the group, I might ask the members to "try on" that rocking and to give voice to how it feels.

An additional way therapists can call attention to the present moment is through maximization (Hoey, 2005). When using maximization, the group leader identifies an aspect of the patient's expression that requires further exploration and amplifies it through dramatic action. For example, in a scene in which a group member confronts a bully, she might utter the line, "Leave me alone!" The leader, understanding that these are significant words, can intervene by having her repeat the words several times, growing louder and stronger each time. Or, the leader might choose to have others in the group stand behind her and join in saying the line. Another example of maximization occurs when the leader freezes a scene and asks the characters to verbalize how they are feeling "inside" during a crucial moment of interaction. This intervention helps to connect here-and-now affect to language in a way that assists traumatized children in reflecting on and describing their internal, lived experience (Hart, 2011).

A Return to Self-Expression

Much has been written about the loss of voice that results from trauma. This loss, often referred to as *speechless terror*, has both psychological and biological origins (Fisher & Ogden, 2009). Many traumatized children experience impairment not only in their capacity to express emotions, but also in identifying and regulating these states (Lanius, Bluhm, & Frewin, 2013). The loss of connection to and control over affect can consequently contribute to a diffuse sense of self and a pervasive feeling of disempowerment.

Yet, in the face of the silence that trauma renders, children still seek opportunities to symbolically represent their stories. Even when they are able to access language to describe their memories, these words are often insufficient to capture the complexities of traumatic events. The abilities to capture complexity and play with time are two significant advantages that the arts hold over linguistic forms of representation used in traditional "talk therapy" (Ramachandran, 2011; Stern, 2010).

Drama, in specific, can act as an emotional release valve (Miranda, Arthur, Milan, Mahoney, & Perry, 1998) that assists patients in beginning to reclaim their voice through the safety of metaphor and character. I have witnessed this phenomenon time and again: children who cannot find their voice in discussion but begin to speak when handed a puppet or when given a character to play; kids unable to talk about their past trauma who can express it through role play; adolescents who remain quiet and guarded until handed a prop microphone and asked to report on the events of the group. With self-expression titrated by an empathic, attuned therapist comes the gradual breathing-out of the trauma experience.

One exercise I have adapted with success for young children was first articulated by Casson (2004). In this piece of dramatic work, group members are asked to pretend to be pet owners in a veterinary office. Each is asked to create an imaginary pet that is sick and to bring it to the doctor's office. The kids talk to the doctor about the pet's physical illness, as well as its feelings. The quality of the interaction between child and animal is often indicative of the amount and quality of caregiving that child has had in her own life. For example, in groups of children who have been abused, it is not uncommon for the children to treat the pet abusively. However, when they articulate the animal's illness to the doctor, they frequently give voice to their own symptoms and worries. As the doctor, I (or my co-leader) engage the members in identifying how to help the animal feel better and, together, we try to provide the pet what it needs to heal—an *in vivo* experience of active response to traumatic disempowerment.

Older children frequently enjoy role-playing a talk show or television interview on the topic of kids' fears (or a similar topic that provides appropriate distance from the direct experience). In a group for traumatically bereaved older children, members worked with partners to create a "goodbye" scene between two characters. Each pair was asked to role-play the scene multiple times with a different emotion attached to the goodbye—worry, anger, silliness, sadness, jealousy, and so on.

A key element of any drama therapy process is the therapist's facilitation of scene work: pausing the scene when the action becomes too intense; encouraging cognition if the scene is too affectively charged by asking for the characters' inner thoughts (or utilizing a similar intervention if the scene is too distant and requires a deeper exploration of affect); engaging the group in suggesting new directions or strategies for a character who is stuck; reversing roles if a patient could benefit from exploring a new perspective or requires distance; suggesting multiple endings for a scene in order to imagine different options characters have; projecting a scene into the past or future. The possibilities are numerous, but require a skilled facilitator who is interested in the use of role play for more than didactic purposes, who understands the multidimensional therapeutic benefits of the creative act. Although the group leader does indeed provide direction, she must balance this with engaging patients in collectively creating their own scenes and stories. As she does this, she begins to return the patients to their own sources of self-expression.

The act of creation exists in dialectical tension with the destruction that often results from trauma (Dokter, Holloway, & Seebohm, 2011). Engaging the group in creative tasks and purposeful action can provide a sense of possibility and future that helps members to metabolize the past while mitigating retraumatization and engendering a collective sense of accomplishment and shared meaning (Saul, 2014). In my groups, children have collectively built a safe parent, safe school, safe boyfriend, ideal hospital, perfect town, and loving family when their experiences in life have been the opposite. In a boys' group in a residential facility, the members worked to create a video drama that articulated their experiences of mental illness and displacement from families (Haen & Brannon, 2002). Even the act of creating a scene within a group can offer a sense of possibility when the members are all invested and engaged (Nash & Haen, 2005).

CONCLUSION

Like trauma, the experience of acting somehow defies linguistic representation. It is difficult to capture, in the simplicity of words, all that happens when people harness their imaginations and step into role. It is an absorbing experience that can access possibility, indomitable spirit, and connection. Most drama therapists enter the field after experiencing the power of creativity as theater artists. Having recognized the resulting changes within themselves, they endeavor to learn how to harness this force to similarly help others.

Guided by research advances in parallel fields, drama therapists can utilize what they know intuitively—that working with children through the imagination provides a means to safely integrate the damage wrought by traumatic events. In the dramatic space, victims become conquerors, midgets become giants, and children who feel cornered can learn to see many pathways. Robert Edmond Jones, a theater artist, recognized the transcendent possibility of acting and articulated it in his 1941 book *The Dramatic Imagination*. In it, he wrote:

> These players became aware of the profound duality of life at the moment when they spoke their first lines on a stage, and thereafter all their acting was animated by it. They called it giving a good performance. But what they meant was that a spirit was present in them for a time, making them say things that they themselves did not know they knew. . . . The thing that is absent from these records is the thing that never can be recorded, the emotion that these artists aroused in our hearts, the sense of triumph they gave us. Their peculiar power lay in this, that in their impersonations they could show us man's creating spirit, in action, before our eyes. They did not teach or preach about life or explain it or expound it or illustrate it. They created it—life itself, at its fullest and truest and highest. (pp. 156–157)

REFERENCES

Allen, J. G., Fonagy, P., & Bateman, A. W. (2008). *Mentalizing in clinical practice*. Washington, DC: American Psychiatric Association.

Allen, J. G., Lemma, A., & Fonagy, P. (2012). Trauma. In A. W. Bateman & P. Fonagy (Eds.), *Handbook of mentalizing in mental health practice* (pp. 419–444). Arlington, VA: American Psychiatric Association.

Armstrong, V. G. (2013). Modelling attuned relationships in art psychotherapy with children who have had poor early experiences. *Arts in Psychotherapy*, 40(3), 275–284.

Ayalon, O. (2013). CARING—Children at risk intervention groups: BASIC Ph guide for coping and healing. In M. Lahad, M. Shacham, & O. Ayalon (Eds.), *The "BASIC Ph" model of coping and resilience: Theory, research and cross-cultural application* (pp. 61–88). London: Jessica Kingsley.

Barrat, G., & Kerman, M. (2001). Holding in mind: Theory and practice of seeing children in groups. *Psychodynamic Counselling, 7*(3), 315–328.

Blaustein, M. E., & Kinniburgh, K. M. (2010). *Treating traumatic stress in children and adolescents: How to foster resilience through attachment, self-regulation, and competency.* New York: Guilford Press.

Bloom, S. (2005). Foreword. In A. M. Weber & C. Haen (Eds.), *Clinical applications of drama therapy in child and adolescent treatment* (pp. xv–xviii). New York: Brunner-Routledge.

Bromberg, P. (2011). *The shadow of the tsunami and the growth of the relational mind.* New York: Routledge.

Caldwell, C. (2012). Sensation, movement, and emotion: Explicit procedures for implicit memories. In S. Koch, T. Fuchs, M. Summa, & C. Müller (Eds.), *Body memory, metaphor and movement* (pp. 255–265). Amsterdam: Benjamins.

Casson, J. (2004). *Drama, psychotherapy and psychosis: Dramatherapy and psychodrama with people who hear voices.* New York: Brunner-Routledge.

Curran, L. A. (2013). *101 trauma-informed interventions: Activities, exercises and assignments to move the patient and therapy forward.* Eau Claire, WI: Premier.

D'Andrea, W., Ford, J., Stolbach, B., Spinazzola, J., & van der Kolk, B. A. (2012). Understanding interpersonal trauma in children: Why we need a developmentally appropriate trauma diagnosis. *American Journal of Orthopsychiatry, 82*(2), 187–200.

Dix, A. (2012). All the better to see you with: Healing metaphors in a case of sexual abuse. In L. Leigh, I. Gersch, A. Dix, & D. Haythorne (Eds.), *Dramatherapy with children, young people and schools: Enabling creativity, sociability, communication and learning* (pp. 83–90). New York: Routledge.

Dokter, D., Holloway, P., & Seebohm, H. (2011). *Dramatherapy and destructiveness: Creating the evidence base, playing with Thanatos.* New York: Routledge.

Ecker, B., Ticic, R., & Hulley, L. (2012). *Unlocking the emotional brain: Eliminating symptoms at their roots using memory reconsolidation.* New York: Routledge.

Ehlert, U. (2013). Enduring psychobiological effects of childhood adversity. *Psychoneuroendocrinology, 38*(9), 1850–1857.

Emerson, D., & Hopper, E. (2011). *Overcoming trauma through yoga: Reclaiming your body.* Berkeley, CA: North Atlantic Books.

Fisher, J., & Ogden, P. (2009). Sensorimotor psychotherapy. In C. A. Courtois & J. D. Ford (Eds.), *Treating complex traumatic stress disorders: An evidence-based guide* (pp. 312–328). New York: Guilford Press.

Ford, J. D., Albert, D. B., & Hawke, J. (2009). Prevention and treatment interventions for traumatized children: Restoring children's capacities for self-regulation. In D. Brom, R. Pat-Horenczyk, & J. D. Ford (Eds.), *Treating traumatized children: Risk, resilience, and recovery* (pp. 195–209). New York: Routledge.

Ford, J. D., Fallot, R. D., & Harris, M. (2009). Group therapy. In C. A. Courtois & J. D. Ford (Eds.), *Treating complex traumatic stress disorders: An evidence-based guide* (pp. 415–440). New York: Guilford Press.

Fosha, D. (2001). Trauma reveals the roots of resilience. *Constructivism in the Human Sciences*, 6(1–2), 7–15.

Galatzer-Levy, R. M. (1991). Considerations in the psychotherapy of adolescents. In M. Slomowitz (Ed.), *Adolescent psychotherapy* (pp. 85–100). Washington, DC: American Psychiatric Association.

Gil, E. (2010). Children's self-initiated gradual exposure: The wonders of posttraumatic play and behavioral reenactments. In E. Gil (Ed.), *Working with children to heal interpersonal trauma: The power of play* (pp. 44–63). New York: Guilford Press.

Goldstein, T. R., & Winner, E. (2012). Enhancing empathy and theory of mind. *Journal of Cognition and Development*, 13(1), 19–37.

Goodman, R. F., Chapman, L. M., & Gantt, L. (2009). Creative arts therapies for children. In E. B. Foa, T. M. Keane, M. J. Friedman, & J. A. Cohen (Eds.), *Effective treatments for PTSD: Practice guidelines from the International Society for Traumatic Stress Studies* (2nd ed., pp. 491–507). New York: Guilford Press.

Green, J., McLaughlin, K. A., Berglund, P. A., Gruber, M. J., Sampson, N. A., Zaslavsky, A. M., et al. (2010). Childhood adversities and adult psychiatric disorders in the National Comorbidity Survey Replication I: Associations with first onset of DSM-IV disorders. *Archives of General Psychiatry*, 67(2), 113–123.

Haen, C. (2005a). Group drama therapy in a children's inpatient psychiatric setting. In A. M. Weber & C. Haen (Eds.), *Clinical applications of drama therapy in child and adolescent treatment* (pp. 189–204). New York: Brunner-Routledge.

Haen, C. (2005b). Rebuilding security: Group therapy with children affected by September 11. *International Journal of Group Psychotherapy*, 55(3), 391–414.

Haen, C. (2011). The therapeutic use of superheroes in the treatment of boys. In C. Haen (Ed.), *Engaging boys in treatment: Creative approaches to the therapy process* (pp. 153–175). New York: Routledge.

Haen, C., & Brannon, K. H. (2002). Superheroes, monsters and babies: Roles of strength, destruction and vulnerability for emotionally disturbed boys. *Arts in Psychotherapy*, 29(2), 31–40.

Haen, C., & Weber, A. M. (2009). Beyond retribution: Working through revenge fantasies with traumatized young people. *Arts in Psychotherapy*, 36(2), 84–93.

Hart, S. (2011). *The impact of attachment: Developmental neuroaffective psychology*. New York: Norton.

Harvey, S. (2011). Physical play with boys of all ages. In C. Haen (Ed.), *Engaging boys in treatment: Creative approaches to the therapy process* (pp. 91–113). New York: Routledge.

Haste, E., & McKenna, P. (2010). Clinical effectiveness of dramatherapy in the recovery from severe neuro-trauma. In P. Jones (Ed.), *Drama as therapy: Vol. 2. Clinical work and research into practice* (pp. 84–104). New York: Routledge.

Hodermarska, M., Haen, C., & McLellan, L. (2014). Exquisite corpse: On dissociation and intersubjectivity—implications for trauma-informed drama therapy. In N. Sajnani & D. R. Johnson (Eds.), *Trauma-informed drama therapy: Transforming clinics, classrooms, and communities* (pp. 179–205). Springfield, IL: Charles C Thomas.

Hoey, B. (2005). Children who whisper: A study of psychodramatic methods for reaching inarticulate young people. In A. M. Weber & C. Haen (Eds.), *Clinical applications of drama therapy in child and adolescent treatment* (pp. 45–65). New York: Brunner-Routledge.

Holmes, J. (2010). *Exploring in security: Towards an attachment-informed psychoanalytic psychotherapy*. New York: Routledge.

Irish, L., Kobayashi, I., & Delahanty, D. L. (2010). Long-term physical health consequences of childhood sexual abuse: A meta-analytic review. *Journal of Pediatric Psychology, 35*(5), 450–461.

Irwin, E. (2005). Facilitating play with non-players: A developmental perspective. In A. M. Weber & C. Haen (Eds.), *Clinical applications of drama therapy in child and adolescent treatment* (pp. 3–23). New York: Brunner-Routledge.

Jennings, S. (2011). *Healthy attachments and neuro-dramatic play*. London: Jessica Kingsley.

Johnson, D. R. (1986). The developmental method in drama therapy: Group treatment with the elderly. *Arts in Psychotherapy, 13*(1), 17–33.

Johnson, D. R., Lubin, H., James, M., & Hale, K. (1997). Single session effects of treatment components within a specialized inpatient posttraumatic stress disorder program. *Journal of Traumatic Stress, 10*(3), 377–390.

Jones, P. (2007). *Drama as therapy: Theory, practice and research* (2nd ed.). New York: Routledge.

Jones, P. (2012). Approaches to the future of research. *Dramatherapy, 34*(2), 63–82.

Jones, R. E. (1995). *The dramatic imagination*. New York: Theatre Art Books. (Original work published 1941)

Kindler, R., & Gray, A. A. (2010). Theater and therapy: How improvisation informs the analytic hour. *Psychoanalytic Inquiry, 30*(3).

Kisiel, C., Blaustein, M., Spinazzola, J., Schmidt, C. S., Zucker, M., & van der

Kolk, B. (2006). Evaluation of a theater-based youth violence prevention program for elementary school children. *Journal of School Violence, 5*(2), 19–36.

Koch, S., & Harvey, S. (2012). Dance/movement therapy with traumatized dissociative patients. In S. Koch, T. Fuchs, M. Summa, & C. Müller (Eds.), *Body memory, metaphor and movement* (pp. 369–385). Amsterdam: Benjamins.

Landy, R. J. (2010). Drama as a means of preventing post-traumatic stress following trauma within a community. *Journal of Applied Arts and Health, 1*(1), 7–18.

Lanius, R. A., Bluhm, R., & Frewen, P. A. (2013). Childhood trauma, brain connectivity, and the self. In J. D. Ford & C. A. Courtois (Eds.), *Treating complex traumatic stress disorders in children and adolescents: Scientific foundations and therapeutic models* (pp. 24–38). New York: Guilford Press.

Leahy, R. L., Tirch, D. D., & Napolitano, L. A. (2011). *Emotion regulation in psychotherapy: A practitioner's guide.* New York: Guilford Press.

Levine, P. A. (2010). *In an unspoken voice: How the body releases trauma and restores goodness.* Berkeley, CA: North Atlantic Books.

Levine, P. A., & Kline, M. (2007). *Trauma through a child's eyes: Awakening the ordinary miracle of healing.* Berkeley, CA: North Atlantic Books.

Levine, S. K. (2009). *Trauma, tragedy, therapy: The arts and human suffering.* London: Jessica Kingsley.

Ludy-Dobson, C. R., & Perry, B. D. (2010). The role of healthy relational interactions in buffering the impact of childhood trauma. In E. Gil (Ed.), *Working with children to heal interpersonal trauma: The power of play* (pp. 26–43). New York: Guilford Press.

Macy, R. D., Macy, D. J., Gross, S. I., & Brighton, P. (2003, Summer). Healing in familiar settings: Support for children and youth in the classroom and community. *New Directions for Youth Development, 98*, 51–79.

Marks-Tarlow, T. (2012). *Clinical intuition in psychotherapy: The neurobiology of embodied response.* New York: Norton.

McArdle, P., Moseley, D., Quibell, T., Johnson, R., Allen, A., Hammal, D., et al. (2002). School-based indicated prevention: A randomised trial of group therapy. *Journal of Child Psychology and Psychiatry, 43*(6), 705–712.

McArdle, P., Young, R., Quibell, T., Moseley, D., Johnson, R., & LeCouteur, A. (2011). Early intervention for at risk children: 3-year follow-up. *European Child and Adolescent Psychiatry, 20*(3), 111–120.

Miranda, L., Arthur, A., Milan, T., Mahoney, O., & Perry, B. D. (1998). The art of healing: The Healing Arts Project. *Journal of Music- and Movement-Based Learning, 4*(4), 35–40.

Muller, R. T. (2010). *Trauma and the avoidant patient: Attachment-based strategies for healing.* New York: Norton.

Nash, E., & Haen, C. (2005). Healing through strength: A group approach to therapeutic enactment. In A. M. Weber & C. Haen (Eds.), *Clinical applications of drama therapy in child and adolescent treatment* (pp. 121–135). New York: Brunner-Routledge.

Ogden, P. (2009). Emotion, mindfulness, and movement: Expanding the regulatory boundaries of the window of affect tolerance. In D. Fosha, D. J. Siegel, & M. F. Solomon (Eds.), *The healing power of emotion: Affective neuroscience, development, and clinical practice* (pp. 204–231). New York: Norton.

Ogden, P., & Gomez, A. (2013). EMDR therapy and sensorimotor psychotherapy with children. In A. Gomez (Ed.), *EMDR therapy and adjunct approaches with children* (pp. 247–271). New York: Springer.

Panksepp, J., & Biven, L. (2012). *The archaeology of mind: Neuroevolutionary origins of human emotions.* New York: Norton.

Pearce, J. W., & Pezzot-Pearce, T. D. (2007). *Psychotherapy of abused and neglected children* (2nd ed.). New York: Guilford Press.

Perry, B. D. (2006). Applying principles of neurodevelopment to clinical work with maltreated and traumatized children: The neurosequential model of therapeutics. In N. B. Webb (Ed.), *Working with traumatized youth in child welfare* (pp. 27–52). New York: Guilford Press.

Perry, B. D. (2009). Examining child maltreatment through a neurodevelopmental lens: Clinical applications of the neurosequential model of therapeutics. *Journal of Loss and Trauma, 14*(4), 240–255.

Porges, S. W. (2011). *The polyvagal theory: Neurophysiological foundations of emotions, attachment, communication, and self-regulation.* New York: Norton.

Ramachandran, V. S. (2011). *The tell-tale brain: A neuroscientist's quest for what makes us human.* New York: Norton.

Ramseyer, F., & Tschacher, W. (2011). Nonverbal synchrony in psychotherapy: Coordinated body movement reflects relationship quality and outcome. *Journal of Consulting and Clinical Psychology, 79*(3), 284–295.

Saul, J. (2014). *Collective trauma, collective healing: Promoting community resilience in the aftermath of disaster.* New York: Routledge.

Schore, A. N. (2012). *The science of the art of psychotherapy.* New York: Norton.

Siegel, D. J. (1999). *The developing mind: Toward a neurobiology of interpersonal experience.* New York: Guilford Press.

Silberg, J. L. (2013). *The child survivor: Healing developmental trauma and dissociation.* New York: Routledge.

Steele, W., & Malchiodi, C. A. (2012). *Trauma-informed practices with children and adolescents.* New York: Routledge.

Stern, D. (2004). *The present moment in psychotherapy and everyday life.* New York: Norton.

Stern, D. (2010). *Forms of vitality: Exploring dynamic experience in psychology, the arts, psychotherapy and development*. New York: Oxford University Press.

Tinnin, L., & Gantt, L. (2013). *The instinctual trauma response and dual-brain dynamics: A guide for trauma therapy*. Morgantown, WV: Gargoyle Press.

Trevarthen, C. (2009). The functions of emotion in infancy: The regulation and communication of rhythm, sympathy, and meaning in human development. In D. Fosha, D. J. Siegel, & M. F. Solomon (Eds.), *The healing power of emotion: Affective neuroscience, development and clinical practice* (pp. 55–85). New York: Norton.

van der Kolk, B. A. (2003). The neurobiology of childhood trauma and abuse. *Child and Adolescent Psychiatric Clinics of North America, 12*(2), 293–317.

van der Kolk, B. A. (2005, May). *Attachment, helplessness, and trauma: The body keeps the score*. Paper presented at the Harvard Medical School conference on attachment and related disorders, Boston.

Van Horn, P. (2011). The impact of trauma on the developing social brain: Development and regulation in relationship. In J. D. Osofsky (Ed.), *Clinical work with traumatized young children* (pp. 11–30). New York: Guilford Press.

Wise, S., & Nash, E. (2013). Metaphor as heroic mediator: Imagination, creative arts therapy, and group process as agents of healing with veterans. In R. M. Scurfield & K. T. Platoni (Eds.), *Healing war trauma: A handbook of creative approaches* (pp. 99–114). New York: Routledge.

CHAPTER 12

Trauma-Informed Art Therapy and Group Intervention with Children from Violent Homes

Cathy A. Malchiodi

Todd is an 8-year-old boy who recently witnessed the physical abuse of his mother by her boyfriend on several occasions. Previous to these incidents, Todd's biological father divorced his mother, Maria, after 3 years of verbally abusing Todd and battering Maria. At the age of 6, Todd attempted to intervene during one of his parents' violent episodes by contacting the police on his mother's cellphone. In response, his father punished him by locking him in a closet for 3 days. He and his mother are staying in a shelter for battered women and their children.

Shareesa is a 12-year-old girl who witnessed her stepfather beat her mother and her younger brother. Earlier in her life, her biological father physically and sexually abused her for 2 years until her mother decided to take her and seek refuge at a shelter for battered women and their children. Shareesa and her mother and younger brother are currently staying at a safehouse for domestic violence survivors and will be moving to long-term housing for battered women in the next month.

Megan is a 10-year-old girl who witnessed her father beat her mother and threaten her with a gun and is a victim of physical abuse by her older brother. Megan also witnessed her father kill the family's dog during a particularly violent and prolonged episode. She is currently in foster care until her mother recovers from her injuries and is able to find a secure place for Megan and herself to live. Megan worries that if she tells anyone else about the abuse she has witnessed and experienced, she will be permanently taken away from her mother.

Tim is the 9-year-old son of two parents in the military; he has a 2-year-old sister. Tim's father has been deployed overseas on at least five occasions and has been in active combat three times. His parents recently separated because Tim's father became violent toward his mother on several occasions; during one incident, Tim's mother had to go to the hospital emergency room because of serious injuries. Tim is now in a children's resiliency-building group designed to support military families who are experiencing stress and interpersonal violence; he still worries that there will be more "hitting," and his teacher reports that he is becoming withdrawn and anxious at school.

Although each of these children has had experiences that could be considered traumatic in nature, all have one experience in common— exposure to violence in their homes, also known as *domestic violence* or *intimate partner violence*. Domestic violence is defined as the use or threat of use of physical, verbal, emotional, or sexual abuse within an intimate relationship with the intention of creating fear, intimidation, or control (Child Welfare Information Gateway, 2013); it is not only an action by men against women and may include assaults by women against men or between same-sex partners/spouses. When there is domestic violence, there is often child abuse; children may be hurt or injured purposively or accidently. In all cases, it is a serious problem in families and is a frequent source of trauma reactions in children.

The negative impact of domestic violence on child victims has been repeatedly acknowledged, but there continue to be few models of intervention developed to address these children's short- and long-term psychosocial needs (Child Welfare Information Gateway, 2013; Malchiodi, 1997; McCue, 2008). Art therapy and play therapy are two widely applied approaches with children from violent homes (Gil, 2011; Malchiodi, 1997, 2014; Webb, 2007) and are an important part of many trauma interventions, including trauma-focused cognitive-behavioral therapy (TF-CBT; Cohen, Mannarino, & Deblinger, 2012) and trauma-informed art therapy (Malchiodi, 2011, 2014) in group formats. There is wide agreement that art and play therapy allow memories and emotions to surface in ways that these children can tolerate and enable the use of make-believe toward therapeutic ends (Klorer, 2008; Malchiodi, 2011). This chapter presents a brief description of the nature of domestic violence, its effects on school-age children, and a model for structured group trauma-informed art therapy.

DOMESTIC VIOLENCE AND CHILDREN

Todd, Shareesa, Megan, and Tim are among the estimated 10 million children who may be exposed to domestic violence each year (Child Welfare Information Gateway, 2013); the exact number is really not known because many events of child exposure are not reported. In all cases, each child has witnessed violence in his or her home and seen his or her mother beaten by an intimate partner or husband. Because children can be witnesses and recipients of domestic violence, "exposure to domestic violence" is incorrect and does not cover the vast number of ways children experience violent behavior in their homes. "Exposure" or "witness" imply that children are passive bystanders; in many situations, children are active participants who assess their roles in "causing the fight," worry about consequences, and try to protect themselves, siblings, or a parent, grandparent, or other family member. They may take on parental or caregiver roles, attempting to problem-solve or referee conflicts, distracting the abuser, or calling first responders or neighbors for outside help. In brief, children's exposure to domestic abuse includes, but is not limited to, the following experiences (Child Welfare Information Gateway, 2013; National Child Traumatic Stress Network, 2014):

1. Hearing or witnessing an episode of violence or loud conflict.
2. Seeing the aftermath of an episode, such as injuries or arrival of police.
3. Being used as part of the violence, such as a shield against an abusive parent or caregiver.
4. Intervening in an attempt to prevent family violence.
5. Experiencing repercussions of a violent episode.
6. Being forced to watch or participate in abuse or battering.
7. Being used as a pawn to convince an adult victim to return home or to a relationship.
8. Experiencing accidental harm during an attack on an adult victim.
9. Being coerced to remain silent about family violence and to maintain the family secret.
10. Being encouraged or forced to abuse a parent through threats and/or abuse to a pet.
11. Stating the child's misbehavior is the reason the parent or caregiver is abusive.

Exposure to domestic violence can result in a wide range of emotional, psychological, cognitive, social, and behavioral problems for children. Research indicates that children who are exposed to domestic violence may incur any or all of the following.

Emotional, Social, and Behavioral Problems

Children who are exposed to domestic violence may display more fear, anxiety, anger, low self-esteem, excessive worry, and depression than nonexposed children. They also may be more aggressive, oppositional in their behavior, withdrawn, or lacking in conflict resolution skills and often have poor peer, sibling, and other social relationships. They are often particularly watchful of others (hypervigilance) because events have led them to believe that people can be dangerous, volatile, or unpredictable. Others may have attachment difficulties throughout childhood, and many suffer from sleep problems, eating disorders, somatic symptoms, and/or bedwetting or other regressive behaviors. These children are diagnosed more frequently with separation anxiety, obsessive–compulsive disorder, and conduct disorder than children who are not exposed to family conflicts (Child Welfare Information Gateway, 2013; Malchiodi, 1997; McCue, 2008; National Child Traumatic Stress Network, 2014).

Cognitive Problems

Children exposed to family violence may perform poorly in school, have lower cognitive functioning, and have limited problem-solving abilities. They also may have difficulties in concentration and comprehension due to repeated traumatic experiences.

Long-Term Problems

As adolescents and adults, children exposed to domestic violence have more depression and trauma-related symptoms. They also may accept violence as normal to interpersonal interactions and may believe in gender stereotypes that support beliefs of male dominance in relationships. Domestic violence is believed to have intergenerational aspects, and perpetrators of domestic violence who were abused as children are also more likely to maltreat their own children later in life (Child Welfare Information Gateway, 2013).

Variability

The impact of domestic violence can be mediated by a number of factors, including type of experience with violence (witnessing, single direct assault, or multiple direct assaults), children's adaptive skills, age, gender, time elapsed since exposure, and exposure to other traumatic events. Research also suggests that children who experience physical violence from family members are more likely to have posttraumatic stress than those who simply witness abusive events (Child Welfare Information Gateway, 2013; McCue, 2008).

Similarity

Children who have long-term exposure to domestic violence have striking similarities to children who survive wars and other conflicts. For example, interparental conflicts wax and wane in their severity and may be sporadic or daily. Like children who are in the midst of wars, children from violent homes are witnesses to, and recipients of, physical harm, unstable conditions, and volatile situations. There may be destruction of property, displacement, loss, and separation of family members. On occasion, children may be imprisoned or even held hostage. As a result, they develop thoughts, perceptions, and beliefs consistent with their experiences of conflict and react to disputes and disagreements between adults as stressful and possibly dangerous due to what they have learned from interactions between parents or caregivers.

Resiliency

Finally, despite exposure to domestic violence, some children are remarkably resilient and show few reactions as a result of their experiences. In other words, whereas some children react adversely to stressful circumstances, others recover quickly from exposure to violence when they return to safe living arrangements. Mediating factors for resilience to domestic violence include the level of exposure to violence, personal characteristics of the child, and the extent and quality of parental/adult support (National Child Traumatic Stress Network, 2014).

TRAUMA-INFORMED ART THERAPY

Trauma-informed art therapy (Malchiodi, 2011, 2012a, 2014) is a model for intervention that integrates neurodevelopmental knowledge and the sensory qualities of all the arts within trauma intervention. It includes five principles: (1) using sensory, arts-, and play-based approaches to self-regulation; (2) applying a neurodevelopmental approach to stabilize the body's responses to stress; (3) identifying the body's reactions to stressful events and memories; (4) using arts- and play-based interventions to establish and support safety and positive attachment; and (5) capitalizing on strength building through arts- and play-based therapies to normalize and enhance resilience (Malchiodi, 2011, 2014). In brief, this approach takes into consideration how the mind and body respond to traumatic events, recognizes that symptoms are adaptive coping strategies rather than pathology, and helps individuals move from being survivors to "thrivers" (Malchiodi, 2011). In particular, it is an approach used to assist the individual's capacity to self-regulate affect and moderate the body's reactions to traumatic experiences to set the stage for eventual trauma integration and recovery.

A TRAUMA-INFORMED ART THERAPY ENVIRONMENT

Providing safety and self-regulation creates the foundation for effective group trauma-informed art therapy with children who have experienced interpersonal violence (Malchiodi, 2011). Safety and self-regulation begin with establishing a setting and therapeutic relationships that support these goals (Steele & Malchiodi, 2012). The environment includes not only the physical surroundings the children encounter, but also how helping professionals respond in trauma-informed ways. The Sanctuary Model® (2014; Bloom, 2009, 2010) is a seminal example of a trauma-informed environment that teaches necessary skills for maintaining and cultivating nonviolent lives and systems; this model has been widely applied to group intervention in shelters and other agencies that deal with trauma and interpersonal violence. It also uses sensory-based, culturally sensitive practices to ameliorate the impact of trauma and is based on understanding how mind and body respond to traumatic events.

Levine and Kline (2008) propose that a child must experience the following in order to feel safe and to be able to self-regulate: (1) my body is safe; (2) my feelings are safe; (3) my thoughts, words, and ideas are safe; and (4) things I make are safe. These principles are essential to providing trauma-informed art therapy in residential groups as well as outpatient groups for children from violent homes. They can be summarized as the following trauma-informed art therapy practices that define a trauma-informed environment:

1. *Establish a sense of control.* Consider how children who have experienced interpersonal violence perceive their environment and relationships; in most cases, they are hyperaware of possible danger or harm. It is important that helping professionals provide opportunities for children to feel in control of the therapeutic environment; for example, therapists can give children the opportunity to arrange seating in the art and play therapy room or let them share in determining group routines for art making. To help children feel safe during sessions, practitioners can help them establish cues (e.g., hand signals for "time out" or "slow down").

2. *Maintain consistency.* Children from violent homes have typically experienced an inconsistent and often chaotic home life. Predictable rituals for beginning and ending art and play therapy sessions are essential; for example, each group should start with a familiar art or play activity that establishes a routine. Also, helping professionals can support consistency by being predictable in their own responses and actions during sessions.

3. *Reduce sensory overload.* Art and play therapy present many stimulating materials, props, and toys; however, children who have been traumatized are overactivated by too many sensory stimuli and choices. Limit materials and props during initial sessions until young clients can self-regulate and adjust to the environment when confronted with new experiences or media. Use art materials that are more easily controlled, such as felt markers, pencils, and precut collage materials or self-soothing activities (simple coloring, doodling, or familiar crafts) that reduce sensory overload and increase relaxed alertness.

4. *Support experiences of mastery.* A key reason for introducing art and play in trauma-informed practice is to support a sense of mastery. Overly complicated directives with multiple steps can be too overwhelming; choose activities that are success-oriented with high engagement and a low potential for frustration. Also, stress reduction strategies that address the physiological aspects of the traumatic stress of exposure to violence at home can provide a sense of mastery over fear, panic, and worries that many children experience.

5. *Be culturally sensitive.* Getting to know the various cultural backgrounds of children is a key trauma-informed practice. Ethnicity is not the only consideration. Tim, described in the beginning of this chapter,

comes from a military culture; other children may come from specific religious or community values. Children constitute a "culture"; they feel respected in an atmosphere that communicates their worldviews and values their perspectives. In all cases, culturally diverse art and play materials are an important component of trauma-informed practice.

6. *Provide reassurance.* Working with children who have experienced or witnessed violence challenges the therapist's ability to help them feel safe through sensory and verbal cues. Levine and Kline (2008) underscore the importance of looking for physical cues that indicate trauma responses (fight, flight, or freeze) such as rapid breathing, hyperarousal, or withdrawal. Because art and play experiences are sensory in nature and may tap implicit responses to trauma, it is particularly important to observe children's somatic reactions to these activities. Finally, reassurance also includes reinforcing that what has happened at home or between parents or caregivers is not the child's fault and that what happened is not "happening right now."

7. *Instill and enhance resilience.* From the beginning of intervention it is important to reinforce with children that although they have been victims of situations out of their control, they are also survivors with capabilities of thriving. Art and play activities that support self-empowerment, positive relationships, and positive contributions are essential. Identifying and supporting resilience in children from violent homes is key to their success throughout childhood, adolescence, and beyond (Malchiodi, 2011).

Finally, the following items are helpful to have in group trauma-informed art and play environments:

1. Tables and comfortable chairs for children.
2. Pillows and floor mats for relaxation activities.
3. Art materials (paper, cardboard, oil pastels, felt-tip markers, collage materials including precut magazine images, colored paper, fabrics and yarns, child-safe scissors, stapler, tape, white glue, glue sticks, clay, tempera paint, and brushes).
4. Puppets (multicultural family puppets, assortment of animal puppets, finger puppets, and rescuer puppets such as police, doctors, or other first responders).
5. Children's books for quiet reading time and therapeutic storytelling.
6. Board games for recreation and therapeutic games for group work (e.g., Ungame or the Talking, Feeling, and Doing Game).

7. Building blocks or Legos for construction.
8. Snacks for breaks and stickers or other tokens as treats.

Some therapists favor generic play materials and toys rather than figures that are associated with story characters from movies or cartoons because they allow children to use their imaginations to project their own experiences. Gil (2011) notes that specifically and purposively selected play materials are key to supporting children's expression about difficult experiences involving abuse and family violence. For example, she provides access to a set of play figures depicting a court scene because many children who have been exposed to violence may end up testifying in court and seeing a perpetrator on trial. In my experience, in short-term, time-limited situations, more generic materials support children's adaptive coping skills when they feel the need to remain guarded about what are often "family secrets" and uncomfortable disclosures. In settings where children are seen over a longer period of time and in individual sessions, specific materials, props, and toys are important to in-depth work with issues inherent to interpersonal violence and parents/caregivers who hurt children or each other.

GROUP INTERVENTION: STRUCTURE AND CHALLENGES

Group intervention is a popular strategy for addressing the trauma of school-age children's exposure to domestic violence (Child Welfare Information Gateway, 2013). Therapeutic programs for these children have mostly been available in shelters for battered women or homeless families or in agencies providing services to women and their children. Most structured groups for children exposed to domestic violence are time-limited and usually run 6–10 sessions. They often have psychoeducational components, including discussion of family violence, development of personal safety plans, and understanding feelings associated with trauma. A group format is effective for most children because it helps them realize that others have had the same or similar experiences and that they are not alone in their feelings of fear, anger, worry, sadness, or guilt. For example, 10-year-old Megan (described in the beginning of this chapter) learned by listening to other children that she was not the cause of her abuse and that talking about what had happened with the art and play therapist will not cause her to become separated from her mother.

Nevertheless, there are some challenges to group intervention with this population. Groups for children from violent homes are, at best, variable in the number of sessions; that is, because of the nature of a shelter, agency, or other therapeutic setting, the number of group sessions in which children may be available to participate is unpredictable. In some domestic violence shelters, children may be seen for as few as one or two sessions; in outpatient or mental health agency settings, children may participate in 6–10 sessions on a weekly basis. In many cases, group participants change frequently, with new children admitted and others terminating their participation without notice. In brief, consistent participation is one of the greatest challenges in working with this population.

Because the number of sessions for participation is often limited, another challenge is the type of art and play intervention offered and the pace of treatment. Introducing emotionally loaded topics in sessions may not be of service to children who may only attend a limited number of times. In brief, using materials and directives in a careful and controlled manner is one solution to this challenge. For example, I use drawing and magazine photo collage, two materials that are more easily contained and controlled, when the task is to focus on more emotionally charged topics and uncomfortable feelings; for older children, writing in a journal or workbook is another variation. The general principle is to provide an experience that allows for more control because it taps executive functioning rather than lower, sensory parts of the brain.

In contrast, in providing activities that are intended to support resilience and experiences of self-soothing and self-regulation, I use more sensory-based materials such as clay, paints, fabric, tactile papers, yarns, feathers, and glitter. In thinking about interventions, Levine's (Levine & Kline, 2008) concepts of titration and pendulation are helpful. *Titration* refers to exposing individuals to small amounts of distress or uncomfortable emotions; *pendulation* refers to moving back and forth between less comfortable and more comfortable emotional and somatic states. Titration and pendulation are more easily accomplished with materials that are contained and controlled when addressing distress (e.g., "What happened?" or "Draw a picture of a worry") than more flexible and multisensory media. The latter is more appropriate when children are directed to activities meant to promote relaxation and stress reduction and to enhance a sense of accomplishment and mastery (for a more detailed discussion of the therapeutic applications of art materials, see Malchiodi, 2012b).

A MODEL FOR TRAUMA-INFORMED ART THERAPY GROUP INTERVENTION

Judith Herman (1992), a well-known expert on the trauma of abuse and domestic violence, describes a three-part trauma recovery model that is applicable to developing group intervention with children from violent homes. Her model includes (1) establishing safety, (2) telling the trauma story, and (3) restoring connection between traumatized individuals and their communities. Over the years I have modified Herman's model to adjust to the pace of children's experiences, the setting for group intervention, and the reality of domestic violence, which often does not follow a linear path from safety to stable reconnection with caregivers. In group work, just as in individual therapy, it is essential to honor the pace of individual children who may not be ready to engage in all activities described in the next sections. The activities included in each stage are simply recommended guidelines to be adapted depending on the composition and type of trauma experienced by child participants.

Early Sessions: Establishing Safety and Supporting Self-Regulation

Initial group sessions emphasize the development of trust and safety and learning self-regulation skills. No child who has come from an abusive situation, whether a victim of physical assault or a witness, will be able to recover from trauma, be comfortable with self-disclosure, or learn new skills without first feeling secure. Children who come from violent homes often are fearful or anxious about the environment and any unfamiliar children and adults, including the therapist. Also, for those children whose participation is limited to only one or several sessions, the self-regulation skills presented in these early sessions are internal resources that they can use once they leave a shelter or therapeutic program.

On a practical level, it is imperative to discuss confidentiality during initial interviews for entry into the group and during the first several group meetings. Children should know and understand that the therapist will not repeat their words to parents or caregivers without their permission but that the therapist will keep those adults informed about what issues children are working on in therapy and their general progress. Children should also know and understand that certain disclosures that come up in the group—such as intent to self-harm, threat of harm from others, or threat of harm to others—cannot be kept confidential. Additionally, during the initial session, group rules are introduced. In work with children from violent homes, it is also important to discuss rules about physical contact and to state clearly that hitting or other forms of physical assault and verbal abuse (name calling, bullying, and insults) are not acceptable; art products and other creative expressions are given the same respect. These rules can be placed on a colorful poster, signed by the children to reinforce the group's contract and displayed in the group meeting room. Overall, trauma-informed practice underscores that therapists support group members' needs for safety and control in choosing what to talk about in the group in order to build trust.

Activities during initial sessions of the group include:

- Creating a safe place for a small toy animal, using art materials (see Figures 12.1 and 12.2).
- Creating a "safety hand," with names and contact information of people to call in case of emergency or danger of violence.

Materials: Small rubber duck toy, small paper plate, collage materials (tissue paper, colored paper, feathers, fabric, yarn, beads), natural materials (twigs, leaves, acorns), scissors, glue, felt marking pens, and glitter glue.

Instructions: You will be making a safe space for a duck. You can use a paper plate as the base for a home for your duck and decorate it either using drawing materials or collage materials. If you choose to use collage materials, have fun with the fabrics, feathers, pipe cleaners/chenille stems, colored tissue paper, and glitter.

> **Can You Make a Home for Your Duck?**
>
> Your duck needs a home!
>
>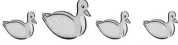
>
> Where does your duck live?
>
> Where would your duck live to be happy and feel safe?
>
> Does your duck live alone or does your duck live with other ducks?
>
> What does your duck like to do? How does your duck have fun?
>
> *Make a drawing or build a home for your duck!*
>
>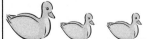

FIGURE 12.1. Creating a safe place for your duck.

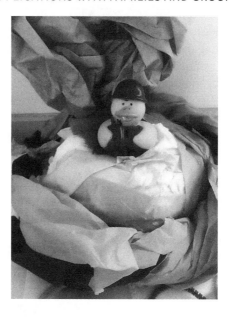

FIGURE 12.2. Example of a "safe place for your duck" activity.

- Making a drawing of a worry and learning to use scaling techniques such as a "feelings thermometer" or "how big is my worry" to identify how bad the worry is.
- Using a body outline to indicate "where my worry is in my body," using colors, shapes, and lines.
- Creating a three-dimensional paper house with collage images of safety and peace.
- Practicing several relaxation activities, such as deep breathing and yoga poses or mindfulness exercises (as described in Rappaport, Chapter 14, this volume).
- Free time for arts, crafts, and play during each session to allow for spontaneous expression and self-soothing.

In brief, activities during this phase provide experiences that address personal care and safety and provide opportunities for expression of feelings about events associated with violence or abuse, according to children's pace. The focus is on supporting children's abilities to learn self-care and self-regulation through identifying resources, situations that create worry or anxiety, how the body reacts to stress, and strategies for reducing stress when uncomfortable feelings arise.

Middle Sessions: Telling the Trauma Story

The second phase of the group, telling the trauma story, involves activities to encourage self-disclosure and the sharing of personal experiences. Children should now have some resources with which to self-regulate and reduce stress. During these sessions, children are encouraged to talk about how domestic violence has affected them, if they feel comfortable doing so. The overall goal is to help children address the trauma of violent events and to begin to regain their abilities to experience and enjoy life even though bad things have happened. James (1989) summarizes this brilliantly as follows: "The goal is to have traumatized children reach the point where they can say something like, 'Yes, that happened to me. That's how I felt and how I behaved when it happened. This is how I understand it all now. I won't really forget that it happened, but I don't always have to think about it either'" (p. 49).

Although this stage in intervention underscores the trauma narrative and associated experiences, many children still need to feel in control of what they disclose and express. Structured interventions during this phase include:

- Creating a magazine picture collage of what it feels like to be powerful and powerless.
- Creating a "strength tree" to illustrate strengths, contributions, and personal courage (see Figure 12.3).
- Reading therapeutic storybooks about domestic violence.
- Drawing something about "what happened" (domestic violence, abuse, or other traumatic events) and drawing "what would make what happened get better."
- Drawing "who/what makes me worried (afraid, angry) since it happened."
- Making "how hands can help or hurt" posters.
- Learning about negative and positive self-talk and practicing simple cognitive-behavioral techniques to reduce negative thinking.
- Practicing scaling techniques such as feelings thermometers and "success towers."
- Engaging in free time for arts, crafts, and play during each session to allow for spontaneous expression and self-soothing.
- Learning relaxation and stress reduction activities to decrease experiences of worries or other uncomfortable feelings in the body.

Materials: For a two-dimensional strength tree (see illustration below)—one sheet of 12″ × 18″ white or colored construction paper for the background; drawing materials such as felt markers or oil pastels; collage materials (scraps of colored paper, tissue paper, glitter glue, feathers, fabric, yarn); white glue and glue sticks; scissors. For a three-dimensional strength tree, one sheet of cardboard or small paper plate for the base; brown paper sandwich bag for tree (see illustration below).

Instructions: You can either draw an image of a tree (don't worry what your tree looks like; just try to include roots at the bottom and branches or leaves on the top) or use collage materials to create your tree image. You can also use a paper bag to make a three-dimensional tree by gluing the bottom of the bag to a paper plate; when it is dry, twist the bag into a trunk and cut the top to make branches. You can use paper and other materials to add leaves.

To make your tree "strong," think of three people who helped you—perhaps a parent, grandparent, brother or sister, friend, teacher, minister, or counselor. Write or make pictures of these three people and put them on the roots of your tree. Now think of three things you are good at or things you have done to help others. Write or make pictures of these three things in the top of the tree.

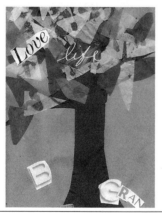 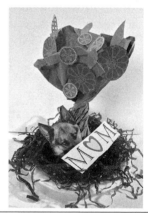

FIGURE 12.3. Creating a strength tree.

During this phase, the therapist models how to be supportive of group members, reassures group members that domestic violence is not their fault, and acknowledges each child's unique contributions to the group. Because discussing traumatic events or feelings can produce anxieties or trigger stress reactions, free time for art making and play becomes particularly important during these sessions. Children need to release tension accumulated after disclosing or discussing abuse or may simply require time to relax after talking about uncomfortable experiences or recalling traumatic memories.

Final Sessions: Transition and Termination

Herman (1992) notes that the final stage of trauma recovery involves restoration of connections with important people in the individual's life. For children from violent homes, this may be a complicated circumstance for many reasons; some may have been separated from a parent or caregiver, or a parent or caregiver may have abandoned a child or may have died. In some cases, however, children may be separated from parents or caregivers for reasons of safety and concerns of exposure to additional violence. All of these challenges cannot be addressed in this chapter, but are obviously important to treatment.

Ideally, nonabusive parents or caregivers are available to participate in the group alongside the children in some of the final sessions. Social support and positive attachment are key factors in enhancing resilience, and parents/caregivers are the most important connection to the child's current and future emotional reparation and recovery; participating in creative arts therapies together is one way to enhance connection (Malchiodi, 2014). In a practical sense, their active participation gives the therapist the opportunity to help parents learn additional information about maintaining a safe and stable home environment for themselves and their children. As long as exposure to violence or lack of safety at home continues, children cannot begin the process of reparation from the trauma of exposure to domestic violence. Many of the activities used during the first phase of the group to help children feel safe and secure can be adapted or repeated in child–parent sessions.

During these joint sessions, it is important to let children take the lead by encouraging them to share accomplishments and achievements. Because of their previous experiences with the group, child participants are now "experts" on art and play therapy. They are the authorities on their experiences within the group; this is a trauma-informed principle that enhances a sense of contribution and empowerment. The final several sessions of the group also focus on termination—preparing to say goodbye to the other participants and the therapist and to end the group. Endings can be particularly difficult for children from violent homes because of previous negative experiences of separation or abandonment by parents, caregivers, or other family members. Therefore, termination should be carefully and sensitively planned so that children understand not only its significance, but also that, despite the group's ending, no one will be abandoned, and support is available if needed in the future.

Interventions during this stage include:

- Sharing of self-selected artwork, skills learned, and accomplishments from previous sessions by children with parents/caregivers.
- Child–parent dyad engages in co-creating art expressions (e.g., a strength tree) or in structured play activities together.
- Child–parent co-create "safety hands" to reinforce and rehearse plans for emergencies or dangerous situations and/or co-create an "escape route" picture.
- Child–parent digital photographs taken, to be included in co-created collages to reinforce positive connection.
- Child-created drawing or collage about the "past, present, and future," summing up the progress made during the group.
- Termination activities, including group photos.
- Drawing worries and using scaling techniques to compare current worries to those expressed in early sessions.
- Reviewing and practicing relaxation and mindfulness skills.
- Having a group celebration during the final session and receiving portfolios of artwork, photos of group members, goodbye cards, and a certificate of completion.

CASE EXAMPLE: TIM

As described earlier in this chapter, 9-year-old Tim witnessed his father battering his mother on several occasions, and his mother separated from his father as a result. Because Tim's father was in the military, he was referred to a children's resiliency group I facilitated for a large military base. Unfortunately, many of the children referred to this group came from families who were challenged by the stress of multiple deployments of one or more parents, posttraumatic stress reactions, alcohol abuse, traumatic brain injury, and in some cases, domestic violence. Tim had been referred to a family advocacy program (FAP), but his mother felt he needed additional assistance and that he would enjoy art and play activities. She observed that Tim had become much more anxious, was not sleeping well, was less independent, and was not performing up to age level in school—all common outcomes for children who experience multiple deployments of a parent and marital conflict (U.S. Department of Defense, 2010). In fact, Tim's pediatrician was worried that he had higher than normal blood pressure for a child his age; since he was not overweight, she attributed it to his level of stress, noting, "Tim is excessively hyperalert to his surroundings and is easily startled." Tim's reactions, in fact, were similar to those of combat military with post-traumatic stress, particularly in terms of hyperarousal, sleeplessness, and impaired cognitive functioning.

Tim was cautious and somewhat withdrawn during the first several sessions of the resiliency group; he seemed watchful and, at times, dis-sociative when other participants became noisy or anxious. He shared very little about himself except to say that he was "proud of his father's service to his country" and that he worried about his younger sister lately because "she was crying a lot since their dad did not live with them anymore." Rather than pressing Tim for more disclosure about the family violence, I spent some extra time with him at the end of each group, practicing relaxation and mindfulness activities to help him self-regulate; he particularly enjoyed mindfulness techniques that were physically challenging, such as balancing a peacock feather on the end of his index finger and standing with one foot on a balance disk (a semi-soft disk) while breathing in and out to specific rhythms.

During the fourth session, the participants were given a plastic duck and asked to create a "safe place for your duck" (Figure 12.1) using assorted materials (colored tissue paper, glitter, feathers, twigs, beads, chenille stems) and a paper plate for a foundation. The ducks provided for this activity come decorated with various armed services hats and clothing (toy manufacturers make ducks in different colors, costumes, and themes). Unlike previous sessions, Tim responded with excitement, jumping out of his seat to grab one of the ducks and materials to get started. His duck environment (Figure 12.2) was elaborate; he used a little of each of the different materials provided and even gave his duck some additional military clothing. After the children completed the activity, each child shared a story about his or her duck in a small group of two or three children. Tim shared the following about his "Captain Duck":

> "Captain Duck wants to come home cuz he has been away a long, long time. He sometimes reads the Bible and makes believe he is at home. This gives him better feelings. He is a brave duck who is proud to be a soldier. His children draw pictures of him when he is in Iraq and make believe that he comes to life. They also make believe that he and their Mother Duck are like parents in the mov-ies and they all live together."

The activity seemed to act like a release valve for Tim, and although it did not eliminate all of his anxiety and startle responses, he kept his duck with him, bringing it to each subsequent session and sharing the story about Captain Duck on several occasions. His narrative communicated many of the mixed feelings and wishes that his parents would someday reunite. As he retold the story, he also added his concerns about Captain Duck's "temper" and the time that "Mother Duck" was injured and some of the fears he had about a possible recurrence of violence at home. For Tim, like many children who witness violence at home, this simple activity provided a way to tell a story from a third-person perspective, creating a measure of safety in disclosure. The activity also provided a way to have a conversation with Tim about personal safety and what he could do to "feel better" when he was anxious or experiencing sleeplessness.

Tim's mother attended three of the final sessions of the resiliency group, and along with other parents, joined in activities with their children. During one session, they were asked to create a "strength tree" (Figure 12.3) together; this activity became an important turning point for Tim and his mother, both as a source of resilience and as a way to strengthen their connection to each other. They created a three-dimensional tree with a large brown paper bag and decorated it with numerous "good things about each other." To the mother's surprise, Tim wanted to put a large leaf on the tree with the words "my mom is very brave" on it. When I asked Tim if he had anything else to say to his mom about her courage, he quickly volunteered, "She kept my baby sister and me safe when dad got scary. My dad is brave, but our mom is just as brave." Tim was also gratified to learn that his mother was very proud of his own bravery during so many stressful and challenging times over the last 2 years of family conflict.

Tim's parents eventually entered a relationship-building program for couples via the military base, and Tim's father started treatment for anger management and posttraumatic stress reactions that contributed to his violence. After many months of hard work, the couple reunited; Tim's father was reassigned to duty in the United States, which relieved the family of the stress of future multiple deployments for the short term. Tim continued to participate in groups for military children, and although he still experienced some problems in learning, he was able to concentrate more effectively, and his teachers and doctor reported that he was generally less anxious and more outgoing. For children such as Tim who have experienced violence in their homes, continuing to support stress reduction and resilience are important "maintenance" practices to help them adjust to new challenges throughout childhood and adolescence.

CONCLUSION

Art making and play are the natural activities of childhood. Unfortunately, domestic violence often robs young survivors of a normal childhood, taking away the very experience of being a child. Purposeful art and play activities, within a trauma-informed structure, can help these children reconnect with these experiences and restore the sense of spontaneity through providing opportunities for creative self-expression and imagination.

Brief treatment through group trauma-informed art and play therapy may not result in complete recovery from exposure or abuse, but it can establish the foundations necessary to reduce stress-related symptoms and enhance resilience to future crises. For some children from violent homes, positive changes occur relatively easily and are noticeable to parents, teachers, and helping professionals over the short term. For others, behavioral changes occur slowly or may be delayed by additional trauma. For these children, group intervention can be an important step along a longer journey toward healing. In all cases, individual personality, capacity for resiliency, personal histories, amount of exposure to interpersonal violence, parental support, and the availability of additional trauma-informed intervention affect each child's potential for emotional reparation and recovery.

REFERENCES

Bloom, S. (2009). Domestic violence. In J. O' Brien (Ed.), *Encyclopedia of gender and violence* (pp. 216–221). Thousand Oaks, CA: Sage.

Bloom, S. (2010). The mental health aspects of IPV: Survivors, professionals and systems. In A. Giardino & E. Giardino (Eds.), *Intimate partner violence, domestic violence, and spousal abuse* (pp. 207–250). St. Louis, MO: STM Learning.

Child Welfare Information Gateway. (2013). *Definitions of domestic violence.* Washington, DC: U.S. Department of Health and Human Services, Children's Bureau.

Cohen, J. A., Mannarino, A. P., & Deblinger, E. (2012). *Trauma-focused cognitive-behavioral therapy for children and adolescents*. New York: Guilford Press.

Gil, E. (2011). *Helping abused and traumatized children*. New York: Guilford Press.

Herman, J. (1992). *Trauma and recovery*. New York: Basic Books.

James, B. (1989). *Treating traumatized children*. New York: Free Press.

Klorer, P. (2008). Expressive therapy for severe maltreatment and attachment disorders. In C. A. Malchiodi (Ed.), *Creative interventions for traumatized children* (pp. 43–60). New York: Guilford Press.

Levine, P., & Kline, M. (2008). *Trauma-proofing your kids*. Berkeley, CA: North Atlantic Books.

Malchiodi, C. A. (1997). *Breaking the silence: Art therapy with children from violent homes* (2nd ed.). New York: Brunner-Routledge.

Malchiodi, C. A. (2011). Trauma-informed art therapy and sexual abuse in children. In P. Goodyear-Brown (Ed.), *Handbook of sexual abuse* (pp. 341–354). Hoboken, NJ: Wiley.

Malchiodi, C. A. (2012a). Art therapy with combat veterans and military personnel. In C. A. Malchiodi (Ed.), *Handbook of art therapy* (pp. 320–334). New York: Guilford Press.

Malchiodi, C. A. (2012b). Art therapy materials, media, and methods. In C. A. Malchiodi (Ed.), *Handbook of art therapy* (pp. 27–41). New York: Guilford Press.

Malchiodi, C. A. (2014). Creative arts therapy approaches to attachment issues. In C. A. Malchiodi & D. Crenshaw (Eds.), *Creative arts and play therapy for attachment problems* (pp. 3–18). New York: Guilford Press.

McCue, M. L. (2008). *Domestic violence: A reference handbook*. Santa Barbara, CA: ABC-CLIO.

National Child Traumatic Stress Network. (2014). Children and domestic violence. Retrieved February 3, 2014, from *www.nctsnet.org/content/children-and-domestic-violence*.

Sanctuary Model®. (2014). Sanctuary in shelter. Retrieved February 2, 2014, from *www.sanctuaryweb.com/shelters.php*.

Steele, W., & Malchiodi, C. A. (2012). *Trauma-informed practices with children and adolescents*. New York: Routledge.

U.S. Department of Defense. (2010). *The impacts of deployment of deployed members of the Armed Forces on their dependent children: Report to the Senate and House Committees*. Washington, DC: Author.

Webb, N. B. (Ed.). (2007). *Play therapy with children in crisis* (3rd ed.). New York: Guilford Press.

PART IV

Creative Interventions as Prevention

CHAPTER 13

Bullying, Trauma, and Creative Art Interventions
Building Resilience and Supporting Prevention

Margaret M. McGuinness
Kathy J. Schnur

In the practice of art therapy with children, we frequently hear about bullying experiences. We believe that bullying, especially during childhood, creates long-lasting negative feelings and memories resulting in palpable trauma. When working with those who have experienced bullying in individual sessions, we found an unmet need for an art therapy community response inclusive of the bully, the bystander, and the person being bullied. As a result, we designed a project called Drawing the Line, Building Resiliency and Creating Art to (1) increase awareness of bullying, (2) focus on prevention, and (3) build resilience using the sensory–motor activities necessary for healing trauma. This project has been applied to work with individual children ages 10 years and older who self-reported helpless feelings and were coping with anxiety as a result of their exposure to increased incidences of suicide and suicidal gestures in their community. According to a Centers for Disease Control and Prevention (CDC; 2013) report, suicide-related behaviors are higher among youth involved in bullying, The CDC linked bullying perpetrators and bullying victims to higher suicidal behaviors in adolescents.

This chapter provides brief overviews of bullying and its effects on children as well as a resiliency-based intervention to address the multiple cognitive, emotional, and social impacts of bullying. A case example is included to demonstrate principles and practices of using sensory-based methods as a form of art therapy intervention to resolve the effects of bullying. Finally, we describe our community project—Drawing the Line, Building Resiliency and Creating Art—and present recommendations for a strengths-based art therapy and trauma-sensitive approach focusing on the community crisis of bullying, using sensory activities to build resilience.

THE IMPACT OF BULLYING

Much work is being done about the problem of bullying and its connection to aggressive and self-harming behaviors. For the purpose of our project, the three parts of the bully experience are defined here as the perpetrator being the person who engages in bullying behavior toward another; the person being bullied is the victim and refers to the experience of being the target; and the bystander is the person(s) who are witnesses or aware of these behaviors.

There once was a prevalent belief that being bullied tested one's character, but recent neuropsychological research now shows that it negatively affects self-esteem (Graham & Juvonen, 1998), especially in children whose brains are still developing. It is now well accepted that bullying is about power and control in relationships. It can be direct or indirect, physical or verbal. It is most often repetitive and deliberate.

The rapid development of Internet technology, cellphones, instant text messaging, blogs, and e-mails has changed the face of bullying. Shariff (2009), a Canadian educator who has studied the legal problems of cyberbullying, says the constant connectivity of technology has created an easy means to verbally assault one another, include or exclude individuals socially, and quickly affect large numbers of people. This unseen aspect protects the perpetrator (often anonymous), thereby leaving the victim feeling trapped and helpless. Bazelon (2013) believes the impersonal power of the Internet, with its printed words and images, escalates the meanness. Additionally, the faceless aspect of cyberbullying decreases the connections needed to reinforce empathy. This permanent electronic trail results in serious, negative psychological effects as the person being victimized is continuously retraumatized by rereading the hurtful words, and/or reviewing the images, and/or losing connection to his or her social network. The anonymity of the bully makes it harder for the victim to reframe the event, which is a necessary step in healing from trauma.

The trauma of being bullied causes cognitive, emotional, and physical changes in behaviors. D'Andrea, Ford, Spinazzola, and van der Kolk (2012) maintain that for some children, the trauma of bullying also results in neurobiological brain changes that negatively impact their sense of safety. They suggest that a combination of verbal abuse and violence is strongly associated with emotional dysregulation, which impacts the functioning of the limbic system. The resulting symptoms of increased heart rate, increased blood pressure, decreased sleep, and disinterest in activities of daily living are similar to those in the diagnosis of posttraumatic stress disorder (PTSD). However, at present, there is no specific diagnosis for the trauma of being bullied, and the consequences of bullying are often misdiagnosed. Van der Kolk suggests in this text the conflicting symptomologies of PTSD and trauma such as being bullied would change if a diagnosis of *complex trauma* were available.

Currently, children who are bullied can be given the diagnosis of PTSD or acute stress disorder (ASD), depending on their age and the length of time from the incident(s). Regardless of diagnosis, the experience of being bullied leaves children feeling helpless and isolated; this decreased sense of safety, combined with the loss of trust, creates a negative sense of self-worth (Aideuis, 2007) resulting in stress. Blanche (2005) studies violence and finds traumatic stress from repetitive abuse affects some children more than others. By definition, bullying is a form of repetitive abuse.

Children who have a disability or are impaired have a higher incidence of being bullied (Safran, 2002). Humphrey and Symes (2010) maintain that some children are at increased risk of becoming victims of bullying and incurring the residual effects. Their study examined the frequency of bullying incidents among children, both those in special needs programs and those who are mainstreamed in the inclusive educational system used today. Focusing on children diagnosed on the autism spectrum, they found that poor social skills were linked with increased victimization. Children who are perceived as different tend to be bullied (Safran & Safran, 2008). The resulting anxiety, problems with self-regulation, and cognitive difficulties are easily observed in school settings (Safran & Safran, 2008).

BULLYING AND RESILIENCY

Antonovsky (1996) developed a "salutogenic" approach to recovery, in which practitioners learn to identify the strengths that lead to health rather than the pathologies that lead to disease. This strengths-based approach focuses on the value of facilitating successful coping skills when clients are faced with life's stressors. The core concepts of this approach encourage finding meaningfulness and comprehensibility while increasing manageability and resiliency skills. Developing a positive and meaningful sense of identity permits an individual to make healthy choices and improve quality of life—important resiliency factors (Sheedy & Whitter, 2009). In 2011, the Substance Abuse and Mental Health Services Administration (SAMHSA) called on art therapists in the mental health field to develop child programs that integrate a salutogenic approach focusing on resiliency skills. Prescott, Sekender, Bailey, and Hoshino (2008) list the building blocks of resilience as self-reflection, perspective taking, connection, flexibility, and self-regulation. Focusing on resilience and looking for a proactive response to bullying, we utilized a trauma-informed approach in developing our community project (described later in this chapter).

Feeling safe, engaging in repeated activities that promote self-empowerment (mastery), and finding consistent peer support (connection) are crucial to developing resiliency to trauma. Blanche (2005) cites health programs that use strengths-based approaches to support a type of natural resilience. Hansen (2011) agrees that resiliency plays a key role in mental health and that it can reduce anxiety by creating a type of flow experience of a more ordered consciousness. During art therapy sessions, we have observed that engaging in the exploration and use of sensory-based art materials to make art creates a flow state in children that helps them access and process their feelings about their bullied experiences without becoming overwhelmed.

Resiliency skills are developed by learning to build relationships and understand other children's experiences. Iacobini and colleagues' (2005) work outlines a fundamental building block linking how watching actions of others and understanding intentions happens in the mirror neuron system. Franklin (2010) links the mirror neuron system with the response of empathy, suggesting that an individual can feel "as-if" what is being experienced by another as his or her own experience. He suggests that this link via the mirror neuron system extends to the art therapist and the client in shared art-making experiences, concluding that adult role modeling is important for learning to respond empathically. Stanbury, Bruce, Jain, and Stellern (2009) suggest that an empathy-focused program can reduce school bullying incidents. Following a protocol of storytelling and imagination-guided exercises, students showed an increase in both compassion and empathy that was associated with a reduction in bullying behaviors. Badenoch (2008) notes that empathy is related to "the ability to resonate internally and accurately with another person's state of mind" (p. 30).

Relationship building is also referred to as *attunement*; Schore (2003) maintains that attunement begins when the child feels safe and starts to build a relationship with the caregiver. Siegel (cited in Badenoch, 2008) states that attunement is achieved right brain to right brain and is necessary for building empathy

Children who have more characteristics of resilience handle the trauma of being bullied more easily than those with fewer resources. Resilience allows healthy function despite trauma (Healey, 2002). The ability to bounce back from adverse situations presupposes a strong belief system that recovery is possible, thereby instilling hope, an essential element for those healing from trauma. Similarly, Healey (2002) defines resiliency as self-protective attitudes that result in a set of behaviors and actions that enable coping with life's disappointments and challenges. Healey utilizes Antonovsky's (1996) salutogenic approach to establish three core concepts of resiliency that can be applied to bullying:

1. Comprehension that bullying is an adverse situation.
2. Manageability of clients' self beliefs that they have the skills to meet the challenge.
3. Meaningfulness, or the hope to derive meaning (personal narrative) from the demands confronted, based on the understanding that the deficit lies within the bully and not themselves, allowing for a positive and resilient outcome.

Healey (2002) feels that teaching resiliency-fostering strategies can provide effective proactive responses for victims, irrespective of the anxiety related to the experience, as well as provide a buffer for the stress and anxiety related to the traumatic experiences of peer abuses.

THERAPEUTIC INTERVENTIONS

In his neurosequential model of therapeutics, Perry (2006) cites three main principles necessary for treatment of trauma in children:

1. Therapeutic interventions must be relevant to the emotional age of the child and be repetitive to stimulate neuronal development.
2. A healthy, stable, predictable, and safe environment must be maintained for therapy to progress.
3. Treatment must be rewarding for the child, culminating in a positive experience.

Nonverbal therapeutic interventions useful for processing trauma and creating connections may include physical activities such as dancing, drumming, and singing, which use rhythms that maintain consistent heartbeat. These activities increase the brain's ability to maintain attention and create attunement by activating both hemispheres of the brain (Berrol, 2006). Because the child is having fun and attunes to the rhythmic beat, he or she invisibly gains a level of synchronous and responsive attention to both verbal and nonverbal cues. Sharing matching movements with others fosters a feeling of connection, which may increase empathy as clients explore dance and movement as a healing process. Berrol (2006) connects earlier work with mirror neurons and understanding others' intentions in her use of dance therapy promoting empathy. Berrol cites prior experiments by Italian neuroscientists of mirror neurons in both animal and human brains becoming activated by primates and humans watching identical movement. Berrol finds participants in her dance therapy groups respond to sensory–motor stimuli from the music, the other dancers, and the audience. She also states that dance links processes in the prefrontal cortex (the thinking, cognitive part of the brain) with those in the limbic (emotional) system. She postulates that this affect attunement increases emotional connections and empathy. This increased interconnectedness is demonstrated in dance or movement for all to see by observing similar facial expressions in participants and the imitation of matching rhythmic pattern and spatial shapes.

Self-regulation is a higher cognitive skill that is essential to resilience and can be measured in art therapy (McGuinness & Schnur, 2013). Other nonverbal creative experiences can also foster self-regulation in children. Masten (2001) finds that the self-regulation of breath work reduces anxiety and strengthens connection through repetition and rhythm. Children reported a decrease in anxiety symptoms when we taught them a form of regulated breathing before accessing possible traumatic memories of being bullied.

Prescott and colleagues (2008) focus on the creative power of art to build resiliency, stating, "Resiliency and the creative process are reciprocal:

Not only is creativity an aspect of resilient behavior; it also fosters resilience" (p. 157). Creativity empowers, promotes, bridges, and heals. Creating art in a group setting helps participants process conflict arising from the task and encourages connection to others, promoting mutual respect, empathy, and security (Gibbons, 2010). We utilize art making and other nonverbal sensory-based interventions to promote resiliency and build empathy, as demonstrated in the following case example.

CASE EXAMPLE: PETER

Peter, age 10, was a child who had been bullied. Attending a private school with small classes, he experienced problems fitting in with the other children. An only child, he came to individual art therapy sessions accompanied by his mother. Mom reported a fellow student had physically bullied Peter at recess about 1 month previously. When Mom picked Peter up the afternoon of the incident, he was not feeling well, and when he told her about the incident, Mom noticed that his pupils were unequal in size. Immediately she took Peter to a local emergency room where it was confirmed that he had received a concussion from the abuse. Mom was frustrated about the lack of response she received from the school officials when reporting the concussion incident and perplexed about Peter's interactions with his peers.

Believing that something else might be going on and looking for ways that could help their socially awkward son, Peter's parents contacted a psychologist for an extensive psychosocial assessment. Peter had been previously diagnosed with attention-deficit/hyperactivity disorder (ADHD) and sensory processing disorder. The current report showed that although Peter had a high-average IQ and that he responded like a 4- or 5-year-old in social skills. Final diagnosis was that Peter displayed symptoms that indicated he was on the autism spectrum disorder scale with a diagnosis of Asperger syndrome with a specific impairment in reciprocal social behavior. There was also some evidence of PTSD. Because of his higher IQ and low social skills, both his mother and the diagnosing psychologist thought that Peter was having difficulty making sense of the bullying incident.

Initial Art Therapy Sessions

When Peter was seen for his initial art therapy session, he showed signs of extreme anxiety consistent with hyperarousal, a common response to a traumatic event. At the same time, he also appeared detached and unclear about the recess incident, a dissociating response to the traumatic event. When asked about it, he said, "I can't remember, but I guess some one of us needs to leave the school now, and I guess it will be me." This statement indicated to the therapist that Peter felt the incident made him feel socially unacceptable and compounded his sense of low self-esteem.

Peter was aware that his parents were exploring the option of transferring him to his local public school where additional services would be available to him. Additionally, in the public school Peter would not be mainstreamed into the regular program but put into a special program where social skills would be emphasized and accommodations would be made. Peter was anxious both about changing schools and anxious about not changing schools. This anxiety was evidenced in the first session both by Peter's artwork and by his nervous repetition of the words, "I'm thinking, I'm thinking, I'm thinking," indicating his inability to recall the details of the trauma. Peter's initial artwork filled every inch of the 22″ × 18″ white paper with pencil drawings of people, animals, and buildings all with stories to tell, but Peter had no voice with which to tell his story. The overall impression of this entry drawing was one of chaos.

Because of Peter's high anxiety, Mom had to stay very close to provide safety early in the course of treatment. At the beginning, Mom sat in for weekly sessions and occupied herself as Peter worked. Breathing exercises were taught in session to Peter and Mom to help with self-regulation, and they were instructed to practice the exercises at home daily, whether needed or not. Practicing them frequently helped store them in memory and allow easy access when needed.

Subsequent Art Therapy Sessions

Peter's treatment plan included reducing his anxiety by using sensory–motor art-based activities. Very quickly, Peter became interested in using clay to build a series of connected caves. Peter displayed no sensory issues when using clay. It was important to him that the caves be connected to each other from the inside, creating perfect "hiding spots." Small figures were made out of clay but were not durable for repetitive play. Because of this, Peter suggested he bring in his favorite action figures from home for play with the caves. Peter did not exhibit problems with attention in these initial sessions. Soon his anxiety began to decrease and his focus and trust increased, allowing his mother to sit in the waiting room during his sessions.

When the caves were dry enough to handle, Peter asked to put his caves into the sandtray that was available in the art room for sandplay. In the safe place of the sandtray many conflicts took place (see Figure 13.1). Week by week, new figures appeared, objects changed places, good guys fought bad guys, and the caves were deconstructed and reconstructed. Battles always ended in either Peter or the good guys winning. Working through the battle stage of play, the figures often sought safety inside the caves, regrouped, then ventured out when new assaults occurred. Turner (2005) posits that caves often symbolize wombs in which rebirth can happen and security can be established. She also maintains that inner work (unconscious) can become outer work (conscious) through the use of caves. During the work with Peter, the therapist allowed him to use the sandtray to contain his feelings, and the art was both expressive and fun.

Additionally, as his trauma story unfolded and was reenacted in the sandtray, new adaptive responses emerged without verbalization. After spending one whole session blowing the sand around the figures to create a violent sandstorm, Peter became very loud and verbal, combining guttural sounds with words to emphasize the ongoing work. Before this session he verbalized very little, but shortly after this session, he demonstrated appropriate vocalizations and storytelling in most sessions.

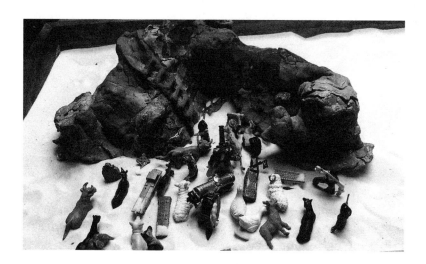

FIGURE 13.1. Bullying reenactment in sand tray.

At a point when Peter had consistently showed signs of improvement, he was asked to repeat the initial art experience of making a large pencil drawing, drawing the subject of his choice. In this task, Peter was able to focus on his ideas and work independently for a much longer period of time than initially seen. As his anxiety decreased, his executive function skills increased, as demonstrated by his ability to attend, plan and organize, and self-regulate work into scenes encased in bubbles, much like a cartoon, creating a cohesive storyline. It was mutually decided by Mom and Peter that it was time to work on social skills after this session.

Working on social skills in individual sessions progressed to the point where Peter joined another boy, who worked in clay, in a small social skills group. Being able to experience making friends in a small group setting led Peter to feel secure enough to join a special interest group outside therapy. Using clay, sandplay, and storytelling, Peter reenacted his memories through sensory play and art making. He was able to communicate his angry feelings through the sandtray battles. As his anger decreased, he was able to build additional caves and safe places for his figures to seek rest between battles. By repeatedly enacting battles and building additional caves, Peter found safe places to regroup his figures, and through his play he demonstrated that he could arrange military-like battles and try various planned strategies as his play became more organized. Peter had begun to reframe his experience as his verbalization increased, and he told the therapist that he just wanted to be a "normal boy." Eventually Peter did not need to talk about the bullying incident any more, and the focus of the sessions became ways to make new friends.

Summary of Interventions and Outcomes of Art Therapy

Peter used the sandtray and the caves as symbols to reenact his trauma, allowing him to achieve mastery and control of the bullying incident. Gil (2011), who has done extensive work with traumatized children, believes that mastery and control are primary goals when working with children who have experienced posttraumatic stress.

As a nonverbal treatment, art therapy allowed Peter to make a complex cave system as a strong container for both his angry feelings about being bullied and his anxiety about attending a new school—all without words. The caves became a safe place that he fortified and changed when he felt anxious. He experienced that although the caves often broke, new, stronger and sometimes better structures could be made. This seemed to help Peter realize a new school might also be a better fit for him. As he rebuilt his structures, his frustration tolerance was increasing in his play as well as in his outside activities. Finally, the therapist was a witness to the pain that Peter felt by being bullied, which he was demonstrating in the aggressive play. Eventually his play became organized and less chaotic as he achieved mastery over his trauma. Peter demonstrated empathy for others when he left his caves for therapy play by other children in the practice.

Finally in a safe place, Peter needed to explore the skills necessary to connect with others and make new friends. Under the guidance of the therapist, he joined another boy in sessions. Initially, both boys worked in individual clay projects side by side, sharing process and stories. It was not long before Peter suggested they make a new clay project together, indicating to the therapist a renewed spirit of trust in others. Therapy became much less frequent and ended as the boys tested their newly found skills out in the community and school social group settings.

DRAWING THE LINE, BUILDING RESILIENCE, AND CREATING ART: A COMMUNITY PROJECT

The primary focus of our art therapy community project is to increase awareness of bullying through unique interactive opportunities that encourage child involvement and creativity, while allowing the children to share their stories about bullying and being bullied, and gaining insight into their own feelings in a community setting. First designed as an open studio workshop, we initially worked with teenagers, ages 12–18 years, in response to a national program on mental health awareness in children. At that time, the goal of our project emphasized raising awareness about bullying and the connection to suicidal behaviors, focusing on how words can be hurtful. In hindsight, we found that using art making with a "words are hurtful" theme failed to get teens to share experiences.

At parental request, we adjusted our target population to include younger children and developed a more sensory-based project, one designed from a trauma-informed expressive arts therapy approach (Malchiodi, 2010). Through trial and error, we found that children (ages 9–14 years) were the most developmentally willing to share and the happiest to participate. In this age group we found deficits in understanding empathy, a key to building resilience. By building a therapeutic relationship in which children can comfortably explore the complicated issues of bullying, we share information about where and when to seek support and make sure the children understand that it is never okay to feel so badly that they consider self-harm or harming others.

We use sensory-based activities to demonstrate resiliency, explore trauma, and understand empathy, and we change the format as needed. We employ various activities that are fun, meaningful, age-appropriate, and that engage children cognitively, emotionally, and physically. Some of the activities are designed to self-regulate emotions, and some are created to encourage a safe and playful bodily response to the traumatic feelings of being bullied. All explore both prevention and intervention ideas. We readily share our findings in presentations with parents and caregivers within the community. In brief, we have created a strengths-based, salutogenic (healthy), art therapy, trauma-informed approach focusing on the community crisis of bullying and using sensory activities to build resilience.

STRUCTURE OF THE PROGRAM

The Circle

Gathering in an informal circle allows participants to see and be seen equally, enabling normalization of sharing trauma-related stories. We introduce ourselves and briefly explain what we as art therapists do in the community and why we are with them today.

Square Breathing/Self-Regulation

Because trauma work can trigger emotions, self-regulation of emotions is a necessary skill. Finding a quick way to demonstrate sensory self-regulation of emotions can be difficult. We start by talking about breath work and teaching how to modulate instant reactions to events—to delay that instant knee-jerk reaction—by using a pause. We rely on changing the sympathetic nervous system response of fight, freeze, or flight reaction into a parasympathetic nervous system one of relaxation and receptivity as a way to self-regulate.

Relaxation techniques, including breathing exercises, are taught to persons experiencing the symptoms of anxiety and panic attacks. One exercise that is easy to teach to children to help them modulate their emotions is square breathing. Using the drawn image of a square, explain to the children that they need to:

1. Breathe in for a count of four.
2. Hold the breath (inspired) for a count of four.
3. Breathe out for a count of four.
4. Hold the breath (expired) for a count of four.

The idea is to be rhythmic in the counting. If each count takes 1 second, then the exercise takes 16 seconds. Try encouraging a "four pack" and draw four adjoining squares. Doing this combination takes slightly more than 1 minute. Breathing in this rhythmic way can clear the mind of fearful, anxious thoughts. Ask children to focus on their body and how they feel physically, mentally, and emotionally after the square breathing. Like any form of meditation, this technique works best when practiced regularly, so it is important to encourage daily practice for best results. It helps when practicing to visualize drawing the square to the count of four. The visualization helps the mind stay focused on the process.

It is also important to explain that the process of holding the breath is important to self-regulation. The act of holding and pausing between breaths gives us the little bit of space that is often necessary to calm emotions. Pausing creates time to reflect on emotions, to step back from the cascade of emotions before becoming overwhelmed. The pause teaches control and interrupts the reactive process.

Animal Analogy to Explain Trauma Response

Utilizing the analogy of animal behavior, we explain the normal responses of the trauma of being bullied by creating a game. Three animals are chosen to define the trauma responses of freeze (rabbit), flight (eagle), and fight (cat), in accord with the animals' natural behavioral patterns. Participants are randomly given a picture card of one of those animals and are asked to form animal groups. Each group is given center stage and asked to nonverbally convey the behavior of the group's animal. The individuals who are not in the group are asked to quietly observe the behaviors. Finally, the participants are asked to construct a living community expression of their chosen animal, using bodily forms of expression. After everyone has "performed," we encourage discussion of the observed behaviors. Allowing participants to playfully explore typical animal responses, they make the connections to freeze, fight, or flight and we link those connections to trauma. By having the sensory experience of trauma reactions in this neutral context, children's resistance to discussing their personal experiences of being bullied usually decreases.

Cognitive–Sensorimotor Skills

Initial resistance to sharing negative personal experiences within groups is to be expected. It is important to encourage participation in the short amount of time allotted for the program (1 hour and 30 minutes to progress through several activities with groups of up to 20 children at a given time).

We include a physical and cognitive skills activity in the circle with a beach-ball-inspired game we call the Bully-Ball. The balls are readily available in a variety of subjects and have easily answered prompts printed on them. For example:

1. "Have you ever seen someone bullied?"
2. "What did you do when someone bullied you at school?"
3. "Do your parents talk to you about bullying?"

Participants engage in throwing the ball to each other. The recipient reads and responds to questions about bullying. Ever maintaining a safe space, we allow the reader to "pass" on the question if he or she does not have an answer ready. The game continues until all have participated to their comfort level. Cognitive learning is heightened as proprioception and balance are activated through the large motor skills of the activity of playing "catch," allowing the central nervous system to self-regulate (Figure 13.2).

Next, we divide the large group into smaller groups of 6–10 to participate in the sensory-based activity centers: painting their hand tracings for a community tree (Figure 13.3), signifying their "Stop Bullying" pledge; and creating an individual "take-home" art piece of a leaf-inspired jewelry item (Figure 13.4) as a reminder of what was accomplished. Children work at different speeds in art-making activities. To accommodate this variability, we end in a free activity—"Draw what a bully looks like to you"—which the children can take with them or leave for us. Allowing for choices and for performing at their different comfort levels promotes community interaction and connection.

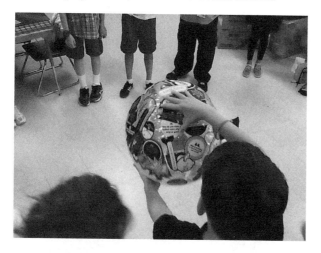

FIGURE 13.2. Sensory activities facilitate conversations about trauma.

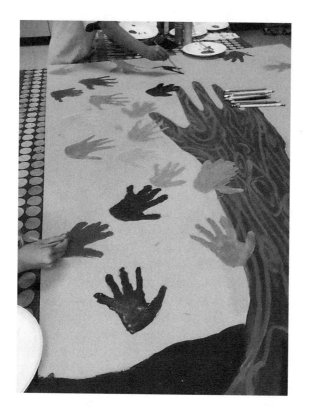

FIGURE 13.3. "Stop Bullying" pledge tree.

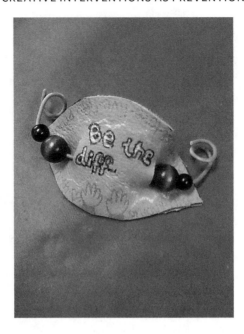

FIGURE 13.4. Visual take-home reminder to stop bullying.

Discussion and Evaluation

Returning to the circle, the group engages in processing the activities and each subgroup creates a pledge to not bully. This pledge is written on the roots of the community tree mural. Younger children are more concrete in their pledge, saying, "I will be kinder and not use hurtful words." Older children respond in more abstract forms, using concepts about social exclusion or cyberbullying, such as "I will not exclude," and adults use modeling words and behaviors such as, "I will be aware of my own actions." To end this discussion, we have groups recite their pledges out loud to reinforce the message. In our visits at various sites with this project, we have found a deficit of the understanding of empathy, so we conclude with an empathy-focused directive.

Empathy Building

Empathy is often referred to as walking in another person's shoes. We designed an activity using sensory work to demonstrate this core concept of empathy through a technique appropriate for all levels of development. Recalling the animal analogy, we ask participants how they know when to feed or play with their pets, as pets cannot speak. Responses tend to note how the animals feel hungry when they go to their food bowls and move them around, barking or mewing, or bored when their pet stands at the door, pawing. The children appeared receptive to our acknowledgment of their capacity to understand what their pets needed through connecting specific behaviors observed to patterns of hunger, boredom, and so on; caring for a pet brings about feelings of empathy. From this beginning, we connected that observing someone doing something, we find ourselves imitating the movement, such as learning a karate move or a dance step. When presented with a challenge to listen to a selection of current music and to observe and follow along with a chosen partner's movement, they may learn more about empathy.

Empathy Dance

1. Form small groups (two to four dancers), choosing a leader for each group.
2. Use various styles of music and ask each leader to begin to move to the music.
3. Followers have to mimic the movements as best as possible, paying attention to how their body feels in the process.
4. The music is halted when switching of leadership until all have the opportunity to lead.

By discussing what it was like for participants as leader and follower, we begin to cull a working definition of empathy. For most participants, initially imitating was difficult, but as each began to keenly observe the leader, the rhythms of the music allowed them to anticipate moves more easily. As observers, we found this activity resulted in happy reactions. Shared laughter filled the air as participants practiced giving total attention to each other, watching and letting each other know they had been seen and understood by nonverbal imitation. Using this simple sensory experience to embody the idea of what it might be to walk in another person's shoes by experiencing what another experiences was a success. How better to understand empathy than to experience it directly by sharing what another is feeling as a bodily response?

CONCLUSION

This chapter describes a strengths-based, salutogenic, trauma-informed approach to art therapy, working in private sessions with bullied children and working in the community to raise awareness of bullying, using sensory activities to support resilience. Creating a focus on healthy responses, we normalized the complex behaviors caused by bullying, creating a safe place to talk about bullying actions and reactions.

During the sensory-based group activities, especially during the Bully-Ball activity, we listened to stories of how children perceive bullying in their homes, on the school bus, and on electronic media. Regardless of the details, the stories demonstrated how bullying creates negative feelings. Regardless of the diagnostic criteria, today's children face bullying in ways never before felt, both in terms of intensity and frequency. When given the opportunity to explore creative art interventions in a supported and safe venue for self-expression, we found that children willingly participated in a process that can increase their natural resilience. Using sensory-based activities in a group program or with an individual in art therapy bypasses verbal resistance and provides a safe place for the emotional recall of personal bullied/bullying experiences.

REFERENCES

Aideuis, D. (2007). Promoting attachment and emotional regulation of children with complex trauma disorder. *International Journal of Behavior Consultation and Therapy, 3*(4), 546–547.

Antonovsky, A. (1996). The salutogenic model as a theory to guide health promotion. *Health Promotion International, 1*(1), 11–18.

Badenoch, B. (2008). *Being a brain-wise therapist: A practical guide to interpersonal neurobiology.* New York: Norton.

Bazelon, E. (2013). *Sticks and stones: Defeating the culture of bullying and rediscovering the power of character and empathy.* New York: Random House.

Berrol, C. F. (2006). Neuroscience meets dance/movement therapy: Mirror neurons, the therapeutic process and empathy. *Arts in Psychotherapy, 33,* 302–315.

Blanche, A. (2005). *Transcending violence: Emerging models for trauma healing in refugee communities* (Contract #280-03-2905). Alexandria, VA: National Center for Trauma-Informed Care, SAMHSA.

Centers for Disease Control and Prevention. (2013). CDC findings show higher suicide-related behaviors among youth involved in bullying. Retrieved May 21, 2014, from *www.cdc.gov/media/releases/2013/a0619-bullying-suicide.html*.

D'Andrea, W., Ford, J., Spinazzola, J., & van der Kolk, B. (2012). Understanding interpersonal trauma in children: Why we need a developmentally appropriate trauma diagnosis. *American Journal of Orthopsychiatry, 82*(2), 187–200.

Franklin, M. (2010). Affect regulation, mirror neurons, and the third hand: Formulating mindful empathic art interventions. *Art Therapy: Journal of the American Art Therapy Association, 27*(4), 160–167.

Gibbons, K. (2010). Circle justice: A creative arts approach to conflict resolution in the classroom. *Art Therapy: Journal of the American Art Therapy Association, 27*(2), 84–89.

Gil, E. (2011). *Helping abused and traumatized children: Integrating directive and nondirective approaches.* New York: Guilford Press.

Graham, S., & Juvonen, J. (1998). Self-blame and peer victimization in middle school: An attritional analysis. *Developmental Psychology, 34*(3), 587–599.

Hansen, L. (2011). Evaluating a sensorimotor intervention in children who have experienced complex trauma: A pilot study. *Honors Project,* Paper 151. Available at *http://digitalcommons.iwuedu/psych_honproj/151.*

Healey, J. (2002). Resiliency as a critical factor in resisting bullying. Retrieved November 7, 2013, from *http://bscw.rediris.es/pub/bscw.cgi/d497958/Resiliencia.pdf.*

Humphrey, N., & Symes, W. (2010). Perceptions of social support and experience of bullying among pupils with autistic spectrum disorders in mainstream secondary schools. *European Journal of Special Needs Education, 25*(1), 77–91.

Iacoboni, M., Molnar-Szakacs, I., Gallese, V., Buccino, G., Mazziotta, J. C., & Rizzolatti, G. (2005). Grasping the intentions of others with one's own mirror neuron system. *PLoS Biology, 3*(3), e79.

Malchiodi, C. A. (2010). Trauma-informed expressive arts therapy. Retrieved November 7, 2013, from *www.psychologytoday.com/blog/the-healing-arts/201203/trauma-informed-expressive-arts-therapy.*

Masten, A. (2001). Ordinary magic: Resilience processes in development. *American Psychologist, 56*(3), 227–238.

McGuinness, M. M., & Schnur, K. J. (2013). Art therapy, creative apperception and rehabilitation from traumatic brain injury. In C. A. Malchiodi (Ed.), *Art therapy and health care* (pp. 252–265). New York: Guilford Press.

Perry, B. (2006). Applying principles of neurodevelopment to clinical work with maltreated children. In N. B. Webb (Ed.), *Working with traumatized youth in child welfare* (pp. 27–52). New York: Guilford Press.

Prescott, M., Sekender, B., Bailey, B., & Hoshino, J. (2008). Art making as a component and facilitator of resiliency with homeless youth. *Art Therapy: Journal of the American Art Therapy Association, 25*(4), 156–163.

Safran, D. (2002). *Art therapy and AD/HD: Diagnostic and therapeutic approaches.* London: Jessica Kingsley.

Safran, D., & Safran, E. (2008). Creative approaches to minimize the traumatic impact of bullying behavior. In C. A. Malchiodi (Ed.), *Creative interventions with traumatized children* (pp. 132–166). New York: Guilford Press.

Schore, A. N. (2003). *Affect regulation and the repair of the self.* New York: Norton.

Shariff, S. (2009). *Confronting cyber-bullying: What schools need to know to control misconduct and avoid legal consequences.* New York: Cambridge University Press.

Sheedy, C. K., & Whitter M. (2009). *Guiding principles and elements of recovery-oriented systems of care: What do we know from the research?* (Publication No. (SMA) 09-4439). Rockville, MD: Center for Substance Abuse Treatment, Substance Abuse, and Mental Health Services Administration.

Stanbury, S., Bruce, M. A., Jain, S., & Stellern, J. (2009). The effects of empathy building program on bullying behavior. *Journal of School Counseling, 7*(2), 1–27.

Turner, B. A. (2005). *The handbook of sandplay therapy.* Cloverdale, CA: Temenos Press.

CHAPTER 14

Focusing-Oriented Expressive Arts Therapy and Mindfulness with Children and Adolescents Experiencing Trauma

Laury Rappaport

Focusing-oriented expressive arts therapy (FOAT) is a mindfulness-based approach that I developed by integrating Eugene Gendlin's (1981, 1996) mind–body Focusing method with the arts therapies (Rappaport, 2009, 2010, 2014b). FOAT is based on over 30 years of clinical experience with a range of clients with varying types and causes of trauma. FOAT is especially suitable for children and adolescents who have experienced trauma because its foundational principles are predicated on the needs for safety, empathy, and trust building and its techniques are somatic and sensory-based. FOAT also cultivates a compassionate inner witness aspect of self that can stand outside overwhelming experiences, access an inherent place of well-being, and provide access to one's own inner wisdom. Integrating mindfulness practices with FOAT empowers children and adolescents with self-care methods designed to reduce disturbing symptoms of trauma, such as hyperousal, hypervigilance, and a state of alarm; enhance feelings of calm and groundedness; and increase positive emotions. FOAT and mindfulness practices also access inner strengths and resources, nurturing qualities of resilience to work through and integrate the more difficult experiences associated with the trauma, so that the child or adolescent can move forward and live a meaningful, satisfying life (Weiner & Rappaport, 2014).

This chapter includes an overview of FOAT and describes how its theory and methodology provide a trauma-informed approach for working with children and adolescents. It also describes the significance of incorporating a phase-oriented treatment model in working with trauma and presents a new three-phase model based on FOAT theory and practices. The foundational principles and main methods of FOAT are described and integrated into the treatment phases: (1) establishing safety and cultivating resilience; (2) processing the trauma and accessing inner wisdom; and (3) integrating the healing process and fostering the life-forward direction. Highlights from my work with a 12-year-old girl who suffered traumatic loss and grief are integrated throughout the descriptions of the three phases to demonstrate the methods and healing process over time.

FOAT: A TRAUMA-INFORMED APPROACH

FOAT addresses essential components for trauma-informed care, including the client's need for safety; the importance of working with the body to self-regulate; the significance of the therapist's relationship and attunement with the child or adolescent to help cultivate healthy attachment; and the use of sensory experiences in the creative arts to process the trauma, access strengths, and develop feelings of competence (Blaustein & Kinniburgh, 2010; Malchiodi, 2008; Steele & Malchiodi, 2012). In addition, FOAT is a self-empowering approach that (1) cultivates resilience as it helps clients learn to trust their inner knowing, and (2) accesses an unfolding "life-forward direction" (Gendlin, 1981, 1996) toward well-being.

FOAT with Trauma and Children

FOAT is rooted in Gendlin's (1981, 1996) Focusing and the expressive arts, which are both used with children and for trauma (Bowers, 2007; Doi, 2007; Morse, 2003; Santen, 1990, 1999, 2007; Stapert & Verliefde, 2008; Turcotte, 2003). Since FOAT is a newer approach to the arts therapies field, the research is still limited, but preliminary studies are promising. Lee (2011) conducted a research project on FOAT, using bookmaking with children in a homeless shelter to enhance resilience. She used the Social Emotional and Assets Resilience Scale—Children

(SEARS-C) as well as qualitative and art-based measures. Although there were only five participants, the SEARS-C showed an overall positive change in the pre–post scores. In addition, the qualitative results indicated increases in the children's sense of self. Lee also used the Draw-a Person in the Rain (DAPR) art-based assessment (Hammer 1997; Oster & Crone, 2004) as a pre–post artistic measure, in attempt to notice indicators for stress hardiness or vulnerability. Although the DAPR is not a valid or reliable instrument, it is interesting that all of the post drawings showed an increase in images for protection—such as the addition of an umbrella, a protective person, or a tree covering; these images may indicate an increased sense of safety. Weiner's (2012) study on FOAT and mindfulness with adolescents (a prevention program at a summer camp) also demonstrated decreases in stress and increases in well-being. Other FOAT studies have been conducted with adults and also indicate how FOAT can be taught to create safety, increase self-compassion, promote emotion regulation, and reduce stress (Castalia, 2010; McGrath, 2013; Weiland, 2012).

Phased Treatment and FOAT

Herman's groundbreaking book *Trauma and Recovery* (1992) espoused the necessity of phase-oriented treatment: (1) establishing safety, (2) remembering and mourning (working through the trauma), and (3) reconnecting with ordinary life. Since then, other trauma experts have also maintained the importance of phase-oriented treatment (Luxenberg, Ogden, Minton, & Pain, 2006; Spinazzola, Hidalgo, Hunt, & van der Kolk, 2001; van der Kolk, McFarlane, & Weisaeth, 1996).

For many years, I used Herman's model as a guide and integrated FOAT within her stages for treatment. As I continued to revise this chapter, I realized that although I generally follow her model, I emphasize other aspects within each of her phases that are important for cultivating resiliency. This chapter describes a Focusing-oriented expressive arts three-phase model for trauma work. As with all phased treatment models, the treatment is not linear and does not progress simply from one phase to another. A phase may progress, regress, and/or overlap. Phase 1, establishing safety and enhancing resilience, needs to be attended to throughout treatment. Over time, Phase 1's "establishing safety" progresses into the need to "maintain safety" throughout the treatment. In addition, Phase 1's "cultivating resilience" needs to be reinforced throughout treatment as well.

CLINICAL APPLICATION: FOAT-PHASED TREATMENT

Phase 1: Establishing Safety and Cultivating Resilience

As previously stated, the goal during Phase 1 is to create an atmosphere of safety for the client and to enhance resilience. Conveying safety and respect begins with the foundational principles of FOAT and includes two main FOAT approaches during this phase—theme-directed FOAT and Clearing a Space with the Arts (described below).

FOAT Foundational Principles

FOAT is based on foundational principles that serve as guidelines for establishing and maintaining safety throughout treatment. These principles include fostering safety; presence; listening, reflection, and mirroring; grounding; the Focusing Attitude; and clinical sensitivity.

SAFETY

Cultivating the client's sense of safety is paramount in all therapeutic work but is especially sensitive when working with children and adolescents who have experienced trauma. Through FOAT, safety is fostered in three critical areas: in the therapeutic relationship between therapist and client, in the client's sense of self, and in the external world. These three areas of safety are further clarified in the other FOAT principles described below, as well as through the case vignette.

PRESENCE

The compassionate, respectful, and trustworthy qualities of a therapist transmit an atmosphere of healing presence. This presence is instrumental in helping to create a sense of safety for clients and is essential in trauma-informed relationships (Steele & Malchiodi, 2012). To be a Focusing-oriented arts therapist, it is first essential to learn Focusing for oneself. The therapist is then able to transmit a quality of compassionate presence that is learned through the Focusing Attitude (described below). In regard to staying present, it is important for therapists to ask themselves several questions: Am I aware of challenges within me that get in the way of listening or being able to be present with traumatic material? Am I able to convey compassion and understanding without getting lost in my client's experience? Am I able to take care of myself so that I am not overcome by vicarious trauma?

LISTENING, REFLECTION, AND MIRRORING

To cultivate safety and empathic attunement, experiential listening and reflection are integrated into the FOAT process to mirror verbal, nonverbal, and artistic forms of communication. Experiential listening includes taking in the whole of the client (verbal, nonverbal, and artistic communication), listening for what is important, and succinctly reflecting back the heart of what the client is saying (see Rappaport, 2009, for guidelines). It is essential that the listening responses of the therapist reflect not only the words but the nonverbal communication as well. In this way, the child or adolescent feels deeply understood, with a sense of empathy and compassion, and the child's internal experience can move forward. As expressive arts therapists, we can also reflect the child's or adolescent's experience through artistic reflection and movement mirroring. There are times when it may be appropriate for therapists to show, through drawing or art, that they understand the client's experience. In addition, therapists can mirror, through gesture, movement, and the quality of energy, that they understand the client's experience. Listening, artistic reflection, and mirroring demonstrate an attunement to the young client and help to repair attachment wounds, which is important for healing from trauma.

GROUNDING

It is important to know that the child is able to calm and to ground themselves in the present moment. As an essential aspect of emotion regulation, grounding skills can be taught through a variety of exercises, including mindfulness skills, such as awareness of the breath; body awareness (e.g., noticing the sensation of one's feet on the ground or of sitting in a chair); yoga, chi gong, creative movement, and other expressive arts activities.

FOCUSING ATTITUDE

The Focusing Attitude is a "friendly, curious attitude" toward the felt sense of an experience (Gendlin 1981, 1996; Rappaport, 2009). This attitude is especially important when working with traumatic material, as clients are often overwhelmed, flooded, disassociated, frozen, or afraid of the feelings associated with their experience. I always appreciated that Gendlin would say, "We can't always be welcoming of difficult feelings, but we can try to be friendly to them." The Focusing Attitude of friendliness and nonjudgment extends to creative expression as well.

CLINICAL SENSITIVITY

It is essential that therapists adapt FOAT methods to each specific child or adolescent. Although Focusing and mindfulness can be done with eyes closed as a way to notice sensations and experiences in the body, it is not always appropriate to do so. I recommend beginning with eyes open, and once the child or adolescent feels safe and can ground their experience, then it may be comfortable to close the eyes.

Mindfulness Skills: Grounding and Inner Witness

During Phase 1, mindfulness exercises help children and adolescents to use the breath as a way to calm and center themselves while learning how to observe and witness their emotions, sensations in the body, thoughts, and experiences outside of themselves. I often teach children and adolescents a variety of mindfulness exercises, including mindfulness of the bell, mindful breathing, mindful walking, and a "pebble meditation" (Hanh, 2011). The following mindfulness exercise is based on the teachings of Thich Nhat Hanh, who has been my teacher for many years. Required materials include a bell; markers, crayons, and oil pastels (for teens); and precut peaceful magazine pictures and words.

Mindful Breathing and FOAT

"Find a comfortable way of sitting and take a nice deep breath into your body and out of your body."

Inviting the Bell

"To begin, I'd like to share with you the sound of this bell. I learned this from a great teacher of calmness [Thich Nhat Hanh]. Instead of 'hitting' the bell, he teaches us to say, 'Let's invite the bell.' That sounds more peaceful . . . doesn't it? Before inviting the full sound of the bell, he teaches how to wake up the bell . . . which is also helpful for waking us up and getting ready to really hear the bell. First I am going to gently touch the bell with this little stick and stop it . . . so that the sound doesn't continue ringing. Then I'll take a couple of breaths and invite the sound of the bell fully. As you hear the sound, just notice it . . . and also enjoy breathing in . . . and breathing out during it."

Mindful Breathing

"We're going to be noticing our breath as it comes in the body and moves out of the body. This is important as it helps us to focus our attention and also to become calm and peaceful. Some children/teens like to notice the breath as it comes in through the nose and out through the nose or mouth. Some like to notice their belly as it rises when you breathe in . . . and flattens as you breathe out. Choose whatever works for you. As you begin to notice your breath, you'll also begin to notice thoughts in your mind and feelings or sensations in your body. You may also notice sounds in the room or outside. As we focus on our breath, I'll guide you to notice those thoughts, feelings, or sounds and to let them pass by like the way the clouds in the sky keep moving and changing.

"Take a nice breath into your body . . . and a nice breath out. As you breathe in, say to yourself, 'Breathing in, I'm aware of breathing in; breathing out, I'm aware of breathing out.' [Repeat several times.]

"[Lightly invite the bell] Now, as you breathe in, we're going to breathe in calm; as you breathe out, we're going to breathe out peace. Breathing in, I feel calm; breathing out, I feel peaceful. [Repeat several times.] You can shorten this to: In—calm; Out—peaceful. If you notice thoughts, feelings, or sensations, just notice them and let them pass by like the clouds in the sky."

FOAT Exercise

"[Toward the end of the exercise, invite the children/teens to express their felt sense of their experience.] Now take a moment and bring your awareness to your body. Notice how it feels inside . . . it may be calm, or jumpy, or peaceful. Just notice it and be friendly to it as it is. See if there's a color, shape, or image that matches how it feels in your body. When you're ready, be aware of being in this room. You can wriggle your toes and feet, and stretch your arms and hands. If your eyes are closed, you can gently open them. When you're ready, use the art materials to create and express how the mindful breathing felt in your body."

Variations

"The felt sense of the experience can be expressed through a gesture, sound, or writing (e.g., see if there's a movement, sound, or
word that expresses how it felt inside your body doing the mindful
breathing)."

CLIENT EXAMPLE: KATELYN AND MINDFUL BREATHING

Katelyn is a 12-year-old girl whose mother brought her for expressive
arts therapy after her healthy father died unexpectedly from a heart
attack. There was no warning and so the sudden death was traumatic—
leaving Katelyn with overwhelming feelings of both fear and grief. I first
met with Katelyn with her mother for the entire session since Katelyn
said that she wanted it that way. They both told me what had happened
and shared that Katelyn is having feelings of anxiety and panic. I told
them it is understandable since it was a shock for Katelyn's dad to have
a heart attack and to die unexpectedly.

    I shared that I could teach both of them a method to help with
the anxiety and panic and asked if they would like to learn it together;
this way, they could practice together. They both agreed. I led them
both through the mindful breathing exercise, presented in the preced-
ing material. After the guided Focusing, I showed them the art materials, including paper with predrawn circles (like mandalas), a basket
of peaceful images, another basket with healing words, and markers.
Katelyn chose two images, a butterfly and a flower, and a piece of
paper with the words, "Be calm and carry on." Katelyn glued the butterfly in the center of the circle and then cut the words, placing "calm"
above the butterfly and "and carry on" underneath it. She added the
word "breathe" so that her art read "Breathe calm and carry on." She
placed the flower underneath the mandala, all held on a piece of yellow
designed scrapbook paper (see Figure 14.1).

    I asked Katelyn if she wanted to share anything about the mindful
breathing and art experience. She said, "I really liked the sound of the
bell. It was so peaceful that it helped me to calm down. After a little
while, I noticed that my heart got quieter. Sometimes it's been pound-
ing. I liked finding the pictures and words that matched my experience
and I enjoyed making it."

    Katelyn's mother also found the experience helpful. I asked them
if they would like to take their art home because it can be a helpful

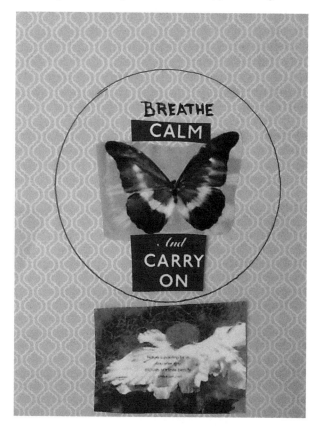

FIGURE 14.1. Mindful breathing.

reminder to breathe in calm and breathe out peace. Sometimes just looking at the art can help bring a sense of calm.

Focusing Attitude: Self-Compassion

Teaching children and adolescents about the Focusing Attitude helps them to know that whatever they feel is okay. I use various materials to help concretize the Focusing Attitude, such as have different precut samples of gingerbread-shaped people, animal shapes made of construction paper, and small assorted wooden shapes (circles, hearts, footballs, squares). I invite the child or adolescent to imagine a person or animal who will be their champion, giving them a positive message that however they are or whatever they feel is okay . . . that all feelings are welcome—whether they are sad, happy, afraid, scared, angry, funny, and so forth.

After the introductory session with Katelyn and her mother, I met with Katelyn individually. I talked with her about feelings—how we all have feelings of sadness, hurt, anger, fear, happiness, love, and so on—and that is helpful to create something that helps to know that all feelings are welcome, whatever they are. Therapy is about learning how to notice those feelings and to experience them in a way that is safe.

Focusing Attitude with Gingerbread Figure (or Animal Shape)

"Using the gingerbread figure [or animal shape], decorate it in a way in which it gives a message that all feelings are welcome here. Sometimes we know of someone in our life who shows us that . . . or sometimes we have a pet. We can also imagine what it would be like to have a superhero, person, pet, or other animal give us that welcoming message. It's something that can be a reminder when you look at it. When you're ready, choose a shape and make your Focusing Attitude figure and message."

Katelyn picked up one of the cutout gingerbread figures and traced it onto a sheet of orange paper. She made a girl who looked a little like her, added a smile, rosy cheeks, and a big heart, and wrote inside a dialogue bubble: "Everything you feel is okay. Welcome!" (see Figure 14.2). After, I said to Katelyn, "She has such a big heart [reflecting on her art]. It looks like she can help bring some caring, since I know things have been painful with the loss of your dad." She said, "Yeah—she reminds me of a care bear!"

Clearing a Space with the Arts: Finding the Right Distance and Well-Being

Clearing a Space with the Arts is a fundamental approach of FOAT. It is especially useful for teaching children and adolescents how to notice feelings and experiences that are in the way of feeling "All Fine," and to gain a healthy distance from them. It also helps them to find the place

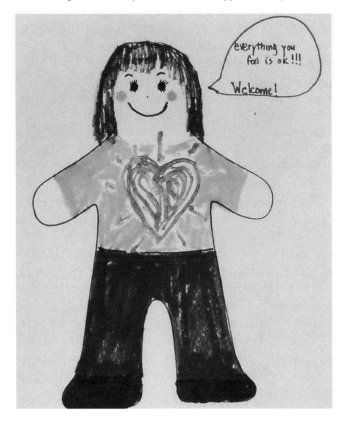

FIGURE 14.2. Focusing Attitude.

within themselves that is "All fine" or whole—separate from the trauma. There are four different approaches to Clearing a Space with the Arts (Rappaport, 2009, 2014a) that range from concrete imagery (use of art without guided Focusing) to nondirective imagery that includes listening to the bodily felt sense and allowing spontaneous imagery to image. In the early stages of trauma treatment, the Clearing a Space with the Arts using concrete imagery is most appropriate.

Clearing a Space with the Arts: Concrete

Clearing a Space

"We all have feelings and experiences that feel stressful or painful. First, what we are going to do is make a safety box to hold all of those feelings. You can decorate your box in any way you'd like. [Offer materials based on the child's or adolescent's interests and needs.] After you finish the box, we can take a look and see what feelings and experiences you would like to put in there. Then you can use other art materials and draw, paint, sculpt, and/or write anything that you want to put in there."

All Fine Place

"[After completion of above] Now, you can put the box away . . . anywhere in this room that you'd like . . . so that it feels at a comfortable distance from you. Then, we're going to take a moment to notice how it feels inside when you set all of those things in the box, place it at a distance that feels good, and you take a vacation from it for a couple of minutes. Okay? When you're ready, let me know. If you'd like to close your eyes for this part, let me know . . . or you can keep them open, whichever you'd like.

"Bring your attention inside to your body . . . and imagine there's a light that shines in there. Notice how it feels inside your body now—the place that is "All fine," separate from the things you placed in the box. Be friendly to whatever is there. It may be jumpy, or calm, or something else."

FOAT Exercise

"See if there's a color, shape, image, word, phrase, gesture, or sound that matches the felt sense of how it is now. Check to see if it's right. If not, let it go and wait for another color, shape, image, word, phrase, gesture, or sound to come. When you have it, express the felt sense of the symbol through art, movement, sound, or writing."

KATELYN: CLEARING A SPACE WITH THE ARTS

Katelyn used a combination of collage images, tape, and a lock. She glued a magazine photo of a lion and tiger on top of the box and decorated the rest of the box with colored strips of tape. Katelyn found a lock in the materials and taped it to the box to symbolize that she could keep it private (Figure 14.3). After, I reflected, "The lion and tiger look really strong and are going to keep whatever is inside the box safe." She replied with an emphatic, "Yeah!!!"

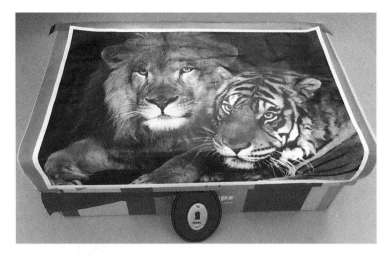

FIGURE 14.3. Clearing a space: outside box.

I then invited Katelyn to use the art materials to represent whatever was in the way of feeling "All fine." She took a large sheet of newsprint paper and tore it into a number of pieces. She crumpled them up, drew on them with a marker, and one by one put them in the box (Figure 14.4). After I asked, "Do you want to tell me what you put in there?" She said that the red piece in the corner is her hurting heart about her dad; two others represented feeling afraid and panicky; and the torn-up papers are about her life being torn apart.

I reflected to Katelyn, "Inside there's your hurting heart missing your dad, feeling and afraid and panicky, and the feeling that your life has been torn apart. Can you be friendly to these [Focusing Attitude]?" Katelyn nodded "yes." I asked her to place the box somewhere in the room that felt like a good location for it. I then invited Katelyn to notice how it feels inside her *now*, with the feelings held safely in the box . . . and to see if there's a color, shape, image, word, gesture, or sound that matches the felt sense.

She took a few moments to listen inwardly, opened her eyes, and went over to the meditation bell. Gently, Katelyn invited the sound of the bell. After listening, I inquired, "It feels calm and peaceful?" Katelyn said, "Yeah . . . it felt good to put those things in the box and put it over there [pointing across the room]. It doesn't feel so depressing."

As can be seen in the aforementioned examples, a FOAT approach seeks to create a sense of safety for the child or adolescent within themselves and enhance resilience factors at the same time. During this phase and the other two phases, it is also helpful to focus on strengths, resources, and other positive factors in the child's or adolescent's life. For example, theme-directed FOAT exercises might address topics such as, "Things I enjoy or have enjoyed"; resources of support; hobbies; family, friends, teachers, and pets. It helps to strengthen resilience and balance the trauma work.

Phase 2: Processing Trauma and Accessing the Body's Wisdom

The goals of safety and resilience-building continue into Phase 2, processing the trauma. The analogy of a sandwich is useful during this phase. Addressing the trauma directly needs to be sandwiched between safety and self-soothing. The primary methodology of Phase 2 integrates Gendlin's Focusing steps into the ongoing moment-to-moment

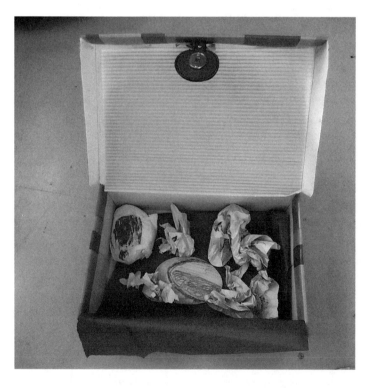

FIGURE 14.4. Clearing a space: inside box.

unfolding of the therapy interaction (Gendlin, 1981, 1996; Rappaport, 2009, 2010, 2014a). The flow of the session stays carefully attuned to the unfolding of the client's experiential process rather than following a prescribed directive. This point is important as this approach delicately addresses the safety necessary for trauma-informed work on relational, somatic, and sensory levels. A summary of the FOAT definitions derived from Gendlin's (1981, 1996) Focusing and methods for working on trauma follow.

FOAT Psychotherapy Process for Working through the Trauma

Integrate Focusing, listening, reflection, and expressive arts in a carefully attuned, moment-to-moment process.

Definitions

Felt sense: sensation in the body.

Handle/symbol: word, phrase, image, gesture, or sound that describes the felt sense.

Resonate: checking the felt sense for a feeling of rightness; checking which arts materials and modalities feel right to match the felt sense.

Ask: an inner dialogue to ask the felt sense (or art) a question.

Receive: hearing the answer that comes from the felt sense in response to a question.

Phase 2 requires that the therapist attune to the delicate balance of assisting the child or adolescent to safely experience feelings without getting lost in them, while providing the tools (learned in Phase 1) and the relationship to be able to step back and witness the experience when needed.

KATELYN: WORKING ON THE TRAUMA

Katelyn was ready to express how she felt about the death of her father. Since she liked the gingerbread cutouts, I asked if she wanted to use them to draw how she felt inside. Katelyn drew a sad-looking girl with a broken heart and a lightning bolt going through it (Figure 14.5). I asked her if she wanted to tell me about the art. The following is an excerpt of our interaction, with notations clarifying the FOAT methods:

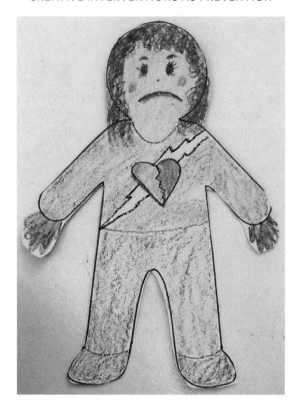

FIGURE 14.5. Felt sense about Dad's death.

KATELYN: I feel like I was hit with a bolt of lightning and my heart is torn apart. I don't know how I will ever be the same. I was so close to my dad. He was everything to me.

THERAPIST: You were shocked and your heart is broken. Your dad was everything to you, and you can't imagine how your life will go on without him [listening response].

KATELYN: Yeah. And no one understands. All my friends are busy with school, going to the mall . . . and I feel alone.

THERAPIST: You feel like no one understands . . . and your friends have no idea what it's like for you [listening response].

KATELYN: Yeah.

THERAPIST: Sometimes it helps to listen inside ourselves to hear what would be helpful. Would you like to try that? (*Katelyn agrees.*) Take a moment to bring your awareness inside to your body [felt sense]. See if you can be friendly to that place where your heart feels broken. You and I can sit down next to her and keep her company [Focusing Attitude]. [Note: With vulnerable places, sometimes it is helpful to say, "You and I can sit down next to her . . ." instead of "Can you sit down next to her?" Including the therapist in the delicate act can provide relational support and attunement.] When you're ready, ask, "What do you need?" [ask]. Just wait and listen. It may come as an image or in words. Just receive what comes [receive].

KATELYN: I saw a picture of my mom . . . and I heard her say, "I'm here . . . we're together . . . and you're safe."

THERAPIST: A picture of your mom came to you . . . and she was reassuring you that you're safe. Would you like to draw that?

KATELYN: (*Chooses a larger gingerbread figure and draws it to represent her mom, with a big heart. She places the two gingerbread figures on a larger sheet of paper and puts them together as if they are holding hands* [Figure 14.6].)

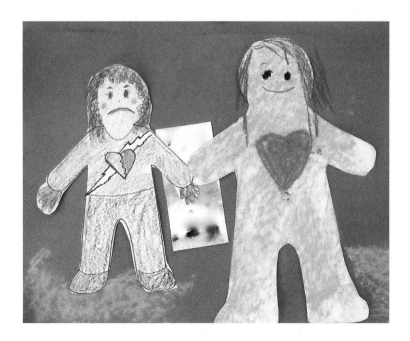

FIGURE 14.6. Asking: What does it need?

THERAPIST: So your mom is there with you . . . and she has a big heart [artistic reflection]. Can you sense how that feels now [felt sense]?

KATELYN: It feels good.

THERAPIST: It feels good to feel your mom with you. Is there anything else you need [ask]? You can go back inside to ask again . . . it's amazing how there's a place in our heart and body that can hear what we need.

KATELYN: (*Closes eyes and listens inwardly.*) My dad is in heaven and I want to see him or feel him still [receive].

THERAPIST: You want to be able to see or feel your dad in heaven [listening reflection]. (*Katelyn nods.*) The heart is one place that can help feel things that we don't see. Many people who have lost someone special often can feel them in their heart. Do you want to try that?

KATELYN: Yes.

THERAPIST: (*guiding Katelyn*) Take a few deep breaths into your body . . . and imagine your dad just as you'd like to see him again. . . . Remember the things you enjoyed about being with him . . . the ways that you spent time with him. . . . See if you can feel him in your heart . . . or some other way.

KATELYN: (*Opens her eyes.*) Yes. I can remember the fun things we would do together . . . and I can see a picture of him in my heart.

THERAPIST: Would you like to draw that?

KATELYN: No . . . I think I'd like to use a real photo of him and use that with the art.

THERAPIST: That's a great idea. If you bring it in, you can do that here next time or you can do it at home if you feel like it.

The gingerbread figure provided a safe container for Katelyn to express the felt sense of the shock and loss from her dad's sudden death. The felt sense can be accessed through mindful awareness of body sensations or through the sensory experience of art making. The skills developed in Phase 1 (mindfulness, Focusing Attitude, Clearing a Space, and "All Fine") helped me to know that Katelyn would be able to listen inside to her felt sense and to ask it a question. I find asking the felt sense "What do you need?" often leads to a form of self-soothing or self-care. It is also possible to ask the art the same question. Then when the client hears the answer, he or she can add to the art making.

I was also impressed that Katelyn knew that drawing her father didn't feel right. She trusted her inner sense to know that she wanted a photograph of her dad that she would bring to work with. In a later session, Katelyn created a memory book with various photos and writings about her dad.

Phase 3: Integration and Life-Forward Direction

The last phase of trauma treatment focuses on an integration of the self before and after the trauma. This phase is especially important for children and adolescents since their sense of self is impacted by their developmental stage. Although integration of the trauma and the life-forward direction occurs in small steps throughout all phases of treatment, the final phase of treatment culminates with an emphasis on living fully in the present with an eye toward the future. During this phase, I often like to focus on themes of "What I want in my future," "My dreams and wishes," and "A toolbox of resources of what I learned through therapy that I want to take with me."

KATELYN: MY LIFE NOW AND IN THE FUTURE

In the last phase of our work together, I congratulated Katelyn on the amazing work that she had done in therapy, how much she learned, and her courage in facing difficult feelings. I offered her a few possible choices for a closing FOAT exercise, and she chose "creating a mandala of my life now and in the future." I led her in a Focusing exercise to notice her life now and what she wanted in the future:

My Life Now and in the Future

"Take a few breaths into your body, noticing your breath as it comes in your body and moves out of your body. Now, let yourself be aware of how your life is today . . . the things that you enjoy . . . the things that have meaning. See if any images come. Now, imagine your life in the future. How would you like it to be? Be friendly to whatever comes [pause]. Now sense how it feels in your body . . . your life now and how you'd like it to be. See if there are colors, shapes, images, or words that match the felt sense inside . . . [pause]. When you're ready, you can open your eyes [if they're closed], and create a mandala of how that feels—your life now and how you imagine it."

Katelyn seemed to enjoy the artistic process of creating a mandala. She incorporated a few new materials—tissue paper, feathers, and stickers along with the familiar magazine images and markers. Katelyn picked up a heart shape and wrote the word *Love* on it. Then she picked up a flower shape and began writing the things that she enjoys in life—karate, reading, drawing, sunshine, friends, piano, the color blue, hockey, movies, and family. She then started to tear the tissue paper and began gluing it to the circle, adding origami papers. Next Katelyn searched through a basket and found magazine images that matched the words on the flower petal. She then placed the heart with *Love* in the center of the flower and glued it as the center of the mandala. Next, she glued the word *Family* and added two heart stickers right next to it, placing one heart sticker and a silver star inside the larger *Love* heart. Katelyn then added one star at the top of the mandala (Figure 14.7).

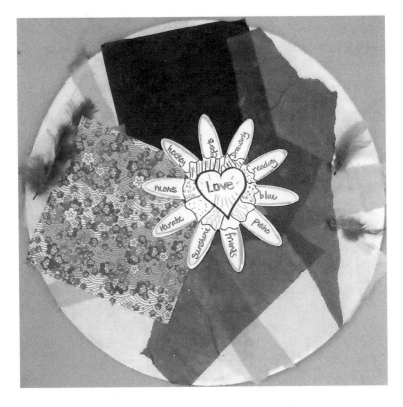

FIGURE 14.7. My life now and in the future.

When Katelyn finished, I asked her if she wanted to tell me about it. She shared that the flower and magazine pictures are the things that she loves to do. She added that the star at the top is her dad and that he is in heaven and always shining down on her. She shared, "I also put the word *Love* with a sticker heart and star inside the heart in the center. I know that I can always listen to my heart and hear my dad . . . and my mom too."

As seen in this phase, Katelyn is able to enjoy her present life; integrate the shock, fear, and sadness; and carry the love of her father and mother with her.

CONCLUSION

As demonstrated throughout this chapter, FOAT addresses the significant components of trauma-informed care with children and adolescents: safety, relationship, attunement, empathy, and the need for sensory and somatic processing. The case of Katelyn demonstrates how safety is cultivated both within the therapeutic relationship and within her own self. The Focusing Attitude, mindfulness practices, and Clearing a Space with the Arts help to develop a witness aspect of self to be able to stand outside of difficult experiences while "being friendly" and sensing them at a comfortable distance through the body or artistic process. A theme-directed FOAT approach harnesses strengths and resources, building resilience. In all of the approaches, the arts externalize the felt sense and deepen the experience of empathy and attunement, as the child or adolescent knows the therapist can literally see what is felt. In addition, listening and reflection enhance the experience of attunement and compassion.

A FOAT-phased treatment model provides a guide for creating safety, cultivating resilience, working through the trauma, accessing the body's wisdom, and integrating the trauma into a new sense of self that can actualize what Gendlin termed the "life-forward direction." Both Focusing and the arts provide access to our inherent wisdom—no matter how young a child is. It is a responsibility of adults working with children and adolescents, especially those with trauma, to empower them to listen inwardly to hear their innate wisdom. As Gendlin (1981) affirms, "Your body knows the direction of healing and life. . . . If you take time to listen to it . . . it will give you the steps in the right direction" (p. 78).

REFERENCES

Blaustein, M. E., & Kinniburgh, K. M. (2010). *Treating traumatic stress in children and adolescents: How to foster resilience through attachment, self-regulation, and competency.* New York: Guilford Press.

Bowers, L. (2007). Focusing enables children to live with fear. *Folio: A Journal for Focusing and Experiential Therapy, 29*(1), 81–91.

Castalia, A. (2010). *The effect and experience of clearing a space with art on stress reduction in sign language interpreters.* Unpublished master's thesis, Notre Dame de Namur University, Art Therapy Department, Belmont, CA. Available at *www.Focusingarts.com.*

Doi, A. (2007). A safe container for passing down a prayer to future generations: My experience with the Hiroshima peace museum. *Folio: A Journal for Focusing and Experiential Therapy, 29*(1), 3.

Gendlin, E. T. (1981). *Focusing.* New York: Bantam Books.

Gendlin, E. T. (1996). *Focusing-oriented psychotherapy: A manual of the experiential method.* New York: Guilford Press.

Hammer, E. (1997). *Advances in projective drawing interpretation.* Springfield, IL: Charles C Thomas.

Hanh, T. N. (2011). *Planting seeds: Practicing mindfulness with children.* Berkeley, CA: Parallax Press.

Herman, J. (1992). *Trauma and recovery.* New York: Basic Books.

Lee, H. (2011). *Focusing-oriented art therapy and bookmaking to promote protective resiliency of children living in a homeless shelter.* Unpublished master's thesis, Notre Dame de Namur University, Art Therapy Department, Belmont, CA. Available at *www.Focusingarts.com.*

Luxenberg, T., Spinazzola, J., Hidalgo, J., Hunt, C., & van der Kolk, B. A. (2001). Complex trauma and disorders of extreme stress (DESNOS) diagnosis: Part II. Treatment. *Directions in Psychiatry, 21,* 395–415.

Malchiodi, C. A. (Ed.). (2008). *Creative interventions with traumatized children.* New York: Guilford Press.

McGrath, J. (2013). *Clearing a space with art and pain.* Unpublished master's thesis, Notre Dame de Namur University, Art Therapy Department, Belmont, CA. Available at *www.Focusingarts.com.*

Morse, D. (2003). Assimilating trauma through focusing. Retrieved January 4, 2014, from *www.Focusing.org/morse_assimilatingtrauma.html.*

Ogden, P., Minton, K., & Pain, C. (2006). *Trauma and the body: A sensorimotor approach to psychotherapy.* New York: Norton.

Oster, G. D., & Crone, P. G. (2004). *Using drawings for assessment in therapy: A guide for mental health professionals.* New York: Brunner Routledge.

Rappaport, L. (2009). *Focusing-oriented art therapy: Accessing the body's wisdom and creative intelligence.* London: Jessica Kingsley.

Rappaport, L. (2010). Focusing-oriented art therapy with trauma. *Journal of Person-Centered and Experiential Psychotherapies, 9*(2), 128–142.

Rappaport, L. (2014a). Focusing-oriented arts therapies and working on the avenues. In G. Madison (Ed.), *Theory and practice of Focusing-oriented psychotherapy: Beyond the talking cure*. London: Jessica Kingsley.

Rappaport, L. (2014b). *Mindfulness and the arts therapies: Theory and practice*. London: Jessica Kingsley.

Santen, B. (1990). Beyond good and evil: Focusing with early traumatized children and adolescents. In G. Lietaer, J. Rombauts, & B. van Balen (Eds.), *Client-centered and experiential psychotherapy in the nineties*. Leuven, Belgium: Leuven University Press.

Santen, B. (1999). Focusing with young children and young adolescents. In C. Schaefer (Ed.), *Innovative psychotherapy techniques in child and adolescent therapy* (2nd ed.). New York: Wiley.

Santen, B. (2007). Into the fear factory: Treating children of trauma with body maps. *The Folio: A Journal for Focusing and Experiential Therapy, 20*, 60–78.

Stapert, M., & Verliefde, E. (2008). *Focusing with children: The art of communicating with children at school and at home*. Ross-on-Wye, UK: PCCS Books.

Steele, W., & Malchiodi, C. A. (2012). *Trauma-informed practices with children and adolescents*. New York: Routledge.

Turcotte, S. (2003). Course handout from the Trauma and Focusing course. Retrieved January 1, 2014, from *www.Focusing.org/turcotte_handout.html*.

van der Kolk, B. A., McFarlane, A. C., & Weisaeth, L. (1996). *Traumatic stress: The effects of overwhelming experience on mind, body, and society*. New York: Guilford Press.

Weiland, L. (2012). *Focusing-oriented art therapy as a means of stress reduction with graduate students*. Unpublished master's thesis, Notre Dame de Namur University, Art Therapy Department, Belmont, CA. Available at *www.Focusingarts.com*.

Weiner, E. (2012). *A mindful art program: Using mindfulness and focusing-oriented art therapy with children and adolescents to decrease stress and increase self-compassion*. Unpublished master's thesis, Notre Dame de Namur University, Art Therapy Department, Belmont, CA. Available at *www.Focusingarts.com*.

Weiner, E., & Rappaport, L. (2014). Mindfulness and focusing-oriented arts therapy with children and adolescents. In L. Rappaport (Ed.), *Mindfulness and the arts therapies: Theory and practice*. London: Jessica Kingsley.

CHAPTER 15

Sounds of Strength

Music Therapy for Hospitalized Children at Risk for Traumatization

Claire M. Ghetti
Annette M. Whitehead-Pleaux

Children experiencing hospitalization may be at risk for traumatization due to sustaining injuries, experiencing an accumulation of traumatic stresses from the hospitalization itself, or because of past histories of nonmedical trauma. A variety of factors contribute to increase the risk of traumatization for hospitalized children, but early supportive interventions may serve to buffer against those risk factors and promote improved outcomes. As a creative arts therapy that promotes body awareness and facilitates and contains nonverbal emotional expression, music therapy is well suited as an early intervention for hospitalized children who are traumatized. This chapter provides an overview of trauma related to hospitalization, principles of trauma-informed music therapy, and examples that illustrate how these principles translate into clinical practice.

OVERVIEW OF TRAUMATIZATION RELATED TO HOSPITALIZATION

Experiencing a significant injury, especially if it is perceived as life-threatening, can have traumatic consequences. Due to their developmental level, some children may harbor misconceptions about the cause of their injury or illness, or may fail to understand aspects of the prognosis or treatment. Because children who have experienced significant burns or other traumatic injuries may be at risk for the development of acute stress disorder (ASD) and posttraumatic stress disorder (PTSD), early screening to detect related symptomatology is of great importance. Prevalence rates for the development of PTSD in children who have experienced accidental injury range from 6 to 45% depending on the nature of the injury and the diagnostic criteria used (Kenardy, Spence, & Macleod, 2006). Drastic changes in lifestyle or body image carry the potential to be traumatizing, and loss of sense of self or loss of identity and abilities may trigger grief responses. Children who have been injured and their families may go through a process of grieving as they adjust to a new way of being and living (Loewy, 2002).

Advances in medical technology have contributed to improved life-saving capability for children and adolescents with severe injury and illness, though sometimes the life-saving interventions themselves may contribute to traumatic stress (Saxe, Vanderbilt, & Zuckerman, 2003). Invasive medical interventions paired with aversive environmental stimuli in intensive care can stress children at a critical point in their recovery (Rennick, Johnston, Dougherty, Platt, & Ritchie, 2002). Children who undergo painful or anxiety-producing medical procedures can experience anticipatory anxiety if such procedures are repeated, and such anxiety can exacerbate feelings of fear and helplessness. Thus, it is not surprising that children with a variety of life-threatening medical illnesses demonstrate posttraumatic symptoms (Saxe et al., 2003).

Instead of experiencing a single, traumatizing injury, some children undergo repeated stressors during hospitalization that carry a cumulative, traumatizing effect. For example, children who have sickle-cell disease will experience recurrent pain crises related to vaso-occlusion, which may either be life-threatening in nature or perceived as such (Hofmann, de Montalembert, Beauquier-Maccotta, de Villartay, & Golse, 2007). Intrusive recollections of past pain crises can confound current experiences of vaso-occlusion, compounding perceptions of pain and fear, and without adequate psychological intervention, unmanaged pain can create stress that precipitates additional vaso-occlusive crises (Hofmann et al., 2007). In addition to exacerbating pain, traumatic stress can also impact children's ability to adhere to medical treatments, which may further complicate their health situation (Saxe et al., 2003).

Children with past histories of traumatic experiences may perceive higher levels of threat from hospitalization and medical treatment. Those who have been subjected to physical and sexual abuse may be provoked and challenged by the physically invasive nature of various forms of medical and nursing care (Saxe et al., 2003). Hospitalization may provoke a resurgence in symptoms, including hyperarousal, intrusive memories, and avoidant behaviors.

A conflux of factors places children and adolescents at risk for traumatization during hospitalization. Developmental level is a crucial factor impacting how children understand, experience, and cope with hospitalization. More specifically, "the appraisal and experience of such critical constructs as pain, disability, life threat, and death is highly developmentally determined and likely affects symptoms and recovery" (Saxe et al., 2003, p. 3). Younger children are particularly at risk for traumatic impacts of hospitalization, especially when they experience heightened separation anxiety or undergo prolonged or frequent hospitalization, both of which may negatively impact healthy attachment and undermine coping efforts. Young children who are severely ill and experience numerous invasive procedures can be traumatized by their hospitalization and may demonstrate psychological difficulties for several months following discharge (Rennick et al., 2002).

Children who undergo higher frequencies of invasive procedures tend to have more frequent intrusive thoughts, demonstrate increased avoidance behaviors, and report more medical fears (Rennick et al., 2002). When children have experienced trauma prior to or during hospitalization, as the length of hospitalization increases, so does their level of event-related distress (Murray, Kenardy, & Spence, 2008). Such increases in distress may be related to the accumulation of invasive procedures, pain issues, or other health-related complications (Murray et al., 2008).

Posttraumatic stress and traumatic stress related to hospitalization can have lasting impacts on children, and warrant early intervention (Murray et al., 2008). Untreated PTSD can adversely impact children's social, psychological, and academic development, and thus early detection and treatment are imperative (Kenardy et al., 2006). Creative arts therapies are particularly helpful in addressing medical-related trauma as they provide opportunities for arousal reduction and affect regulation, sensory processing, externalization, and attachment (Malchiodi, 2008). The creative arts therapist works to decrease the traumatized child's arousal, anxiety, and sense of helplessness, while promoting adaptive coping strategies.

TRAUMA-INFORMED MUSIC THERAPY

Music therapy provides an avenue for eliciting and containing nonverbal expression and a means for integrating the somatic, cognitive, and physiological aspects of trauma responses. Music therapy consists of "a systematic process of intervention wherein the therapist helps the client to promote health, using music experiences and the relationships that develop through them as dynamic forces of change" (Bruscia, 1998, p. 20). The following description of trauma-informed music therapy reflects a translation of Malchiodi's (2012) principles of "trauma-informed art therapy" integrated with the trauma-informed music therapy approach of Behrens (2008, 2011) and our clinical and theoretical approaches developed while working with hospitalized children and adolescents.

Therapies that enable the bypassing of higher-level cognitive and language processing and emphasize awareness of present-moment body sensations and emotions are indicated following traumatization (Behrens, 2011). Music therapy may play an important role in recovery following trauma because it may enable reintegration of sensations and emotions and promote the development of emotional coping abilities that assist in emotion regulation (Behrens, 2011). Within a trauma-informed approach to music therapy, children are better equipped to integrate their fragmented experience of traumatization and to mobilize coping resources to deal with current emotions and experiences. Significant components of trauma-informed music therapy for hospitalized children and adolescents include:

1. Arousal reduction
2. Self-regulation and emotion regulation
3. Facilitation of body awareness
4. Promotion of internal locus of control
5. Facilitation of emotional-approach coping
6. Sensory processing of the traumatic event(s)
7. Externalization and containment
8. Promotion of healthy attachment and supportive relationships
9. Integration of the trauma

An initial step when working with a hospitalized child who has been traumatized is to assess his current coping approaches, viewed within the context of familial and cultural coping preferences. Trauma responses may be considered attempts to cope with overwhelming stressors, and the music therapist will support the child's current coping approaches while partnering with the child to develop more adaptive strategies. The therapist assesses the child's choice to accept or deny the illness or injury, as well as his ability to cope with the physical and emotional sequelae (Loewy, 2002). Assessment of coping preferences and abilities remains an ongoing process that lasts throughout the course of music therapy.

Whether the music therapist engages the child in numerous sessions or in a single session of music therapy, she will use musical and interpersonal elements to promote the development of therapeutic rapport and trust.[1] Foremost, the music therapist provides a "safe containing space" in which the child can freely express his feelings and perceptions (Turry, 2002, p. 48). The music therapist will consider the projected length of treatment and the child's coping abilities and developmental level when determining whether to provide supportive, reeducative, or reconstructive levels of therapy. Music therapists who provide more intensive levels of therapy should have advanced clinical training and should engage in ongoing clinical supervision.

Arousal Reduction

Since children who have been traumatized are likely to experience elevated heart rate immediately posttrauma and are prone to sympathetic nervous system hyperarousal (Kirsch, Wilhelm, & Goldbeck, 2011), arousal reduction is an important preliminary focus for music therapy intervention. Furthermore, when children experience intrusive and distressing memories of a traumatic injury or procedure, or are triggered by traumatic stimuli, they will likely reexperience physiological arousal and psychological distress. If a child is dissociating or having intense traumatic recollections, the music therapist must focus on bringing the child back to the here and now, before addressing higher-level needs. Since music is comprised of sound organized through time, the temporal and rhythmic aspects of music can be structured to promote grounding, orienting, or sedative effects.

When a child is highly aroused and distressed, the music therapist may use live music and therapeutic support to provide a strong sense

---

[1] For clarity, throughout the chapter the music therapist is identified as "she" and the child/client as "he."

of grounding. The music therapist may select an accompanying instrument, such as a guitar, that allows her to flexibly position herself directly in the child's line of sight and at close proximity to the child's head (Whitehead-Pleaux, 2013). Depending on the child's needs, the therapist may lean in close to his head to encourage him to focus exclusively on her. Using a calm and secure tone of voice, she may speak to the child, incorporating his name and giving clear cues and reassurances to bring his attention to the here and now. The therapist can use simple instructions and reassurances such as "Look at me," "Squeeze my hand," "Breathe with me," "What color are my eyes?", "You are safe," and "I am here with you." The therapist's tone of voice and vocal inflection is intentionally used to reduce the child's arousal and convey a sense of safety and security. If the child does not orient to the therapist, she may modify her voice to command the child's attention and promote his response, though she remains supportive and secure in her demeanor and tone. Once a child is able to orient to the music therapist, she may soften her tone and continue to provide supportive verbalizations.

Touch may be a helpful tool for providing orientation and grounding, if a child is receptive. The music therapist may gently, but securely, hold the child's hand, stroke his head, or pat his chest (if he is a baby or toddler) to provide reassurance (Whitehead-Pleaux, 2013). Such uses of touch encourage the child to come back into his body if he is experiencing traumatic memories, or direct the child's attention to more pleasant body sensations if he is undergoing an uncomfortable procedure. The therapist should be mindful of the nature of the child's injury or illness to ensure that touch does not cause discomfort. Touch may be particularly provocative or even contraindicated if a child has a premorbid history of abuse. In such cases, the therapist may be able to incorporate supportive touch, but should do so with sensitivity to ensure that the child does not perceive such touch to be restrictive or hyperstimulating. For example, during a medical procedure the music therapist may aim to hold a child's hand to support and encourage him to keep his hand out of the way of the intervening nurse. Instead of holding the child's hand down against the bed, the music therapist can ask the child to hold her hand and squeeze it if he feels pain. The child feels supported, but not restrained, by such use of touch.

If a parent or caregiver is present and able to provide support to the child during a distressing procedure, the music therapist can coach the caregiver in how to provide grounding and emotional support (Whitehead-Pleaux, 2013). Some caregivers find that their coping resources are overwhelmed at such times, and they are not able to serve as functional supports to their children during painful or anxiety-provoking procedures. The music therapist may serve as the primary supportive presence for the child until the caregiver can resume that role.

If children are hyperaroused but not overwhelmed by distress, the music therapist may employ music-assisted relaxation approaches to reduce arousal. Prerecorded music listening paired with various relaxation strategies significantly reduces arousal due to stress in a variety of populations (Pelletier, 2004). Sedative music paired with verbal suggestions for relaxation, cues for progressive muscle relaxation, autogenic techniques, relaxation imagery, and vibrotactile stimulation are all relaxation approaches supported by the research literature (Pelletier, 2004; Whitehead-Pleaux, 2013). The music therapist can implement a variety of music-assisted relaxation strategies, from passive to actively engaging, to reduce arousal or hyperarousal. *Music-assisted relaxation* can be defined as

> the use of music that has been selected for its characteristics of tempo, fluid and predictable movement of melody and dynamics, and pleasing harmonies. The music therapist utilizes the music to structure and teach deep diaphragmatic breathing, progressive muscle relaxation, and to facilitate imagery. (Bishop, Christenberry, Robb, & Toombs Rudenberg, 1996, p. 92)

Great care must be used when selecting prerecorded music for children who have a history of physical or sexual abuse (Whitehead-Pleaux, 2013). Depending on the child's experiences, male or female voices could trigger unpleasant memories or feelings. Similarly, the music therapist must remain cautious when using prerecorded music with extramusical sounds (e.g., rainstorms, waves on the shore, rainforest sounds) as these sounds can be misinterpreted and trigger trauma memories. The timbre, tempo, instrumentation, texture, novelty versus repetitiveness, and density of the music are important considerations when selecting music for arousal reduction. Because the musical preferences and needs for music-assisted relaxation vary for each child, the music therapist should create individualized music plans.

Music therapists often prefer to use live relaxation music (as opposed to prerecorded music) because live music allows them to maximize relaxation potential by modifying musical elements in accord with client responses. Music therapists frequently rely upon the principle of *entrainment* when providing live relaxation music, a process in which the therapist "first matches the breathing rate or heart rate of the child and then gradually slows down the tempo of the music to encourage deeper breathing or a slowing down of the heart rate" (Bradt, 2013, p. 33). When promoting the reduction of arousal, the therapist may provide sedative music using entrainment while pairing sung suggestions such as "calm . . . calm," matched to the child's inhalation and exhalation to center the child. The therapist can cue the child to breathe progressively deeper and more slowly by singing "Breathing in . . . and out . . ." to a rising and falling melodic phrase. Depending on the child's developmental level, the music therapist may promote diaphragmatic breathing by cueing the child. For example:

> a) imagine having a balloon of your favorite color in your belly that expands as you breathe in and deflates as you exhale; b) imagine blowing air down the whole length of your body (this helps to prolong exhalation which, in turn, promotes deeper breathing); c) imagine blowing a feather and keeping the feather afloat in the air; or d) rest your hands on your belly, take a deep breath in through your nose, slowly and gently, and then release it through your mouth while making a "shhhh" or "ahhhhh" sound. (Bradt, 2013, p. 35)

The music therapist uses musical qualities of tempo, melodic contour, phrasing, and tonality to reinforce the approaches of the various breathing strategies. If the child is highly distressed, the music therapist can provide a simplified focus on breathing as a way to provide grounding and stabilization. As the therapist musically synchronizes with the child's breath, she can model deep inhalations through the nose and controlled exhalations through slightly pursed lips, and fade these cues as the child is able to master the approach. When hyperaroused, the child benefits from succinct instructions for deep breathing with clear modeling of techniques.

In cases when the child is not able to focus on the music therapist and follow cues, the therapist may rely solely upon musical aspects to promote reduction of physiological arousal. The therapist uses entrainment to synchronize to the child's breathing, heart rate, or movement patterns and then gradually modulates to a slower tempo and more relaxed state. Reducing arousal to the level at which the child can remain present and actively engaged in music making during a stressful time or procedure may take several minutes to several weeks of therapy. A child's ability to adaptively cope in such situations depends on the extent of the trauma, the frequency of recurring traumatic experiences, the child's resilience, premorbid factors, and the coping capacity of the child's support network. Progress toward developing adaptive coping strategies can be thwarted by various factors such as infection, medication, sleep disturbances, learned pain behaviors, and fluctuating mood.

Self-Regulation and Emotion Regulation

Individuals who have the ability to self-regulate are able to reduce arousal by way of *emotion regulation*, the internal process of consciously or unconsciously modulating aspects of emotion to achieve a comfortable state of arousal (Diamond & Aspinwall, 2003; Sena Moore, 2013). For hospitalized children who are traumatized, the music therapist can use musical elements to help the child shift to a more comfortable state of arousal. Preliminary evidence[2] supports the use of music listening, singing, and improvising to help regulate emotions, and indicates that music that is in a minor key, dissonant, contains unexpected musical changes, has frequent chord changes, or is considered "unpleasant" can impede emotion regulation (Sena Moore, 2013). When a traumatized child actively experiences intrusive memories, the music therapist can gently direct the child to focus on specific elements of the music (e.g., the melodic line, a particular instrument, a repetitive rhythm) to redirect his attention away from the hyperarousing memory and to the present moment as a means to promote emotion regulation (Sena Moore, 2013).

Musical qualities can be utilized to promote other self-soothing strategies that enable self-regulation. Familiar and preferred music can help provide orientation and promote grounding in the here and now in order to reduce anxiety (Rafieyan & Ries, 2007). The music therapist continues to use a calm and secure tone of voice when speaking or singing familiar songs, and avoids extremes of inflection or emotional variation. The therapist's voice conveys a sense of safety and comfort. Providing orientation and reassurance through familiar music is more important than the specific lyric content of songs at such times, as familiar songs help the child remain grounded in reality. If the song lyrics or music appear to be triggering more psychological distress or dissociation, the therapist will naturally transition into different music. Repetitive rhythm and movement, such as singing a familiar lullaby

---

[2]Readers are referred to Sena Moore (2013) for a comprehensive synthesis of research regarding the impact of music on the neural substrates of emotion regulation.

while swaying to the beat, can promote behavioral, physiological, and emotional regulation. Music therapists can encourage caregivers to pair rhythmic movement with simple, familiar music to soothe and reassure young children.

Facilitation of Body Awareness

The creation of music provides a multisensory experience. As a child immerses himself in music, he can connect with sensory input and build awareness of sensations linked to the present moment. Instruments such as maracas, tambourines, bells, and drums provide a variety of sound qualities and physical textures that provide multisensory stimulation. For example, playing a hand drum provides deep sensory input via auditory, tactile, and kinesthetic modalities. Actively making music enables the traumatized child to build tolerance of experiencing in-the-moment sensory input (Behrens, 2011). A child may choose to connect to a grounding and stabilizing resonance by placing his hand on the body of the therapist's guitar, or by strumming the strings while the therapist frets a consonant chord. Similarly, using a Bluetooth speaker connected to an MP3 player or tablet, the child and/or music therapist can provide centering and stabilizing resonance when the speaker is placed on a targeted area of the child's body. Amplifying recorded music in this way allows the music therapist to utilize a greater range of frequencies, which help the child discern and tolerate different tactile experiences. The child who is engaging in music making remains in control of the sensory experience and can expand upon or cease various forms of stimulation as tolerated.

Promotion of Internal Locus of Control

Hospitalization compromises the autonomy of children and adolescents, and younger children who have recently achieved this milestone can become quite frustrated when their independence is threatened. Children are invited to exercise choice and control within the music therapy context, which can promote reinstatement of internal locus of control (Behrens, 2011). Choices related to how the child engages in music, which music is selected, and what the child wants the therapist to do within the music all provide a sense of control and help to overcome the feeling of helplessness. Similarly, as the therapist helps the child learn and practice various emotion regulation and stress management strategies through the use of music-facilitated approaches, the child can develop a greater internal locus of control. By empowering the child or adolescent in the music therapy context, he can experience a sense of "doing" rather than "being done to" (Rafieyan & Ries, 2007, p. 50). The music therapist promotes mastery by creating situations in which the child can experience success and satisfaction. Children and adolescents are often intrigued by electronic instrument applications that are easily accessible through use of tablets or computers. Such adaptive software enables children to exercise greater independence and control over music making through the use of familiar technologies. The therapist can use instrumental improvisation via adaptive technologies or simple songwriting processes to promote mastery and empower children and adolescents.

Facilitation of Emotional-Approach Coping

Children naturally use music and musical play as a means to express and work through their emotional experiences. Music therapy may provide a context within which children are able to gradually approach challenging feelings and perceptions, and it provides an opportunity to reframe stressful experiences. *Emotional-approach coping* can be defined as the expression, awareness, acknowledgment, and understanding of emotions as a means of coping with stress (Austenfeld & Stanton, 2004). Music therapy that includes an emphasis on emotional-approach coping can enable individuals to approach challenging emotions related to stressful situations, facilitating a process of progressive and gradual exposure that ultimately results in increases in positive affective states (Ghetti, 2013a).

Hospitalized children who have undergone traumatic experiences may benefit from the use of *music-facilitated dramatic play*, a form of "improvised song that incorporates play and dramatic action using props and musical instruments to enable the expression of feelings and the symbolic working through of internal conflicts" (Ghetti, 2013b, p. 160). Given musical and therapeutic support from the therapist, the child spontaneously engages in creating songs and dramatic action that can offer the therapist insight as to how the child conceives of hospitalization and treatment. Subsequently, the therapist can use the music-facilitated dramatic play context to "give the child a supportive means of approaching, working through, and resolving fears and conflicts"—challenges that might otherwise impede coping or thwart self-regulation (Ghetti, 2013b, p. 177).

When a child engages in music-facilitated dramatic play, he may choose to (1) give voice to a puppet or prop while the music therapist provides musical mirroring and accompaniment; (2) use a puppet or prop to create action while the music therapist gives voice to the puppet and provides musical accompaniment; (3) use instruments or voice to create a narrative or accompaniment while the music therapist uses a puppet or prop; or (4) use instruments and/or voice to sing or illustrate a story while the therapist provides musical accompaniment and mirroring (Ghetti, 2013b). The child who has undergone traumatic experiences can use music-facilitated dramatic play as a contained way to process traumatic material, and by approaching and working through difficult emotions, may mobilize strengths.

Sensory Processing of the Traumatic Event(s)

Nonverbal expression enables the working-through of implicit memories—that is, those that are stored in sensations and emotions (Malchiodi, 2008). Music therapists can use musical improvisation to promote somatic experiencing in various forms. A therapist can use *referential improvisation*, a form of clinical improvisation in which the music depicts some nonmusical theme, an emotion, or an experience (Bruscia, 1998). The therapist can ask the child to use instruments or voice to capture what "relaxed" sounds like or what "strength" sounds like, prompting positive somatic experiencing. If the child is ready and if such an approach is clinically indicated, the music therapist can also use improvisatory methods to help the child work through implicit memories of hospital-related traumatic experiences. The child can be encouraged to pair instrumental sounds to particular internal somatic sensations, thereby helping to integrate his somatic experience and, at the same time, providing the therapist with insight into those experiences.

Another intervention that is useful for the sensory processing of a traumatic event is using electronic music technology to create a *sound story* that musically narrates the traumatic medical experiences. Through selection of musical and nonmusical samples, a child can create a composition that musically narrates his experience with a traumatic medical procedure or traumatic injuring event (Whitehead-Pleaux, 2013). Similar to the improvisational method described above, the child is encouraged to choose samples that match or describe his internal somatic sensations. Once the sound story is completed, the therapist and child listen to it together in its entirety, which reduces the segmentation of memories and somatic sensations and integrates the experiences by means of the creative process. Additionally, this sound story can give the therapist a greater understanding of the child's memories, perceptions, and somatic sensations.

Externalization and Containment

Music therapy provides a supportive space that offers opportunities for externalization and creation of narrative, though such experiences should remain client-directed, emerging at the child's pace, based on his coping abilities (Ghetti, 2013b). The music itself can serve as a container for emotional expression, as a child emotes while singing a personally significant song, tells his story through songwriting, beats forcefully on a drum, or projects meaning onto song lyrics. Both the process of music therapy (e.g., improvising with the therapist) and the product of music therapy (e.g., audio recording of an originally composed song) may provide containment for the externalization of feelings. Use of metaphor and projection help the child externalize his trauma experience until he becomes secure enough to identify with the metaphor or projection and integrate it into his own narrative. Children and adolescents may create narratives by engaging in spontaneous improvised song, music-facilitated dramatic play, referential improvisation, or structured songwriting, or they may identify with narratives expressed in the lyrics of preferred songs.

Promotion of Healthy Attachment and Supportive Relationships

One of the devastating impacts of trauma and extended hospitalization on children and adolescents is the atrophying of relationships with family and peers and the severing of connections to life activities that hold meaning for them. Children with severe diseases and injuries require frequent medical treatments that can necessitate lengthy hospital stays. Illnesses, injuries, and medical treatments themselves may impair the child's mobility, limiting his ability to engage in meaningful life activities. Electronic technologies have helped to bridge the gap that can form between the hospitalized child and his family and peers. Websites such as Facebook and CarePages allow the child to connect to loved ones and friends on a daily basis. In addition, the expanded use of cellphones and texting has helped children connect with their support networks. Though they may be beneficial, these electronic and cellular connections do not allow for the full maintenance and development of these vital supportive relationships.

As a result of the stress of illness and hospitalization, children and adolescents may regress in various developmental areas. A toddler who was potty-trained and able to feed himself may require diapers and parental assistance for feeding while in the hospital. A teenager who was actively individuating from his parents may find himself relying upon his parents for his daily care and support. A parent may share his room, sleeping next to him to attend to his every need. Autonomy and sense of privacy are regularly challenged in the hospital environment, and the child or teenager my respond by acting out or demonstrating noncompliant behavior.

The child's needs can become so great that the parents set aside their needs in order to be present and supportive to the child. The parent's life becomes focused solely on the child, to the exclusion of meaningful relationships and activities. As the child heals and recovers, members of the family may realize that they have developed complex and interdependent ways of relating to one another.

Music therapy offers a variety of ways to promote and maintain meaningful connections among children and caregivers. Music improvisations that incorporate the child and parent dyad can help to rebalance the power dynamic and reestablish the child or adolescent in his premorbid developmental frame. The music therapist can assign different roles within the improvisation and select instruments that bring either the parent's or child's musical expression to the forefront while the other acts in a supportive role. These improvisations can develop over time to represent healthy ways of connecting and relating, while letting go of the intense dynamics that developed when the child was in crisis.

In addition to improvisation, songwriting and multimedia productions can promote healthy attachment and supportive relationships whether family members are close or separated. Children can engage in songwriting to express their feelings about important relationships, reflect on happy times together, and plan for future time together (Whitehead-Pleaux, 2013). These songwriting interventions can include lyric substitution using familiar songs or the composition of original lyrics and music. Once the song is created, the child and music therapist can practice it until the child feels ready to record the song. This time of practice can be a time for the music therapist to encourage dialogue about these significant relationships, how the child feels being apart from the individuals, and his hopes and fears about seeing them again. When the child is ready, the music therapist can use electronic music technologies to record the song and save it to a compact disc or MP3 file for the child to share with his loved ones.

Using simple technology to create movies or add impactful visual images to the child's music compositions, the music therapist can work with the child to create a multimedia project that facilitates connection and healthy relationships (Whitehead-Pleaux, 2013). The music therapist can use a song the child composed and combine it with photos or video of the child's choosing. Images can capture the child or his environment, favorite photos from before the hospitalization, or representational images found on the Internet or taken by the child. The addition of visual images to the musical compositions helps to deepen the child's expression regarding relationships and the connection itself between the child and significant others.

Integration of the Trauma

As the child or adolescent begins to gain perspective on his traumatic experiences, he may take steps toward integrating those experiences into an expanded sense of self. The music therapist can engage a child in a discussion of coping approaches, if he is able to evaluate his traumatic experiences, and ask the child to identify what works and what does not. In addition, the two can problem-solve regarding coping approaches to use with future stressors. The music therapist empowers the child to develop his own most adaptive coping approaches, some of which may be musical in nature. The child and therapist can rehearse such approaches in advance of stressful procedures or potentially triggering stimuli.

The child or adolescent can compose original songs, modify song lyrics, or select particular songs that help provide reassurance and express resolve regarding his ability to successfully cope with stressors. Such songs can function as "theme songs" that the child can use during periods of distress to connect to resources and remind him of inner strengths. The child may have composed a series of songs throughout his hospitalization that deal with issues associated with the disease or injury as well as aspects of treatment. The music therapist can work with the child to create an "album" that helps to document, integrate, and expand upon the child's experiences (Whitehead-Pleaux & Spall,

2013). A retrospective examination of the child's healing process, as captured through songs on an album, helps the child gain perspective on those experiences, connecting fragmented parts and promoting integration of disparate experiences. Through the creative process, the child is assisted in integrating his various selves: before hospitalization, during it, and once the medical care is completed.

When a child has undergone a life-changing event such as an extended hospitalization, he may feel alienated from his peers and community, who have limited understanding of what hospitalization meant to him. Music therapists can facilitate reintegration to community by assisting children in composing songs about the hospitalization that can be shared. Alternatively, a child or adolescent can create a multimedia project as a means of explaining his experiences to peers. A multimedia project of this nature could consist of a collection of photos from the hospitalization paired with a precomposed song that the child feels explains his experiences, fears, or strengths. If time allows and the child is able, this intervention can be modified in a variety of ways. The child can compose an explanatory song for a reintegration video or choose representational images to summarize his experiences. The child can compose a song and create a video that acts out the song, asking staff and family to appear in the video. The video might include a tour of the hospital, with interspersed music clips to explore the child's experiences in each area, along with spoken word, narrating the tour. The combination of different creative arts through images, drama, and music can facilitate deep expression and solidify a child's integrated identity as he prepares to go home.

CONCLUSION

Music therapists play a vital role in promoting psychological healing processes in children who are at risk for traumatization due to injury, illness, or hospitalization. By initiating music therapy early in the child's medical treatment, incorporating a trauma-informed approach, and engaging children in a variety of creative music therapy interventions targeted to specific needs, music therapists can provide buffers against the negative impacts of trauma. By engaging in music therapy, children can reduce hyperarousal, regulate their emotions, learn to employ adaptive coping strategies, and contextualize experiences they had throughout the hospitalization, paving the way for both personal and community reintegration. For children with diseases or injuries that require subsequent stressful hospitalizations, building a positive, empowering initial hospital experience will help to mitigate future stress responses to medical care.

REFERENCES

Austenfeld, J. L., & Stanton, A. L. (2004). Coping through emotional approach: A new look at emotion, coping, and health-related outcomes. *Journal of Personality, 72*(6), 1335–1363.

Behrens, G. A. (2008, November). *Using music therapy to understand emotional needs of Palestinian children traumatized by war.* Paper presented at the annual meeting of the American Music Therapy Association, St. Louis, MO.

Behrens, G. A. (2011). Musiktherapie zur Behandlung von traumatischem Stress: Theorie und neueste Forschung [How recent research and theory on traumatic stress relates to music therapy]. *Musiktherapeutische Umschau, 32*(1), 372–381.

Bishop, B., Christenberry, A., Robb, S., & Toombs Rudenberg, M. (1996). Music therapy and child life interventions with pediatric burn patients. In M. A. Froehlich (Ed.), *Music therapy with hospitalized children: A creative arts child life approach* (pp. 87–108). Cherry Hill, NJ: Jeffrey Books.

Bradt, J. (2013). Pain management with children. In J. Bradt (Ed.), *Guidelines for music therapy practice in pediatric care* (pp. 15–65). Gilsum, NH: Barcelona.

Bruscia, K. E. (1998). *Defining music therapy* (2nd ed.). Gilsum, NH: Barcelona.

Diamond, L. M., & Aspinwall, L. G. (2003). Emotion regulation across the life span: An integrative perspective emphasizing self-regulation, positive affect, and dyadic processes. *Motivation and Emotion, 27*(2), 125–156.

Ghetti, C. M. (2013a). Effect of music therapy with emotional-approach coping on preprocedural anxiety in cardiac catheterization: A randomized controlled trial. *Journal of Music Therapy, 50*(2), 93–122.

Ghetti, C. M. (2013b). Pediatric intensive care. In J. Bradt (Ed.), *Guidelines for music therapy practice in pediatric care* (pp. 152–204). Gilsum, NH: Barcelona.

Hofmann, M., de Montalembert, M., Beauquier-Maccotta, B., de Villartay, P., & Golse, B. (2007). Posttraumatic stress disorder in children affected by sickle-cell disease and their parents. *American Journal of Hematology, 82,* 171–172.

Kenardy, J. A., Spence, S. H., & Macleod, A. C. (2006). Screening for posttraumatic stress disorder in children after accidental injury. *Pediatrics, 118*(3), 1002–1009.

Kirsch, V., Wilhelm, F. H., & Goldbeck, L. (2011). Psychophysiological characteristics of PTSD in children and adolescents: A review of the literature. *Journal of Traumatic Stress, 24*(2), 146–154.

Loewy, J. V. (2002). Song sensitation: How fragile we are. In J. V. Loewy & A. Frisch Hara (Eds.), *Caring for the caregiver: The use of music and music therapy in grief and trauma* (pp. 33–43). Silver Spring, MD: American Music Therapy Association.

Malchiodi, C. A. (2008). Creative interventions and childhood trauma. In C. A. Malchiodi (Ed.), *Creative interventions with traumatized children* (pp. 3–22). New York: Guilford Press.

Malchiodi, C. A. (2012). Trauma-informed art therapy and sexual abuse in children. In P. Goodyear-Brown (Ed.), *Handbook of child sexual abuse: Identification, assessment, and treatment* (pp. 341–354). Hoboken, NJ: Wiley.

Murray, B. L., Kenardy, J. A., & Spence, S. H. (2008). Brief report: Children's response to trauma- and nontrauma-related hospital admission: A comparison study. *Journal of Pediatric Psychology, 33*(4), 435–440.

Pelletier, C. L. (2004). The effect of music on decreasing arousal due to stress: A meta-analysis. *Journal of Music Therapy, 41*(3), 192–214.

Rafieyan, R., & Ries, R. (2007). A description of the use of music therapy in consultation-liaison psychiatry. *Psychiatry, 4*(1), 47–52.

Rennick, J. E., Johnston, C. C., Dougherty, G., Platt, R., & Ritchie, J. A. (2002). Children's psychological responses after critical illness and exposure to invasive technology. *Developmental and Behavioral Pediatrics, 23*(3), 133–144.

Saxe, G., Vanderbilt, D., & Zuckerman, B. (2003). Traumatic stress in injured and ill children. *PTSD Research Quarterly, 14*(2), 1–3.

Sena Moore, K. (2013). A systematic review on the neural effects of music on emotion regulation: Implications for music therapy practice. *Journal of Music Therapy, 50*(3), 198–242.

Turry, A. (2002). Don't let the fear prevent the grief: Working with traumatic reactions through improvisation. In J. V. Loewy & A. Frisch Hara (Eds.), *Caring for the caregiver: The use of music and music therapy in grief and trauma* (pp. 44–52). Silver Spring, MD: American Music Therapy Association.

Whitehead-Pleaux, A. (2013). Pediatric burn care. In J. Bradt (Ed.), *Guidelines for music therapy practice in pediatric care* (pp. 252–289). Gilsum, NH: Barcelona.

Whitehead-Pleaux, A., & Spall, L. (2013). Innovations in medical music therapy: The use of electronic music technologies in a pediatric burn hospital. In W. L. Magee (Ed.), *Music technology in therapeutic and health settings* (pp. 133–148). Philadelphia: Jessica Kingsley.

APPENDIX

Resources for Work with Traumatized Children

Bibliotherapy Recommendations

This section summarizes information on children's books used in trauma intervention from the first edition of *Creative Interventions with Traumatized Children* (Malchiodi & Ginns-Gruenberg, 2008). Creative interventions such as drawing, movement, writing, or play therapy often capitalize on the power of storytelling to give meaning to nonverbal self-expression. However, the purposeful use of books in therapy, known as bibliotherapy, and specific story-making techniques are effective interventions, in and of themselves, in work with children who have experienced traumatic events. When applying *reactive bibliotherapy*, the child reads specific stories or books; if they have been appropriately selected, the child will identify with the character or story and will have increased understanding and insight after reading the book. *Interactive bibliotherapy* involves discussion between the therapist and child client to facilitate, reinforce, and integrate concepts gained from reading a particular story. Children who are grieving a loss, struggling with divorce or foster care, or recovering from abuse or neglect can all benefit from the sensitive use of books in therapy.

Here is a brief list of recommendations for bibliotherapy with traumatized children by topic area.

TRAUMA SYMPTOM MANAGEMENT

• *When Sophie Gets Angry—Really, Really Angry* (Bang, 1999) is the now classic story of Sophie, who gets angry and breaks things, but finds a way to handle her feelings. Similarly, *Sometimes I'm Bombaloo* (Vail, 2002) tells the story of Katie who, when she gets angry, stops being Katie and turns into "Bombaloo." The story covers fighting with siblings, using time-out to calm down, and apologizing after becoming Bombaloo.

- *Alexander and the Terrible, Horrible, No Good, Very Bad Day* (Viorst, 1987) focuses on Alexander, who wishes he could move away from his problems after a series of things go wrong in his life.
- *Double Dip Feelings* (Cain, 2001) gives children permission to have more than one feeling at the same time. For children who have contradictory feelings about traumatic events or losses, this book is particularly helpful.
- *When Fuzzy Was Afraid of Losing His Mother* (Maier, 2005) focuses on separation anxiety and encourages children to identify with Fuzzy and his dilemma.
- To help children cope with nightmares, *Jessica and the Wolf* (Lobby, 1990) and *Annie Stories* (Brett & Chess, 1988) are two good resources.

NATURAL AND HUMAN-MADE DISASTERS

- *Sailing through the Storm* (Julik, 1999) is a story that centers on a sailboat on the water of life that is "happily sailing along in calm, blue water. Suddenly there is a big boom. Someone has been hurt, and everything changes. Violence has happened to you, or to someone you know, or even someone you have never met" (p. 12). Speaking directly to children, the story captures a wide range of emotions, including feeling like your "little sailboat is going to sink," and moves in a positive direction, encouraging children to express those scary feelings.
- *September 12th We Knew Everything Would Be All Right*, written and illustrated by first-grade students in Missouri (Byron Masterson School, 2002), was an excellent story for restoring feelings of normalcy to children. The book opens with, "On September 11, 2001, many bad things happened. September 12th was a new day. We knew everything would be all right because . . ." (p. 5). At this point in the story, children can be invited to create their own illustrations and stories about the importance of consistency, routines, and self-soothing activities. This book can also be applied to many situations, including divorce, accident, or disaster.

MOVING, DISPLACEMENT, OR SEPARATION

- *Wemberly Worried* (Henkes, 2000) is about Wemberly, who has some big worries about his new school, and is a great book for children who are going through big changes, including moving to a new house.
- *Talk, Listen, Connect* (Sesame Workshop, 2008) is an excellent print and DVD resource from Sesame Street and has been used by parents who are serving in the military to help their children with transitions, including moves and multiple parental deployments. It is also available via an app and a website (*www.sesamestreet.org/parents/topicsandactivities/toolkits/tlc*).

- *The Storm* (McGrath, 2006) is one of several books published on the topic of Hurricane Katrina; children share their stories, drawings, and paintings, providing honest reflections of what it was like to live through a powerful storm.
- *Night Catch* (Ehrmantraut, 2005) tells the story of how a soldier enlists the help of the North Star for a nightly game of catch with his son; it is a timeless tale of how families stay connected when separated, especially due to military deployment.

RELAXATION AND STRESS REDUCTION

- *Cool Cats, Calm Kids* (Williams, 1996) is a popular book on stress management and relaxation skills that children enjoy. There are nine examples of "cat-recommended" stress reduction techniques, such as "Hold your head high" and "Hang in there."
- *Peaceful Piggy Meditation* (McLean, 2004), *Mindful Monkey, Happy Panda* (Aldefer, 2011), and *Moody Cow Meditates* (McLean, 2009) teach the power of meditation to young children through characters and their stories.
- *A Handful of Quiet: Happiness in Four Pebbles* (Hahn, 2012) introduces children to the practice of meditation through a simple, sensory pebble meditation and the interconnection with nature.
- *Starbright, Moonbeam*, and *Earthlight* (Garth, 1991, 1993, 1997) provide calming imagery and affirmations for elementary school–age children.
- *Yoga Pretzels* (Guber & Kalish, 2006) is a set of yoga and breathing activity cards that can be used to supplement stress reduction and self-regulation practices with children.

DEATH OF A FAMILY MEMBER OR FRIEND

- *When Dinosaurs Die* (Krasny & Brown, 1998) is a book that children of all ages will return to many times; it is an ideal book to share with children in the elementary grades when one of their classmates has experienced a death. Dinosaur characters express the common questions and concerns that children have regarding death.
- *Mick Harte Was Here* (Park, 1995) validates common feelings young people experience after a death and may help their peers empathize with them. The story is told from the point of view of a teen whose 12-year-old brother was killed in a bicycle accident.
- *I Know I Made It Happen* (Blackburn, 1991) is a story about believing one is responsible when bad things occur. In this story, adults explain that bad things do not happen just because a child thinks or wishes them to, and children learn that it helps to share their feelings and to know that the death

of a loved one is not their fault. *A Terrible Thing Happened* (Holmes, 2000) also helps children understand their feelings about death through the story of a raccoon named Sherman Smith. Sherman becomes afraid, angry, and disruptive at school until his teacher, Ms. Maple, helps him understand his feelings through play and drawing.

• *Tear Soup: A Recipe for Healing after Loss* (Schweibert & DeKlyen, 1999) uses the metaphor of making soup to explain bereavement. This story is designed for older children and adolescents, but is also useful with adults and families because of its message.

• *They're Part of the Family: Barkley and Eve Talk to Children about Pet Loss* (Carney, 2001) is part of a series of activity and coloring books in which Barkley and Eve, two Portuguese water dogs, talk about death and related topics. It relates three brief stories: about a dog who developed an illness and was euthanized, a turtle who was found dead one morning, and a cat who was killed in an accident.

• *Sadako and the Thousand Paper Cranes* (Coerr, 1977) describes a memorial activity based on the death of a Japanese girl, Sadako, who died of leukemia in 1955, as a result of the atomic bombing of Hiroshima. The story explains the legend of the crane that was supposed to live for a thousand years and that good health is given to a person who folds 1,000 origami paper cranes. Through this story, children learn a specific activity (origami cranes) to commemorate a loved one as well as how another culture remembers its deceased through a specific ritual for self-healing.

• *Someone Special Died* (Prestine, 1993) and *Anna's Scrapbook: Journal of a Sister's Love* (Aiken, 2001) validate the memories of a person who has died through encouraging children to create a tangible record of the deceased.

RESILIENCE

• *Shoot the Moon: Lessons on Life from a Dog Named Rudy* (Humphrey, 2011) reinforces that it does not matter who you are when it comes to resilience and overcoming life's obstacles. Rudy the dog encourages children to be one's own hero, to find a balance and "just roll" with challenges.

REFERENCES

Aiken, S. (2001). *Anna's scrapbook: Journal of a sister's love.* Omaha, NE: Centering Corporation.
Alderfer, L. (2011). *Mind monkey, happy panda.* Somerville, MA: Wisdom.
Bang, M. (1999). *When Sophie gets angry—really, really angry.* New York: Blue Sky Press.
Blackburn, L. (1991). *I know I made it happen.* Omaha, NE: Centering Corporation.
Brett, D., & Chess, S. (1988). *Annie stories.* New York: Workman.

Byron Masterson School. (2002). *September 12th we knew everything would be all right.* New York: Tangerine Press.

Cain, B. S. (2001). *Double dip feelings.* Washington, DC: Magination Press.

Carney, K. (2001). *They're part of the family: Barkley and Eve talk to children about pet loss.* Wethersfield, CT: Dragonfly.

Coerr, E. (1977). *Sadako and the thousand paper cranes.* New York: Putnam.

Ehrmantraut, B. (2005). *Night catch.* Aberdeen, SD: Bubble Gum Press.

Fox, M. (1994). *Tough Boris.* New York: Harcourt Brace.

Garth, M. (1991). *Starbright: Meditations for children.* San Francisco: HarperCollins.

Garth, M. (1993). *Moonbeam: New meditations for children.* San Francisco: HarperCollins.

Garth, M. (1997). *Earthlight: New meditations for children.* Sydney, Australia: HarperCollins.

Guber, T., & Kalish, L. (2005). *Yoga pretzels.* Bath, UK: Barefoot Books.

Hahn, T. N. (2012). *A handful of quiet: Happiness in four pebbles.* Berkeley, CA: Parallax Press.

Henkes, K. (2000). *Wemberly worried.* New York: Harper.

Holmes, M. (2000). *A terrible thing happened.* Washington, DC: Magination Press.

Humphrey, C. (2011). *Shoot for the moon: Lessons on life from a dog named Rudy.* San Francisco: Chronicle Books.

Julik, E. (1999). *Sailing through the storm: To the ocean of peace.* Lakeville, MN: Galde Press.

Krasny, L., & Brown, M. (1998). *When dinosaurs die.* New York: Little, Brown.

Lobby, T. (1990). *Jessica and the wolf: A story for children who have bad dreams.* Washington, DC: Magination Press.

Maier, I. (2005). *When Fuzzy was afraid of losing his mother.* Washington, DC: Magination Press.

Malchiodi, C. A., & Ginns-Gruenberg, D. (2008). Trauma, loss, and bibliotherapy: The healing power of stories. In C. A. Malchiodi (Ed.), *Creative interventions with traumatized children* (pp. 167–187). New York: Guilford Press.

McGrath, B. (2006). *The storm.* Watertown, MA: Charlesbridge.

McLean, K. (2004). *Peaceful piggy meditation.* Park Ridge, IL: Albert Whitman.

McLean, K. (2009). *Moody cow meditates.* Somerville, MA: Wisdom.

Park, B. (1995). *Mick Harte was here.* New York: Random House.

Patterson, S., & Feldman, J. (1993). *No-no and the secret touch.* Fulton, MD: National Self-Esteem Resources.

Pearson, I., & Merrill, M. (2007). *The adventures of a lady: The big storm.* Book Surge.

Prestine, J. (1993). *Someone special died.* Torrance, CA: Frank Schaeffer.

Schweibert, P., & DeKlyen, C. (1999). *Tear soup.* Portland, OR: Griefwatch.

Sesame Workshop. (2008). *Talk, listen, connect: Deployments, homecomings, changes.* New York: Sesame Workshop.

Vail, R. (2002). *Sometimes I'm Bombaloo.* New York: Scholastic.

Viorst, J. (1987). *Alexander and the terrible, horrible, no good, very bad day.* New York: Aladdin Paperbacks.

Williams, M. (1996). *Cool cats, calm kids: Relaxation and stress management for young people.* San Luis Obispo, CA: Impact.

Wrenn, E. (2001). *The Christmas cactus.* Omaha, NE: Centering Corporation.

Trauma-Related Resources

ARTS THERAPIES AND PLAY THERAPY

Focusing and Expressive Arts Institute provides information and education on focusing-oriented arts therapy that can be applied to work with children, adolescents, adults, and families; see *http://focusingarts.com/focusing-arts-therapy.*

International Society for Traumatic Stress Studies (ISTSS) sponsors publications on the treatment of posttraumatic stress, including *Guideline 17* on creative arts therapies with children and adolescents; see *www.istss.org/ EffectiveTreatmentsforPTSD2ndEdition/4942.htm.*

Trauma-Informed Practices and Expressive Arts Therapy Institute provides information on creative arts therapies and trauma intervention with children and families (see *www.trauma-informedpractice.com/philosophy/creative-arts-therapies*) and distance learning on trauma-informed art and expressive arts therapy.

APPROACHES TO TRAUMA INTEGRATION AND RECOVERY

Child Trauma Academy provides information, training, and research on the neurosequential model of therapeutics (NMT), a developmentally informed, biologically respectful approach to working with at-risk children; see *http:// childtrauma.org/nmt-model.*

Child Welfare Information Gateway provides general information on trauma and children and on trauma-focused cognitive-behavioral therapy (TF-CBT); see *www.childwelfare.gov/pubs/trauma.*

Eye Movement Desensitization and Reprocessing Therapy (EMDR) Institute provides general information and links to publications and research; see *www.emdr.com/general-information/what-is-emdr.html*.

Sensorimotor Psychotherapy Institute (SPI) provides information and education on a body-oriented talking therapy that integrates verbal techniques with body-centered interventions in the treatment of trauma, attachment, and developmental issues; see *www.sensorimotorpsychotherapy.org/about.html*.

Somatic Experiencing® (SE) is an educational and research site that provides professional training in SE and outreach to underserved populations and victims of violence, war, and natural disasters; it is a good place to start to read about Peter Levine's work; see *www.traumahealing.com/somatic-experiencing*.

TRAUMA-INFORMED PRACTICE

Culturally sensitive trauma-informed care refers to the capacity for health care professionals to effectually provide trauma-informed assessment and intervention that acknowledges, respects, and integrates patients' and families' cultural values, beliefs, and practices; see *www.healthcaretoolbox.org/index.php/ cultural-considerations/culturally-censitive-trauma-informed-care*.

Substance Abuse and Mental Health Services Administration (SAMHSA), National Center for Trauma-Informed Care (NCTIC), is a technical assistance center dedicated to building awareness of trauma-informed care and promoting the implementation of trauma-informed practices in programs and services; see *www.samhsa.gov/nctic*.

National Child Traumatic Stress Network (NCTSN) has information on creating trauma-informed systems and a wealth of downloadable information; see *www.nctsn.org/resources/topics/creating-trauma-informed-systems*.

National Trauma Consortium raises public awareness about the prevalence of trauma and its wide-ranging impact on people's lives; see *www. nationaltraumaconsortium.org*.

Sanctuary Model® represents a theory-based, trauma-informed, evidence-supported, whole-culture approach that has a clear and structured methodology for creating or changing an organizational culture; see *www.sanctuaryweb. com/sanctuary-model.php*.

RESILIENCE AND CHILDREN

American Psychological Association provides a comprehensive collection of information on resilience and children; see *www.apa.org/helpcenter/resilience. aspx.*

Positive Psychology Center at University of Pennsylvania provides an overview of resilience in children and strategies to enhance resiliency; see *www. ppc.sas.upenn.edu/prpsum.htm.*

Index